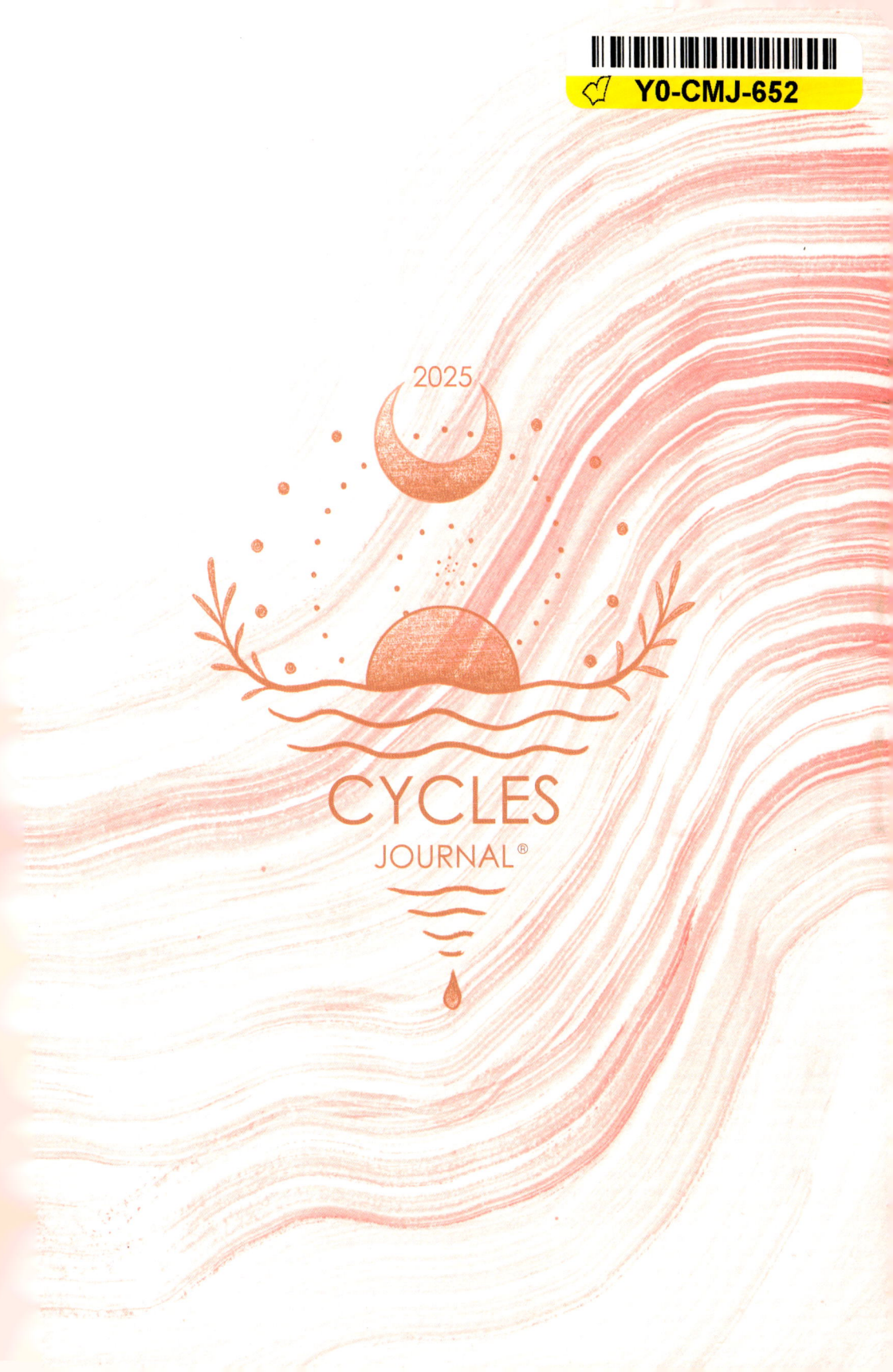

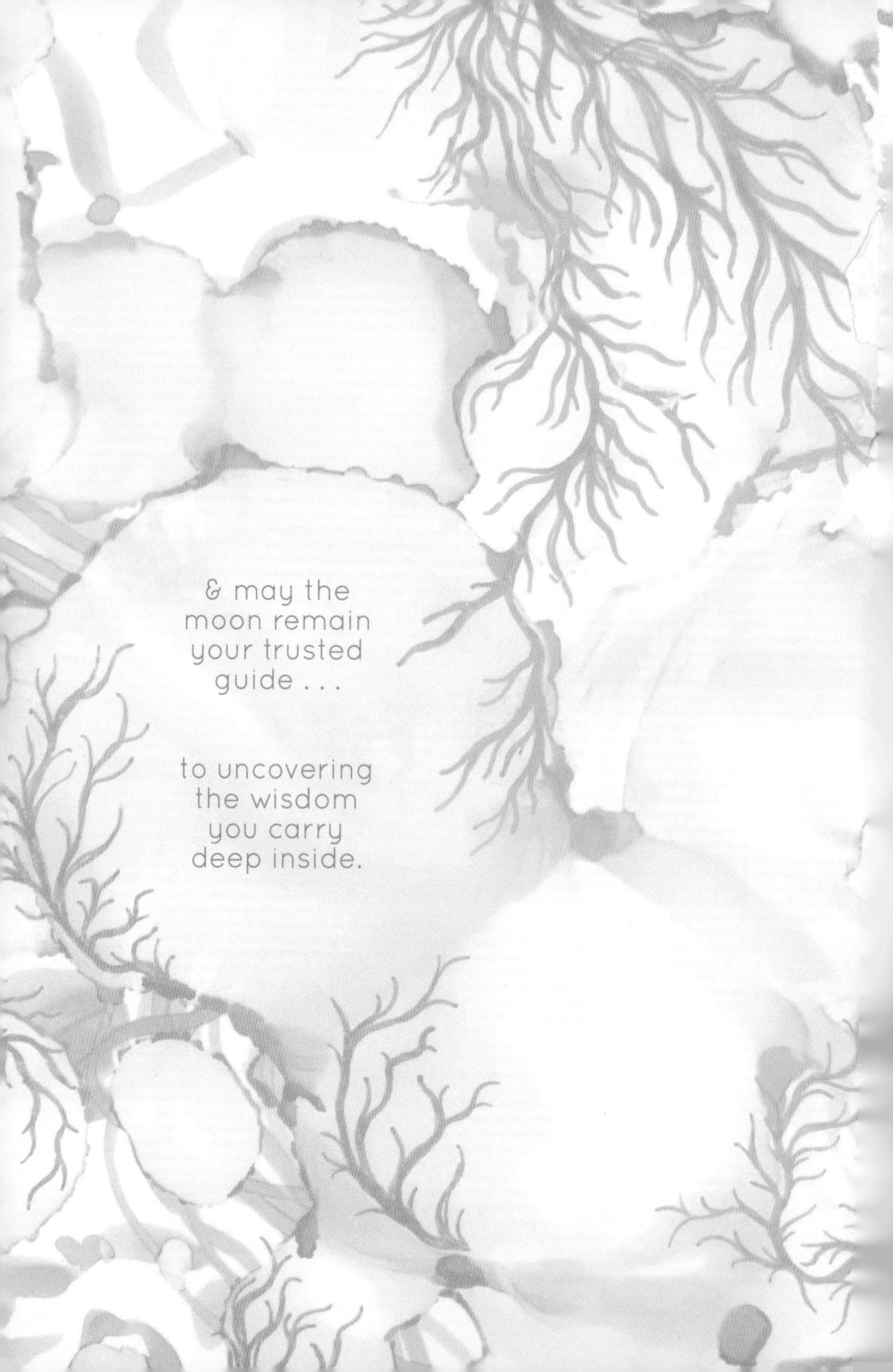

& may the
moon remain
your trusted
guide . . .

to uncovering
the wisdom
you carry
deep inside.

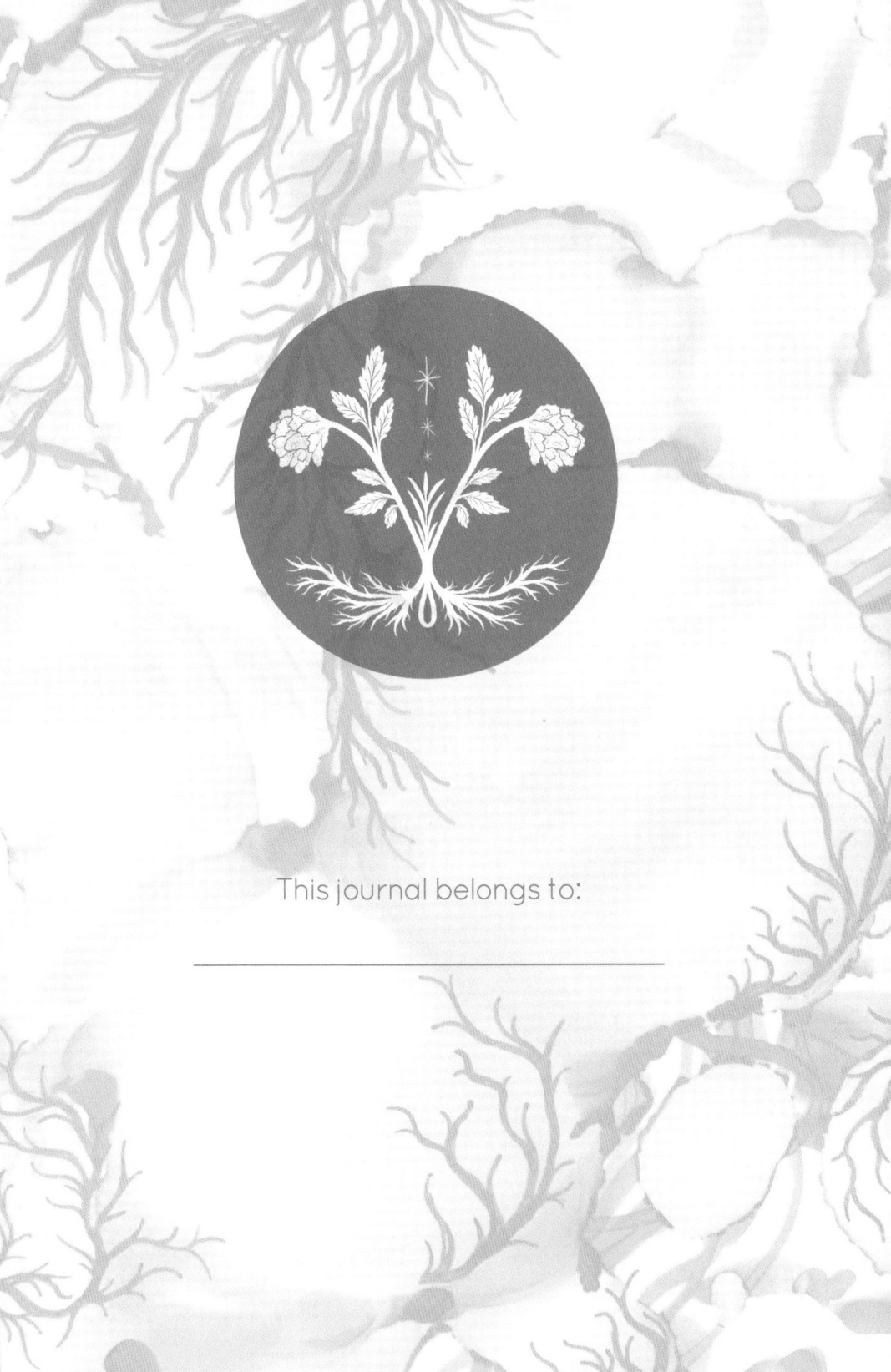

This journal belongs to:
_____

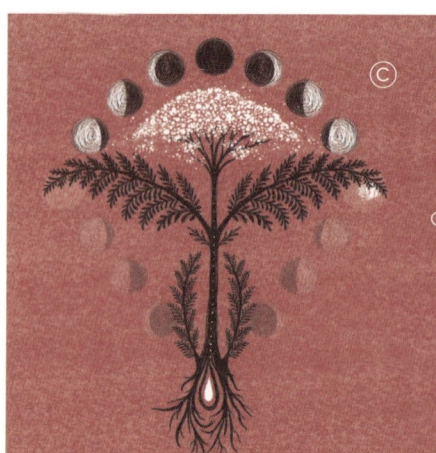

© **CYCLES JOURNAL® 2025**

By Rachael Amber | Cyclical Roots

cyclesjournal.com || cyclicalroots.com

@cyclesjournal || @rachael.amber

Share & tag us!
We love to see your journals
in use & in your sacred spaces.

All rights reserved – Cycles Journal® | Cyclical Nature LLC.
No part of this publication may be reproduced in any form without permission.

All illustrations & designs are © 2025 Rachael Amber Longo, the artist,
unless otherwise stated.

Independently published, originally created & community-funded since 2019.
Cyclical Roots is a feminist, queer, artist-owned business.

Printed in small batches on FSC®-certified paper,
with plant- and oil- based inks & non-toxic adhesives.

ISBN: 978-1-7357127-6-5 • Limited, single print edition.

Browse Our Healing Resource Library

- Free Cyclical Community
- Printable Add On Features + Tools
- Recommended Practitioners
- Free Resources, Tips & Tutorials
- Moonletters, Meditations & More!

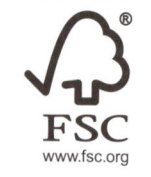

FSC
www.fsc.org
MIX
Paper | Supporting
responsible forestry
FSC® C140526

DISCLAIMER

This book is a stepping stone and general guide that is full of suggestions and not requirements or claims. It is not a replacement for a textbook, medical diagnoses, or your healthcare provider.

All information in this journal is written with research and/or expertise, care, good intention, and experience, but it does not replace what you &/or your healthcare provider agree is best for you. You are encouraged to do your own research and consult your trusted healthcare provider to support the suggestions in this journal! This also serves as a record to share with them.

We (every person involved in this book) do not claim to have cures to any illnesses or to know everyone's situations. We are providing intro-level information in this book; nothing further should be assumed. Everything in this book is to be considered for recreational use at your own risk. We are not to be held responsible for any misinterpretations, medical conditions, or reactions that occur while using this journal.

DEDICATION

This journal is for every cyclical being who holds a physical or energetic womb — a space of endless potential. Thank you for being here. Thank you for being you.

The Cycles Journal Mission

It's time for us to reclaim ourselves and our powerful flows. It's time to mend the parts of our nature we may feel disconnected from or at internal war with.

We are empowering ourselves as unique parts of a blossoming whole.

We are decolonizing and unraveling forced, limiting linear timelines.

We are rebuilding our own beautiful, flowing cyclical way of life.

In this journal, you will...

- Celebrate your fluxes and flows
- Allow space and intention to hear & process your body's wisdom
- Devote time to self-care, love, & empowerment
- Prioritize tracking and integrating your cycle as a regular part of life
- Bring balance into your life by uplifting your inner voice
- Notice your patterns and take some blame off yourself
- Connect deeper to yourself & others through this healing journey
- Follow the moon as a guide & know that you're not in this alone

This journal was created on the unceded land of the Wabanaki Confederacy. We want to take a moment to honor & acknowledge the lineage and origins of cyclical, natural living that Indigenous people have honored pre-colonization and into our present day. May we honor their teachings and do our part to credit and recognize their impact on our wisdom & healing practices. May we recognize our past & present history of living on colonized lands and give back to the Earth and Indigenous peoples. We invite you to take a moment with us to acknowledge, thank and feel in your heart the Indigenous people & land you are practicing & existing on. If you don't know their names, look them up on native-land.ca.

Hello cyclical one,

This journal is a vessel, for you;
a sacred space in which you can connect deeper to yourself.

You have many layers and exist within a web of cycles.
By finding time to spend here to rest, reflect & record
your insight, you can reclaim & connect deeper to all that you already
are and all that you are growing to be. Here and always, you are whole.

This space will help you create a unique map of your body, mind & spirit's patterns and wellbeing. For this linear year and beyond it will serve as a record of your cyclical tendencies, so you can more easily navigate your fluxes and flows as you wax and wane alongside the moon in your own divine timing and natural ways.

I truly believe that by uncovering the patterns that affect us most, we can learn to accept, understand and love ourselves better, and then nothing can stop us from thriving.

Here you can also become more familiar with the space inside of you that holds space for you – your womb space – that extra pocket of potential where you can grow and birth creations, self-love & shared love, intentions, pleasure and anything else you desire. You can learn from and heal with this space, no matter what you have overcome together.

This is a space for healing and forming connections. Remember that you know yourself best – so listen to your body's wisdom over all else. Take the offerings that support you, and leave or adjust anything that doesn't resonate.

It's time to turn inward to listen to your own guidance, and upward to the lunar influence that exists as a part of us all.

I created this for you, for me, and for all of us who need a space of solid ground to hold us within our multidimensional existence and cyclical flows. I am excited to continue to share Cycles Journal and all of the contributions & tools it holds with you & everyone else on this path. May the intentional energy that has been woven into the pages of this expansive edition support you deeply.

I wish you well on this journey of individual & collective healing.

With gratitude from my heart to yours,
Rachael Amber

TABLE OF CONTENTS

Reference, Wisdom & Rituals

Notes on Hemispheres, Timezones, Language & Symbols	6
Menstrual & Lunar Influence	8
The Moon & Astrology	10
Anatomical Diagrams	12
The Menstrual Cycle & Phases	14
Fertility Awareness	16
Sustainable Bleeding	18
Tips & Tricks to Help You Track	20
How to Use This Journal	22
Practicing Cyclical Mindfulness	27
Letter of Devotion & New Year's Intentions	28
Where You're Starting + Prompts/Oracle Spread	30
Tracking Key Replacements	32
Moonthly Overviews	36
Daily + Checkin Pages	62

Articles & Checkins per Lunar Cycle

Navigating Life's Phases: The Wisdom of Planetary Cycles	80
Befriend Your Grief	100
Embodied Activism: Radically Rooted Collective Change	122
The Roots of PMDD	142
Embody your Ecosystems	164
Using Cannabliss for Your Cycles	184
The Xero's/SHero's Journey of the Womb Cycle	204
Moon Sign Medicine: Astrological Tarot Spread	226
How to Make Pelvic Exams More Comfortable	246
Color Wheel Of Emotions	268
Connect with Your Blood Through Self-Pleasure	288
Love Letters From The Land	310
Letter of Reflection & Year's Review	324
Healing Toolkit + Healing Resource Directory	326
How to Reuse Your Journal, About the Creator, What's Next & Notes	332

Notes to keep in mind while using your journal...

LANGUAGE & CONTENT:

In this journal we honor the cyclical nature of all beings. We believe in the beauty of ever-changing, natural fluidity and we acknowledge the energetics & physicalities of the wombspace. As advocates for and members of the LGBTQIA+ community, we honor the full sphere of genders, identities, lineages and bodies.

We do our best to keep this journal's intention focused & language open to be as inclusive as possible. Yet we are all unique beings and this is a reminder that you have full autonomy to take what resonates with you and leave the rest from this space. Please replace or ignore anything that doesn't support your experience. What's true for you will click, and let what's not support someone else.

You know who you are best – may you embrace it fully while also honoring the spectrum of this space & its community. May we all remember our true nature and honor that of others.

BEINGS OF NON-BLEEDING BODIES:

While Cycles Journal has a focus on the wombspace & menstrual cycle, it is built to support & honor non-bleeding bodies & those without a physical womb as well. We all came from a womb, have an energetic wombspace & carry lifeblood within us whether we bleed monthly or not – this is a space to honor that as well as whatever our own current experience may be.

A 28 day menstrual cycle is not required to benefit from the healing tools, resources, rituals & structures within this space. No matter what your cycles look like or what your body is experiencing, this space is here to help you track your physical, mental & energetic wellbeing.

The moon is an anchor for all of us, but especially if we are not bleeding and need a landmark to reference. Therefore, most of the content around menstrual phases is interchangeable with the lunar phases – more on this amongst the following pages.

We welcome and hold space for all bodies & beings; those with irregular or non-existent menstrual cycles, those on birth control, those with regular bleeds, those who are pregnant or postpartum, those who are experiencing menopause or pre- peri- or post-menopause, those experiencing miscarriage or abortion, those who have had a hysterectomy, those transitioning hormonally, & all other experiences that deserve a safe space to track.

We encourage you to include & consider all forms of cycles to support your wholistic understanding of yourself. Menstrual cycles, hormonal cycles, sleep cycles, dream cycles, mood cycles, energetic cycles, & more.

SYMBOL KEY SUPPORT:

Throughout this journal we use symbols of astrology & seasonal shifts to help you easily reference & record in shorthand. You'll learn more about what these mean throughout the next pages. We also created a bookmark "key" for your to use as an easy reference tool as you journey within these pages & beyond.

Download your free printable bookmark key for easy reference:

Lunar Peak Times & Timezones:

Cycles Journal is a cyclical space organized within the linear timeline of the modern world. We source data from astronomical calculations based in the eastern timezone of the northern hemisphere. Regardless of what timezone or hemisphere you are in, this journal's general accuracy & usefulness, along with its reference to lunar influence on our lives, remain intact.

Occasionally, the day of the lunation cycle we highlight may occur the day before or after that of your timezone. This occurs when the moon phase's 'peak' (moon's illumination at 100% full or 0% new) is within hours of midnight in one place or another.

Instead of considering the full & new moons as definitive exactitudes, it's helpful to consider these phases as ranges of influences. The lunar sphere of influence (see pg. 9) of full or new moons can range from 24-48 hours before & after its exact peak time. This serves as an invitation to embrace the intuitive fluidity of our cyclical nature.

Hemispheres & Lunar Perspective:

We all experience the same moon cycle and astrological signs regardless of where we are located on Earth. However, we want to acknowledge the difference in viewpoint from the southern vs northern hemisphere, and give you some tools to be able to use this journal no mater where in the world you are.

This journal is created in the northern hemisphere; the daily lunar phase illustrations reflect the northern hemisphere view of each phase, which would be visually flipped for the southern hemisphere.

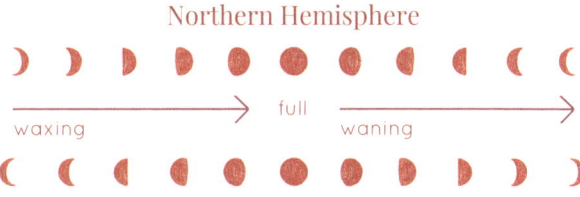

For example, on a given day a person in the northern hemisphere will view the waxing first quarter moon as visually illuminated on the right side. Someone looking at the same moon first quarter moon phase from the southern hemisphere see it visually illuminated on the left.

Energy moves clockwise in the northern hemisphere and the menstrual wheel in this journal reflects this movement. Energy moves counter- or anti-clockwise in the southern hemisphere. For your convenience, we provide via our website a printable version of the menstrual wheel for the southern hemisphere to support you.

Print your southern hemisphere chart to replace pg.14

Cycles Journal would not be possible without our Sponsors...

As an independent publication, we are 100% community-funded through yearly sponsorship & pre-sales. We are ever-grateful to create with & for all of you.

Thank you to all who helped make this edition of Cycles Journal possible:
- Our Featured Collective - Wisdom Offerings Article Pages
- All in the Healing Resource Directory
- All who have helped us spread & share the mission!

With more years of Cycles Journal to come,
please consider joining us for future editions of reciprocal support.

Internal Influence : Menstrual

MENSTRUAL Inner Winter	FOLLICULAR Inner Spring	OVULATORY Inner Summer	LUTEAL Inner Autumn
		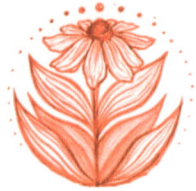	
Allowing flow & space	Emerging & integrating	Aligning with desires & creativity	Slowing down & releasing tension
Plan time for you, nourish yourself, stretch, listen to your internal wisdom, & trust your body.	Maintain connection with your inner voice, allow time to play & experiment, take your time.	Follow, feel, & indulge in what calls to you - self-affirm. Embrace your magnetism & deepen connections.	Prepare for rest, make sure your needs are met. Face your shadows. Ground into what helps you feel at ease.
Be wary of focusing on pain over presence; your body may be requesting help.	Be wary of overloading & disconnecting instead of slowly emerging.	Be wary of disregarding your needs & feelings before others in this extroverted time.	Be wary of burning out by not giving yourself space, time, & relief.

 ## THE ENERGETIC SIDE OF THE MENSTRUAL CYCLE

Alongside the physical & hormonal symptoms of our menstrual cycle phases, there is an energetic side that is a vital part of the whole. As you deepen your awareness & understanding of all aspects of our cycles through this journal, you can also consider the following energies associated with your personal phases.

Nothing exists alone - the phases you experience inside of you are influenced by & directly influence all parts of your existence, environment, mindset, spirit, lifestyle, hormones, & all the rest. Everything is a temporary condition, ever-changing - isn't it beautiful? All of your influences together make up your reality. Becoming aware of your influences helps you understand yourself, find root causes of symptoms, & notice when something is off-balance.

As always, you know your body best. No one can tell you what you experience or how to feel at any given time during your cycle - but these may be helpful in finding or adding to your own explanations.

All of us can tune into the energetic phases of our menstrual cycle to live our lives in cyclical ease rather than linear burn-out; never stopping to listen to what our body needs now or what we should prepare for next.

If you have an irregular or non-existent bleed, which can make it difficult to determine your exact physical phases, focusing on the "seasons" of the inner phases may be helpful. Tuning into your personal energy cycle, you can self-identify your own phases. It's up to you whether you consider your inner winter to be your actual bleed-time, or your energetic menstrual phase instead. Or you can follow the lunar cycle which reflects the same energy. You don't have to bleed to know when your rest phase is here - you just have to tune in and listen.

EXTERNAL INFLUENCE : LUNAR

NEW MOON Renew	FIRST QUARTER Reflect	FULL MOON Embrace	LAST QUARTER Surrender
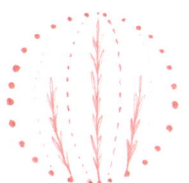		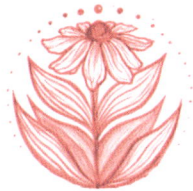	
What do I want to grow and create?	What steps can I take towards this?	How am I embracing change?	What does my body & mind need?
Tune in; internal work. Harness your potential to manifest desires.	Reflect on your needs. Release anything getting in the way.	Creatrix energy, intensity, climax. Harnessing power, giving gratitude.	Release anything else that has come up, honoring your needs.

☾ SETTING INTENTIONS ALONGSIDE LUNAR INFLUENCE ☽

WHAT IS LUNAR INFLUENCE?

The moon is our reminder to turn inwards in the externally focused world we live in. Lunar influence is allowing the phases of the moon to guide you in flowing through your life. Harnessing the lunar cycle alongside or in place of your menstrual cycle can help you build a sense of grounding within a state of constant flow. When we follow the energy and influence that the moon's phases have on us, we can recognize patterns & harness our power to manifest our desires in the creative growth cycle we shift through each day. It's helpful to balance our internal energy through external anchors such as the moon.

HOW DO I MANIFEST LUNAR INTENTIONS I SET?

To manifest is to focus on something with deep belief and intention, to the extent that you shift energy to help it align into your reality. Call it magic, or the law of attraction. You can set intentions to manifest anything from willpower, money or specific opportunities, to a new state of mind. It always requires reflection & release in tandem, along with patience, gratitude, & faith. But it's not just about thinking and hoping - it's about fully embracing, embodying, and taking legitimate steps and actions towards this intention while also working your magic. It's easy to underestimate this power we all innately possess until you try!

SETTING INTENTIONS IN THIS JOURNAL

Each week you'll see the quarter moon phase that is occurring - this is where you'll be prompted to reflect & dive in a little deeper to what you want to focus on. You can follow the prompts or write your own intentions/releases. Doing this alongside our menstrual cycle can be helpful in understanding both our internal & external wants and needs, and the patterns within both.

While both the lunar & menstrual cycle are reflections of all life/death cycles, it doesn't mean that you have to accomplish something or reach a goal each cycle. Some things will take multiple cycles to manifest fully or complete. Be patient with yourself & the natural forces at work.

THE MOON

The moon is our ancestral way-shower – a cyclical cartographer that teaches us how to be our own map-makers as we learn to navigate the inner realm of our wholistic wellness experiences. To be in sync with the moon does not mean your menstrual cycle has to line up with the new moon. Instead you are tuned in to what each phase's alignment means for you. However you align is perfect!

THE MOON IS A REFERENCE POINT

Those of us with inconsistent or non-existent menstrual cycles still have hormonal fluctuations and other symptoms of the cycle. By using the moon as our anchoring guide & reminder, we can track patterns or irregularities within our cycle, even when it may not feel like there is one since tracking from 'Day 1' is determined by bleeding. The new moon can be our Day 1 to ground us with a landmark.

THE MOON IS AN INFLUENCE

Our internal bodies are affected by the moon's pull, just as the tides are, since both we & the Earth are made up of about 70% liquid. Yet, it is scientifically debatable whether the gravitational pull of the moon orbiting the Earth can affect our internal fluids, since we are much smaller than the Earth's oceans.

Scientific specificities can easily overlook underlying energetic occurrences that we cannot fully understand or measure - so we're tracking that here. Subconsciously we react to external stimuli, since we are sensitive beings. Newton's third law of motion states that "for every action, there is an equal and opposite reaction." It reflects Buddhist philosophies of the oneness within duality.

THE MOON IS A MIRROR

We feel our energy and moods shift with the weather - from a rainy day to a sunny day. We vary in sensitivity to these shifts in daytime weather, so therefore we can also tap into to the seasonal shifts of the nighttime. It's not as obvious to us because much of it acts on a subconscious level since the energy of the moon & night is internal as opposed to the sun & day being external.

Regardless, take this all with a grain of salt. The moon can enhance & contribute to our lives, but there are many other factors to consider - our hormones, environment, habits, astrology, and all the other things we track alongside one another here. Our relationship with the moon is unique and individual. The subconscious energy and guidance of the light in the night is always there for us to tap into. It can be helpful in harnessing our creative potential through rituals. May we all find comfort & guidance in the mystery of the moon.

THE MOON YOU WERE BORN UNDER

On the next page we discuss the basics & significance of astrology. While totally optional to follow, it can be useful to be able to compare your moon sign (the astrological sign the moon was in when you were born) to the sign the planets are in currently (transit). Same goes for your sun sign. It can signify tension if it's in the opposite sign, or some harmony and flow when in your same moon sign. If you don't already know your moon sign, astro-charts.com is a great place to find out.

YOUR SUN SIGN & SYMBOL: YOUR MOON SIGN & SYMBOL:

_____   _____
(my outer persona)   (my inner mode of instincts)

Traits

ASTROLOGY

While astrology may not be directly linked to the menstrual cycle, it can be helpful to consider all internal, external, and universal influences alongside one another. We include astrology here to add another layer of comparison – potent yet optional to utilize. Astrology is a complex, multi-faceted area and we are only scraping the very surface by including the moon & sun signs and elements.

We each have an entire birth/natal chart, which maps out how our solar system's planets were aligned when we were born. These relationships create an influence on our natural tendencies and personality. It is one aspect of the "nature" of who you are alongside the "nurture" of how you were raised to be. How the transiting planets (current planetary locations) relate to our charts can be revealing of how it may affect us & society as a whole each day.

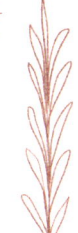

SUN SIGN
changes every 28-31 days, around the 3rd/4th week of every month. The sign that the sun is in can affect the external energy in the world, and also our personal lives depending on how our chart relates to the current placement.

MOON SIGN
changes every ~2.5 days. The phase and sign the moon is in can affect our internal / subconscious energy. On a new moon, the moon and sun will be of the same sign. On a full moon, they are in opposing/balancing signs, making for potent energy.

THEMES & ENERGY OF EACH SIGN:

The signs are archetypal imprints of nature's elements & energies that reflect in our human experience.

- **ARIES:** (fire) activity, motivation, impulses/instincts, vitality
- **TAURUS:** (earth) protection, steadiness, comfort, physicality
- **GEMINI:** (air) communication, ideas, relations, decisions
- **CANCER:** (water) intuition, family/home, emotions, nurture
- **LEO:** (fire) creativity, self-worth, ambition, intimacy
- **VIRGO:** (earth) service, efficiency, presentation, order
- **LIBRA:** (air) justice, balance, exchange, relations
- **SCORPIO:** (water) subconscious, depth, sensuality, transformation
- **SAGITTARIUS:** (fire) knowledge, expansion, movement, travel
- **CAPRICORN:** (earth) structure, stability, logic, work/finances
- **AQUARIUS:** (air) collaboration, mentality, community/society
- **PISCES:** (water) fluidity, dreams, feelings, expression

Download a free printable bookmark key for easy reference:

THE UTERUS / REPRODUCTIVE ORGAN

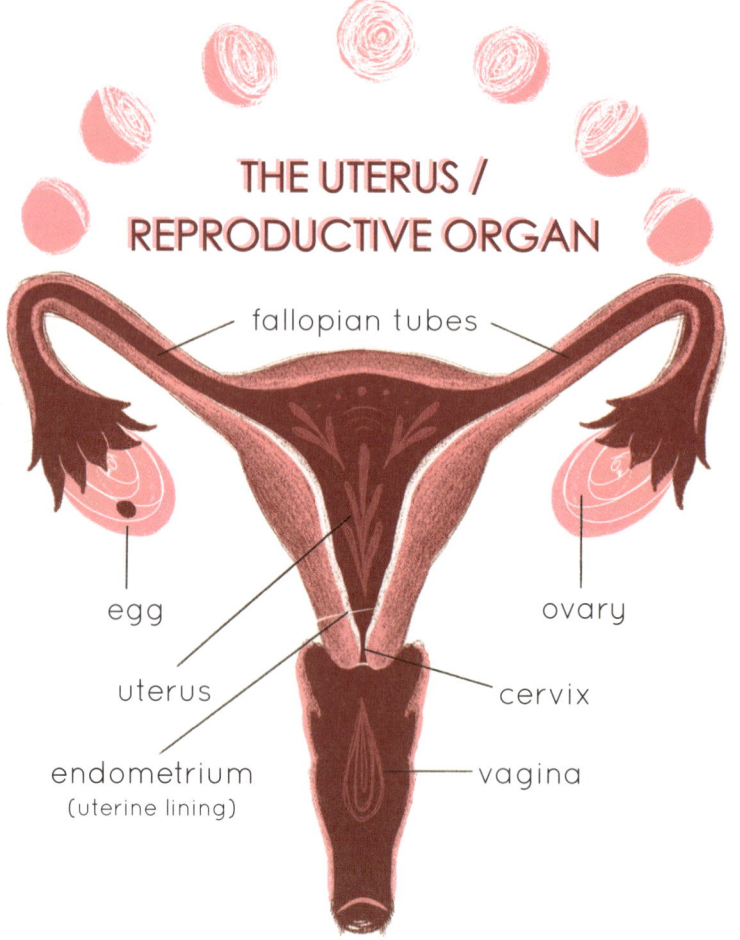

For many of us, what we learned in health class at young ages did not stick. This is likely because the teachings felt non-wholistic, fear-mongering and limited in preventative measures. It only focused on our sexual & reproductive organs' primal, base-level uses of heterosexual intercourse and reproduction, instead of speculating the entire spectrum of possibility.

Our uterus is more than a reproductive organ, although the magnificence of that in itself is not to be discredited or undermined. Our cyclical system represents a heightened link to the cycles within and around us. Everything in life is made up of energy; the blood in your veins flows with energy, the tides rise and fall with energy, you create with energy, the earth spins because of energy. Regardless of the different causes and modalities of these energies, they are all linked at the core of us. Everyone has this link regardless of having a uterus or not – this energetic space is often called the wombspace.

The menstrual cycle directly represents cycles of growth and decay, life and death, high and low, ebb and flow. It is a primary example of how we should be tuning into the patterns in our lives and the power we each hold. No matter our experience, we hold this internal reminder within the lifeblood we all carry. It can be our guide, alongside the moon, to harnessing the patterns of life we are weaved within. We are one with the spinning wheels of life, and it's time we embrace it all. We are on a mission to love ourselves deeper and become the best versions of ourselves — in-tune with our magic and one with the flow.

SELF-EXAM
2-3 days after your menstrual phase

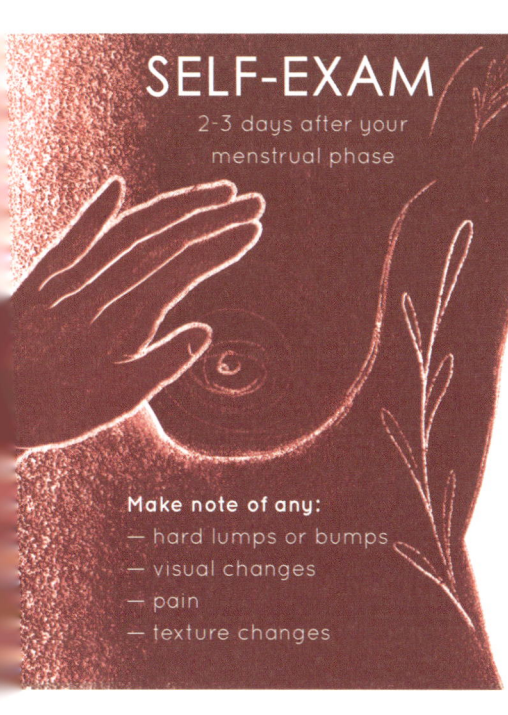

Make note of any:
— hard lumps or bumps
— visual changes
— pain
— texture changes

1. Check yourself in the mirror for any major changes in shape, swelling, redness, darkening, puckering or pulling in of skin, sores, rashes, or scales.

2. Lay on your right side and raise your left arm up to rest on your forehead.

3. With your right hand, use the pads of your middle 3 fingers to feel all tissue:
— start in your armpit
— feel down onto your side
— work your way over to your breast & around it, underneath it, & your collarbone
Work in small, circular motions feeling the surface, then deeper into the tissue.

4. Switch sides laying down and repeat

5. Repeat the above steps while standing

This is a Vulva
(Hint: the vagina is inside!)

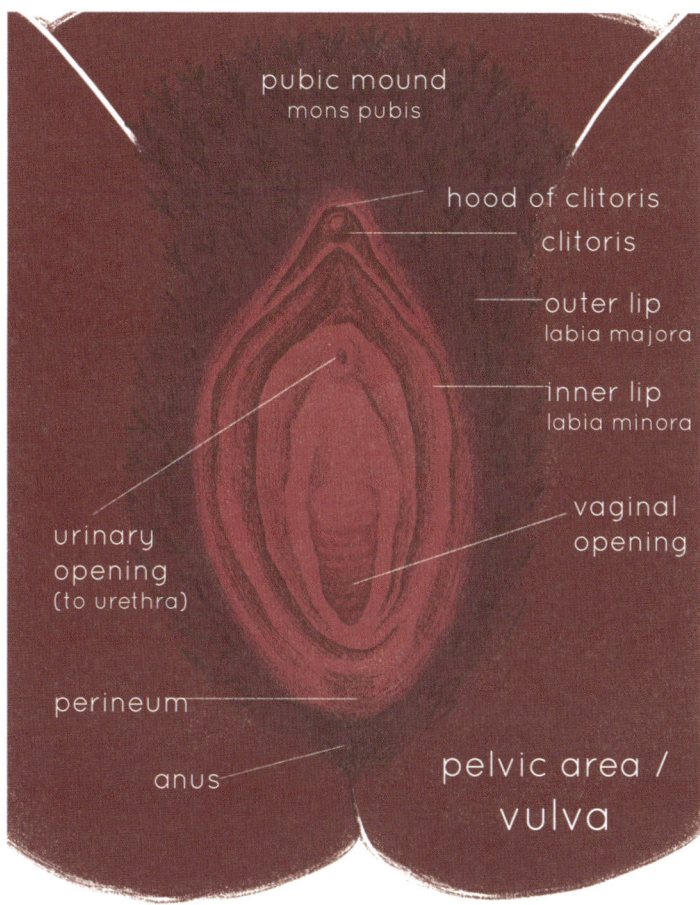

- pubic mound (mons pubis)
- hood of clitoris
- clitoris
- outer lip (labia majora)
- inner lip (labia minora)
- vaginal opening
- urinary opening (to urethra)
- perineum
- anus
- pelvic area / vulva

referenced from Nina Reimer's diagram from "The New Our Bodies, Ourselves" book

13

The Menstrual Cycle: Your Inner Phases

Your menstrual cycle is more than just your period – which is actually just a small fraction of the whole cycle! These are your inner phases; just like the Earth, you are cyclical and have seasons. Paying attention to your whole cycle via tracking will help you notice more of its subtleties, learn when your body needs what based on which phase it's in, and better plan to sync your life to your cycle.

While every body and every cycle is unique, this chart displays a range of what a healthy menstrual cycle looks like. If your cycle is different, irregular, or non-existent – don't panic, just be aware. You can always seek professional support & advice via the Healing Resource Directory in the back of this journal, &/or via your physician(s).

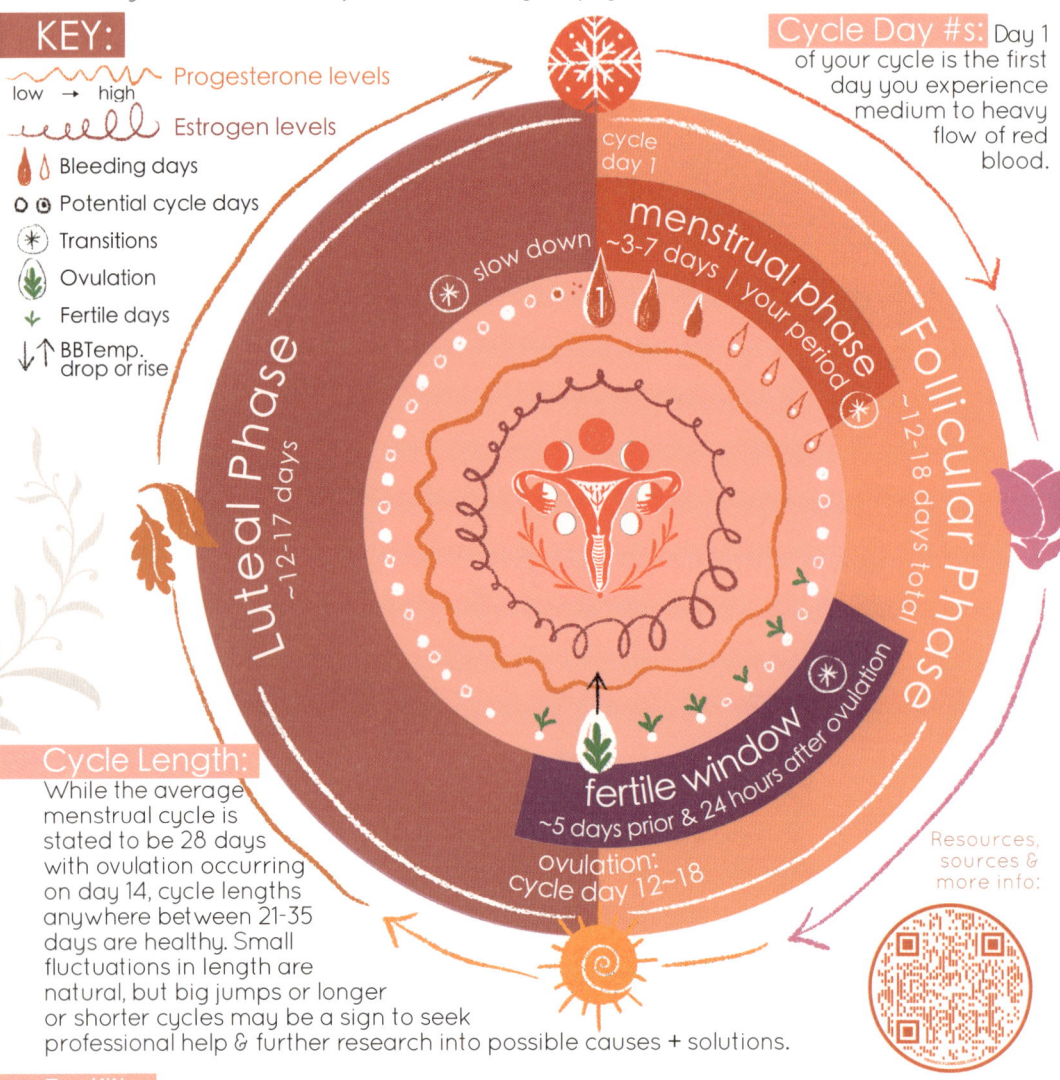

KEY:
- Progesterone levels (low → high)
- Estrogen levels
- Bleeding days
- Potential cycle days
- Transitions
- Ovulation
- Fertile days
- BBTemp. drop or rise

Cycle Day #s: Day 1 of your cycle is the first day you experience medium to heavy flow of red blood.

- menstrual phase ~3-7 days / your period
- Follicular Phase ~12-18 days total
- ovulation: cycle day 12~18
- fertile window ~5 days prior & 24 hours after ovulation
- Luteal Phase ~12-17 days

Cycle Length: While the average menstrual cycle is stated to be 28 days with ovulation occurring on day 14, cycle lengths anywhere between 21-35 days are healthy. Small fluctuations in length are natural, but big jumps or longer or shorter cycles may be a sign to seek professional help & further research into possible causes + solutions.

Fertility: Despite only being fertile for a small window of your cycle, generally 5 days prior to & 24 hours after ovulation, there is always potential for sperm to stick around anytime cervical fluid/discharge is present. Tracking is the best way to remain aware!

Irregular or Absent Cycles: While not bleeding may seem like a perk, your body is lacking an essential function. The hormonal imbalance that is likely a factor can also affect other areas of your health physically, mentally & emotionally. Don't panic, but be aware of this as a signal from your body to pay attention & take action to restore balance. Those near menarche or menopause may experience more cycle variation even while healthy.

Resources, sources & more info:

Phase 1 • Menstrual • Inner Winter • 3-7 days

Uterine Cycle: The uterus sheds its lining (endometrium) when the released egg from ovulation is not fertilized. 2-4 tbsp of vibrant red blood is shed per cycle (approx. 1-2 menstrual cups).

Hormones: Estrogen & progesterone levels remain low.

Common Symptoms:
- increased inflammation
- lower back pain
- mood swings, irritability
- fatigue, bloating, cramps
- headaches, tender chest

Phase 2: Follicular • Inner Spring • ~5-11 days (varies)

Uterine Cycle: The follicular phase is also know as the pre-ovulatory phase. The uterine lining rebuilds as it prepares for the potential implantation of an egg.

Hormones: Follicle Stimulating Hormone (FSH) stimulates egg growth in the ovaries. Estrogen levels rise.

Common Symptoms:
- increased metabolism
- improved moods & energy
- lower body temp. ~96.8-98°F

Phase 3: Ovulatory • Inner Summer • ~2-6 days

Uterine Cycle: Fertile phase (window may vary). More cervical fluid/discharge will be present before & after the egg is released.

Hormones: An abrupt surge of Luteinizing Hormone (LH) triggers egg to release from the ovaries. Body reaches estrogen threshold & decreases after.

Common Symptoms:
- increased libido
- fluctuating moods
- more cervical fluid
- increased appetite
- more autoimmune disease symptoms

Phase 4: Luteal • Inner Autumn • ~12-17 days

Uterine Cycle: The uterine lining thickens and prepares for potential implantation if the egg is fertilized. Follicle that held the egg collapses (corpus luteum) – this prevents the release of any other eggs.

Hormones: Progesterone levels rise. Estrogen levels decrease, then fluctuate.

Common Symptoms:
- higher body temp. ~98.1-99.1°F
- mood swings
- trouble sleeping
- lower immune response
- increased appetite
- swollen/sore, headaches
- skin troubles
- weight gain
- libido shift

Symptoms & Pain:
Menstrual cycle pain has been normalized in our culture – this creates an illusion that we do not have options or the power of choice for our own bodies' health, that we just have to suck it up, and that we have to cover up our symptoms with pharmaceuticals in order to function in a non-cyclical society. We deserve more.

While mild discomfort is common and considered normal, debilitating pain that interrupts your daily life is not normal. Usually pain is a signal from your body that something is off or needs attention; hormonally, nutritionally, physically, environmentally, and/or energetically. We can track our symptoms with our cycle to try to uncover what it is linked to – awareness is the first step. Further pages in this journal offer tips to address pain naturally and nourish your body with food – however it is not a replacement for professional support or diagnosis. We hope that this introductory information can inspire you to further your own research as well, so you can feel empowered to study and know your own body & helpful information that exists.

Fertility Awareness: Natural Birth Control
by Silvia Canelón • Fertility Awareness Educator
@cyclecurious • cyclecurious@pm.me

Through learning to follow our body's cues and signs, we can tell when we are fertile & when we are not. This page is meant to empower you to tune into tracking these methods.

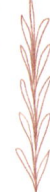

DISCLAIMER: It is not recommended to use the observations described here as a method for birth control without seeking further instruction from the resources provided on these pages or from a certified Fertility Awareness Educator.

FERTILITY SIGNS FROM CERVICAL MUCUS

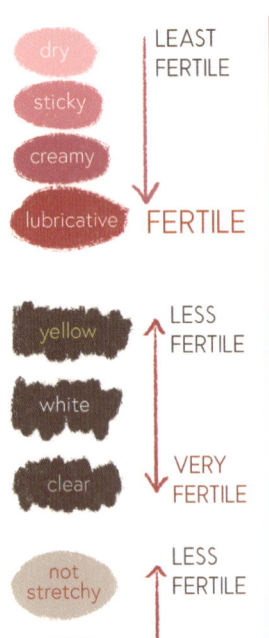

SENSATION: Use tissue paper folded flat before and after you use the restroom and pay attention to how it feels to wipe from front to back. Does it feel dry, smooth, or lubricative? Dry sensations point to least fertile conditions while a lubricative sensation points to the presence of very fertile cervical fluid.

TEXTURE: If you notice the presence of cervical fluid on the tissue, examine it by lifting it off the tissue and feeling it between two fingers. Does it feel dry, sticky, creamy, or lubricative? Dry cervical fluid is least fertile whereas lubricative cervical fluid is most fertile.

COLOR: Does the cervical fluid have a color? Does it look yellow, white, clear? A yellow coloration might point to less fertile quality whereas clear indicates very fertile cervical fluid.

STRETCH: Does the cervical fluid stretch? How much? Less than 1/4 inch, 1/4 - 1 inch, or more than 1 inch? The more it stretches, the more fertile.

moist, sticky, holds its shape, white, opaque

wetter, thinner, slightly stretchy, cloudy

slippery, thin, transparent, stretchy

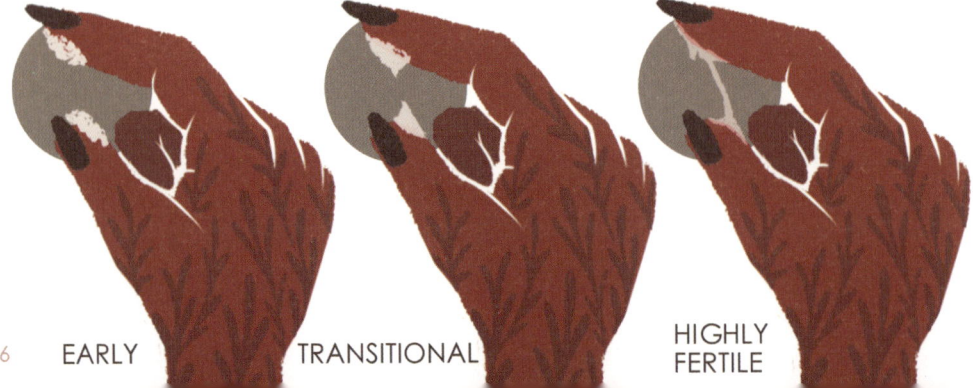

EARLY • TRANSITIONAL • HIGHLY FERTILE

16

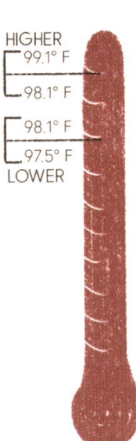

BASAL BODY TEMPERATURE (BBT): Use a BBT thermometer to take your temperature first thing in the morning before talking or getting out of bed: place thermometer under the tongue or in the armpit for at least 5 minutes before reading the temperature.

Make note of temperature on your daily page, and notice deviations:

After ovulation, progesterone levels rise sharply within 24 hours. This increase causes a basal body temperature shift from lower pre-ovulatory temperatures (normally 97.5° to 98.1° F) to higher post-ovulatory temperatures (normally 98.1° to 99.1° F)

CERVIX POSITIONING : Your cervix also responds to the hormonal fluctuations throughout your cycle. A cervix is likely to become straight (vs. tilted), low (vs. high), and soft (vs. firm) with an open (vs. closed) opening as you approach ovulation. You can check regularly by simply inserting a clean finger into your vagina, and feeling upwards.

RULES FOR AVOIDING PREGNANCY NATURALLY

FIRST 5 DAYS RULE:
You are safe the first 5 days of your menstrual cycle, if you've had an obvious temperature shift 12-16 days before.

DRY DAY RULE:
You are safe the evening of each dry day.

PEAK DAY RULE:
You are safe the evening of the 3rd consecutive day after the last day of egg white cervical fluid or lubricative vaginal sensation.

THERMAL SHIFT RULE:
You are safe the evening of the 3rd normal consecutive high temperature and the days remaining until menstruation.

TO OPTIMIZE CHANCES OF CONCEPTION :
Enjoy unprotected vaginal intercourse every day that you have cervical fluid and/or a lubricative vaginal sensation! NOTE: pregnancy is confirmed by 18 days of consistent high temperatures.

RESOURCES:
"Justisse Method User Guide" by Justisse College International
"Taking Charge of Your Fertility" by Toni Weschler

SUSTAINABLE BLEEDING

by Sadie Francis • @onlyintheforest
Environmental Activist, Feminist Advocate & Botanical Artist

Healthy menstruation is, arguably, one of the most important, yet the most overlooked, aspect of our health and the body positivity movement. We who contain wombs have been taught to believe that it is largely an inconvenience: painful, messy, and embarrassing.

For centuries, the patriarchy taught us to believe that bleeding people are "dirty," unholy, and even dangerous. Tampons & pads are bleached for no other purpose than to lend a sense of "white cleanliness," while the toxic by-products, such as dioxin, are absorbed by our bodies.

We can reclaim these sacred cycles by becoming interested, getting informed, and having honest conversations with one another about the best products to use, natural remedies for cramps and infections, and even how to naturally track our fertility cycles.

THE COST

Menstrual hygiene products represent a $5.9 billion industry in the U.S. and $35.4 billion one worldwide. That number is expected to top $40 billion around the world in the next few years, according to Global Industry Analysts.

The "average" person menstruates from the age of 13-51, and each period can last three to seven days. That's about 38 years and 456 periods. Thus, the average menstruator spends $150-$300 a year on feminine hygiene disposables, extrapolated to a cost of between $9,000 and $12,000 over a lifetime.

Yet it never even occurs to most of us to view the purchases that have become integrated into our monthly regime through a critical lens. And, in my experience from talking with others, too many do not seek alternatives simply because of the fact that they didn't think any alternatives existed, when they do!

THE AVERAGE MENSTRUATOR SPENDS $150 TO $300 A YEAR ON REPRODUCTVE HYGIENE DISPOSABLE PRODUCTS, AND BETWEEN $9,000 AND $12,000 OVER A LIFETIME.

THE WASTE

The solid waste accumulating after the use of these products is immense. Over 9 billion tampons are disposed of annually, wreaking havoc on sewage systems all over the world. Tampon applicators, which are not biodegradable, are the most common debris in the ocean, beaches, & in the stomachs of fish and turtles. Over 12 billion pads are disposed of annually, also containing plastics that are not biodegradable. Each pad comes individually wrapped, replete with bleached synthetic fibers imbued with potentially hazardous residues from manufacturing.

These products and their decadent packaging have become an extraneous burden on already overburdened landfills, simultaneously depositing toxic substances into surrounding soil and water.

HONOR YOUR BODY & THE EARTH'S BODY

by Rachael Amber • @rachael.amber

You don't have to be "zero waste" to have an impact. Every little effort to shift from disposable single-use products to reusable products that are both safer & less-costly for ourselves and the Earth makes a difference.

Take a moment to think about the products you use when you bleed; do you use them because they're familiar, comfortable, affordable, accessible, disposable? What are your products made of and where do they go?

Sometimes we use things because it's what we've been told to use or we just didn't know what else was out there. But you have options! The beauty is you can always try new things and potentially find a better way to support your cycle. Or you can confirm that your way is what works best for your body.

SUSTAINABLE vs. DISPOSABLE

While it may cost a bit more up front and require an ounce of your time to clean, these products save you money in the long run and are better for your body, your wallet, & the planet!

These products may be convenient and lower cost up front, but they come with a bigger cost to your body and the environment with all of the hidden chemicals and plastics inside.

MENSTRUAL CUPS

- One-time purchase of ~$25-45
- Lasts ~6-12+ years
- Breaks down to ~$2-4 per year
- You only really need one
- Easy to clean with gentle soap
- Reuse right away
- Comes in multiple sizes & shapes
- Leave it in for up to 12 hours
- No chemicals, toxins, or irritants
- No chance of TSS
- No waste
- Use it to collect blood for other uses

TAMPONS

- Costs ~$8-16 per box, ~$0.40-$1.20 each
- Single use
- Breaks down to ~$150-600 per year
- No maintenance & easy to travel with
- Non-biodegradable waste in packaging & product
- Contains toxins & chemicals
- Fibers can tear internally & irritate
- Wear up to 8 hours
- Risk of Toxic Shock Syndrome
- Stock takes up more space
- More deliveries or trips to the store
- Most are sold by large-scale, male-owned corporations

CLOTH PADS, LINERS & PERIOD UNDERWEAR

- One-time purchase of ~$5-20 per pad or liner, or ~$20-45 per underwear
- Lasts ~3-6+ years
- You only need a few to start or 1-2 if you rotate with other products
- Hand-wash or wash with laundry
- Reuse within ~24 hours or once dry
- Comes in a variety of sizes, absorbencies, styles, & patterns
- No chemicals, absorptive fibers, or irritants. No waste or toxins
- Most period underwear are super cute, comfy, & you can't even tell!

COTTON PADS & LINERS

- Costs ~$5-18 per pack of pads or liners, ~$.10-1 each• ~$150-500 per year
- Single use
- All of the same pros & cons as above

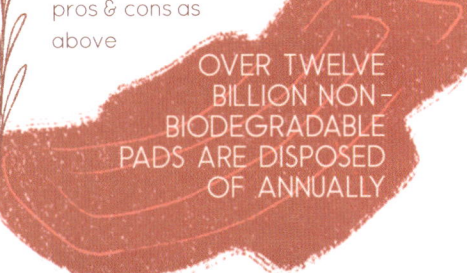

OVER TWELVE BILLION NON-BIODEGRADABLE PADS ARE DISPOSED OF ANNUALLY

Forming Sustainable Habits: Tips & tricks to Help you Track

If you want to get to know your body better and dive deeper into your menstrual cycle awareness, having the intention and desire is the first step!

You already know there is purpose and knowledge in listening to your body & figuring out how it flows – that's why you're here reading this! From here you can begin to form the habit & dedication to make it a regular & easeful part of your life.

First, realize how empowering this is & be proud of yourself by taking the first steps to committing to a life-changing tool in your life; tracking through this space! You're taking matters into your own hands so that you can claim the fullness of your potential. This is a practice in self-acceptance and self-care. We are learning to love what we were told to hate about ourselves. We are learning that our cycles are not a crutch to avoid or get over, but a valuable tool that is full of magic if we learn how to embrace it, understand it, and flow with it!

The more we are able to dedicate ourselves to this practice of keeping track of it all, the more we will get out of it and the more we will have to reflect on. It's normal and okay to miss a few days here and there - you're only human! The goal is to deepen your dedication to yourself and this practice through consistent recordings, but of course this takes practice and perhaps some help to form the habit!

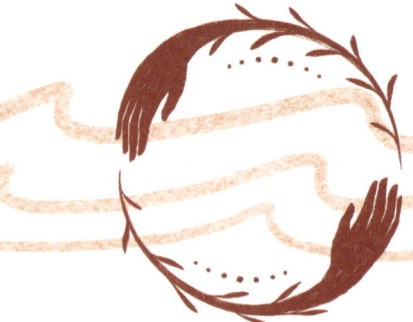

It's not about self-discipline, but self-devotion
The goal is to feel determined to track to find the answers, not to force yourself to do pain-staking work. It's all about finding your rhythm, and being okay with sometimes skipping it for a moment, but knowing we can always come back and find it again when ready. If you miss a few days, just go back and fill in what you can remember, or let it go and keep moving forward!

Be patient with yourself
Forming habits takes time, effort, trial, error, forgiveness & flow. Don't worry if it takes longer than expected or if you miss a handful or chunk of days. The blank space is just holding space for the time you needed away and will always welcome you back.

Leave your journal where you'll see it
Leaving your journal somewhere you'll see it all the time can help you remember to take a moment and spend some time with it. Leave it somewhere along your daily routine; like where you have breakfast or where you meditate before bed. Wherever you'll see it often, and wherever you'll actually use it.

SET A REMINDER ON YOUR PHONE OR CALENDAR!
If you respond well to scheduling, it helps to schedule self-care too so work doesn't take over! Try putting an alarm or calendar reminder in your phone.

PAUSE & CONNECT TO YOURSELF FIRST
Sometimes you just need to ground first and release the resistance of whatever is stopping you from journaling & cycle-tracking. Try meditation, yoga, breathwork, movement; however you like to ground. When we feel connected to our bodies, we can listen better.

UTILIZE YOUR DAILY PLANNER AS AN ALLY
If you use a separate calendar or planner for specific things, then transfer your cycle data into it to keep you reminded of your off days, or make a note to check in here, too.

SOMETHING IS BETTER THAN NOTHING
Just fill in what you can each day - maybe a few keywords that will help you remember what you were feeling & experiencing that you may or may not want to expand on later.

COME BACK TO IT LATER
Not feeling it at all? Skip today! Skip tomorrow if you need to. Maybe in a few days you'll be able to get back to it, and you remember a few things that stood out from the past days you didn't record your symptoms.

FORGIVE YOURSELF AND GET BACK ON IT
If we only beat ourselves up when we don't do what we aimed to do, progress won't be made and self-love sure isn't present. We are only human, and we are building a nurturing, healing practice, not creating harsh discipline.

KEEP PHONE NOTES WHEN YOU DON'T HAVE YOUR JOURNAL WITH YOU
When you're out & about without your journal & notice symptoms or anything significant pop up, take notes on your notes app or send yourself an email with a clear subject line. This way you don't forget, and you can transfer it to your journal later.

ALLOW COMMUNITY TO HELP
When we feel stuck, unsure, or alone, it's easy to spiral without community or loved ones to pull us out of it. Sharing your concerns & observations with others can be super helpful, which is why we created a free space for us all to share & support one another on our journeys: cyclicalcommunity.com

MAKE IT A RITUAL
Better than habit or routine, is ritual. It works similarly, but it's all mindset. If you think of your cycle-tracking as a chore or dreaded habit you're trying to form, chances are you'll just keep forming resistance to dedicating to it. But what if we think of this helpful tool as part of our ritual, or link it to rituals we already do? We can embrace the magic in this.

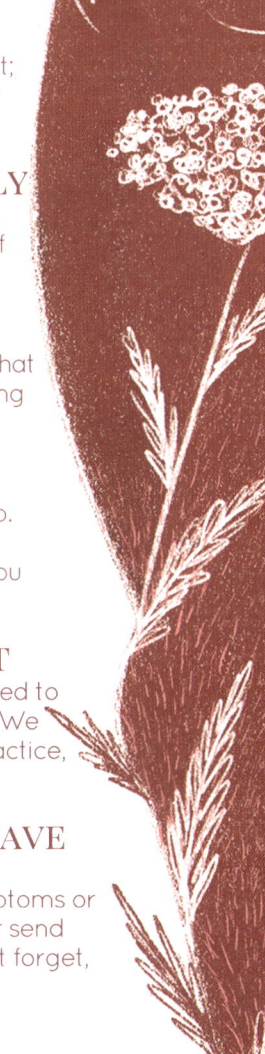

HOW TO USE THIS JOURNAL

MOONTHLY OVERVIEW

Moonth = a lunation or lunar cycle month that begins on the new moon instead of calendar day 1 (how nature keeps time).

MOON CYCLE & SUN SIGN
- The chronological # for this new moon cycle of the year. There are 12 or 13 complete moon cycles each Gregorian/common calendar year.
- The symbol & name for the astrological sign the sun moves into during this cycle.
- The sun sign speaks to the external, collective energy that influences the world & how it aspects your personal astrology.

CALENDAR MONTH
The common calendar month this moon cycle starts during.

EACH CHART STARTS ON THE NEW MOON
- Beginning of the lunar cycle.
- For ease of comparing your menstrual + lunar cycles.
- Use as a landmark if you have an irregular or non-existent bleed.
- Star * signifies an eclipse.

DATE OF MONTH
- Day # of calendar date – corresponds with same date on daily journaling pages.
- Letter day of week above (M = Monday)

CYCLE DAY
If you bleed, write the day # of your menstrual cycle here. Day 1 = first bright red bleed day. Count up from there until your next bleed. Your cycle does NOT have to line up with the new moon. If you don't bleed, the new moon is your day 1.

EXPERIENCES & HABITS TO TRACK + EXTRA SPACE
- In the column beneath each day, you'll track the physical & emotional symptoms you experience.
- You'll fill in the bubble in that day's column per symptom based on how intensely you feel it or how frequently it occurs that day (see key below).
- Follow habits you want to track too. Extra space is provided in each category for you to fill in your own unique symptoms & habits to follow.
- Follow patterns across rows over time.
- All of the moonthly spreads are consecutive in the journal, so that you can easily compare once you've collected a few months of data.
- Don't worry – we remind you each day on the daily spreads to flip to this page. Plus you can keep a bookmark here!

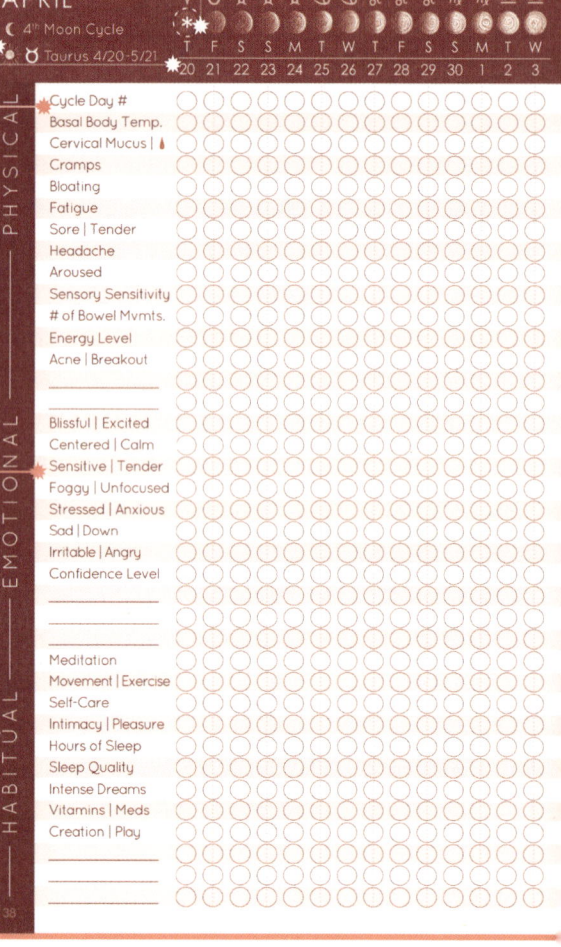

SUGGESTED KEY:
- ⊖ Less • Opposite
- ○ Not occurring
- ⊘ Somewhat • Mild
- ◐ Moderate • Half
- ● Fully Present • Done
- ●! Extreme • Intense

(Or feel free to create your own key instead!)

This chart will help you get into the habit of checking in regularly & noticing patterns as they form or change. In this zoomed out view you can compare all of your internal & external influences in one place! Visit cyclesjournal.com/howto for more info & tips, or scan the QR code:

MOON SIGN + SYMBOL

- The astrological sign the moon is in each day (see pg. 11 for key).
- Changes every 2-3 days.
- Speaks to the subconscious collective energy influencing you.
- Outline highlights the full moon.
- Star ✶ signifies an eclipse.

MOON PHASE DRAWING

- An illustration of the phase the moon is in each day.
- The moon's phases shift when illuminated by the sun – from the dark new moon 0%, to waxing (growing light) phases, the full moon 100%, waning (fading light) phases, until we reach darkness again and a new cycle begins. Quarter moons are 50% illuminated – half light, half dark.
- The moon's phase impacts the tides - and we believe it affects our internal state energetically. We reflect on the growth stages to guide setting intentions on the daily pages.

OTHER DATA

- Calendar month right page starts on
- Traditional full moon names (see blog)
- Any equinox, solstice or eclipse dates

HOW TO USE THIS SPREAD:

1. Each day, find the date at the top.

2. Follow the column below & check each symptom/habit row on the left.

3. Fill in the bubble based on the intensity you experienced of that symptom/emotion or the completeness of the habit (see key).

4. Continue to the daily journaling space for the same date to expand, reflect and deepen your insight, understanding, observations, feelings, ideas, etc.

By the end of the year, you'll have a complete side-by-side record of all your symptoms, patterns, & habits just from these pages alone!

MAY
Full Flower Moon
Eclipse: 4/20 + 5/5

NOTES

★ TRACKING KEY
⊖ Less • Opposite
○ Not Occurring
◐ Somewhat • Mild
◐ Moderate • Half
● Fully Present • ✓
● Extreme • Intense

Use #s or Letters where applicable:

Mucus • Clear, White
Dry • Blood • Spotting

Intimacy • Sex •
Masturbation •
Pleasure w other(s)

USING LETTERS | NUMBERS:

- Use #s instead where applicable, ie: hours of sleep,
- Use letters to specify for Cervical Mucus: C when it's clear, W when white/opaque, D for when you're dry/experiencing none, B for bleeding & S for spotting. Expand on this or adjust as needed.
- Same for Intimacy | Pleasure: Use I for intimacy, S for sex/intercourse, M for masturbation/self-pleasure, & P for pleasure with other(s). Expand on this or adjust as needed.

DAILY SPACE

Each day, you are given half a page to write, reflect, & journal in depth, in addition to the symptom + habit tracking chart on the moonthly overview.

On each new, first quarter, full & last quarter moon, you'll get an extra half page to set & follow your intentions or goals through-out the cycle.

CYCLE PHASE | SEASON

• Circle which inner season/cycle phase you're in; winter/menstruation, spring/follicular, summer/ovulation, autumn/luteal. Reference pg. 14 & make your best inference.
• If you have an irregular cycle, circle the Earth's season or the season you feel inside.

WEATHER | MOOD

The weather can impact our moods, so circle what the weather was like today! Or, circle your internal weather.

REMINDERS

Friendly reminders to tune in first & to check in on the moonthly overview, too. Practicing gratitude (what are you thankful for?) + celebrating (as simple as smiling or doing a little dance) helps affirm healthy habit building + self-connection.

MOON PHASE & SIGN

Astrological sign the moon is in. When there are two signs, it's the current sign 1st, & sign transitioning into.

SUN SIGN

Astrological sign the sun is in.

MENSTRUAL CYCLE DAY

• Record the day # of your cycle (Day 1 = first bright red bleed).
• If you're irregular use the moon phases – new moon as day 1.

BBT | TEMPERATURE

For tracking fertility, take your Basal Body Temp. at the start of each day.

F • JAN 6   Day #: _____

Phase | Season:

○ Breathe & drop in
○ Moonthly tracking
○ Gratitude practice
○ Celebrate yourself!

Physical State
Flow | Fluids

Emotional & Mental State

Self-Care
Sleep | Dreams

FULL MOON IN CANCER

An expansion of nurturing empathy & deeper connection

What is being illuminated?

I give gratitude for what is & what is becoming:

WRITING PROMPTS & SPACE

• Check in with yourself & write about what you're experiencing today physically & any details about your flow/cervical fluid.
• Record how you feel emotionally & mentally.
• Note how well & how long you slept, how you cared for yourself, what you consumed, any dreams, notes on spiritual health...
• Feel free to expand into the space to the right, or use it to plan, write in more depth, etc.

QUARTER MOON PHASE & INTENTIONS

• Quarterly reminders below each new moon, first/last quarter & full moon.
• The astrological sign the moon is in.
• A poetic perspective on the energy of this phase & sign combination.
• Prompts to guide you in setting & following new or existing intentions.

CYCLE REFLECTION

This page will help you record, reflect, follow your patterns & remind you to keep track of your cycle. Learn to increase your cyclical awareness as you plan alongside & around your significant cycle days.

MOON CYCLE

• # new moon cycle of year.
• Start + ends dates of the past/ending moon cycle.
• Reflect & record on this page within these dates, during your cycle, or at end of this lunar cycle.

LAST CYCLE DAY 1

• Record the day of the month you began bleeding this past month. If irregular, your day 1 is the first date of the moon cycle on the left.
• This helps you track the landmark of where your cycle starts within the moon's cycle — circle below.

DAYS TO NOTE

• "Caution days" are those difficult cycle days #s you felt overwhelmed, upset, and may want to block off when planning to avoid overloading yourself & save space for extra care.
• "Bliss days" are cycle days you felt at your best— prime creation days perhaps.
• Note other standout days.
• Use cycle day #s or moon phases here if you can to predict into your next cycle.

OBSERVE PATTERNS, CHANGES & CARE

• A space to discover & keep track of your patterns, their warning signs & landmarks — anything that recurs each cycle or constantly.
• Note any changes or new symptoms here that you want to keep an eye on.
• Reflect on what was nourishing & helpful to you so you can remember what to save space for.
• Keep track of rituals you want to remember.

1st
01 | 21
02 | 19

CHECK IN & REFLECT

Last Cycle Day 1: _____
(new moon if you don't bleed)
(+ now the phase you bleed near)

Use this space to reflect on your experiences & findings from this ending lunar cycle or your last menstrual cycle. Use cycle day #s if you bleed, or moon phases if you don't.

○ ☾ ☽ ● ● ● ● ● ● ● ☾ ○

Caution Days: (days I needed space)   Bliss Days: (days I felt great)

DAYS TO NOTE — Which cycle days stood out?

OBSERVATIONS — Notice any changes or patterns?

SELF-CARE — What was helpful & nourishing?

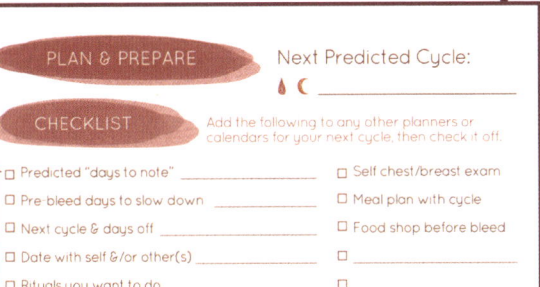

PLAN & PREPARE   Next Predicted Cycle:
                          ♦ ☾ _____

CHECKLIST   Add the following to any other planners or calendars for your next cycle, then check it off.

☐ Predicted "days to note" _____   ☐ Self chest/breast exam
☐ Pre-bleed days to slow down _____   ☐ Meal plan with cycle
☐ Next cycle & days off _____   ☐ Food shop before bleed
☐ Date with self &/or other(s) _____   ☐ _____
☐ Rituals you want to do _____   ☐ _____
☐ _____

PLAN & PREPARE FOR THE NEXT CYCLE

• A checklist of reminders to reflect, predict, & plan with the above info gathered for your next significant cycle days.
• Planning ahead helps us feel more at ease. Count up to predict the next cycle day # these may occur on or near.
• Mark off these dates in this journal & transfer dates into your calendar & any other planners you use.
• Make space for your predicted bleeding days & the days leading up to it — plan to devote to your well-being.

SELF-EXAMS

Refer to page 13 for how to perform your monthly breast exam — best done in the follicular phase (post-bleed).

25

How to use the Cycle Checkins' Open Space

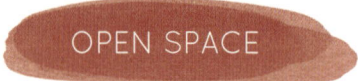 Use this space how you wish, or print out one of our free templates to paste here for BBT charting, dream tracking, or something else:

I wanted to create a space for you to breathe &/or customize as you please. There's no right or wrong way to use this space, but there is an intention behind it.

I've gotten many lovely requests over the years to add features like BBT charts, calendar overviews, dream theme trackers, and more. I've been trying to find a way to include these options for those who want them, while also honoring the spatial limitations of the journal.

Thus I decided to reserve the right page of each Cycle Checkin spread for you to use as you wish. I've created a few free templates of the above requests for you to transfer or paste, and I hope to add more in the future as time allows.

How to use the Phasic Overview & In-Betweens

Phasic Overview & In-Betweens — Use this space to focus on the phases of the moonth and the in-betweens of the peaks.

One way of using this space is to designate one column for your goal-planning, intention-setting or focus per phase/week. Use the other column for reflections, dream themes, nutrition tracking, cards pulls, etc!

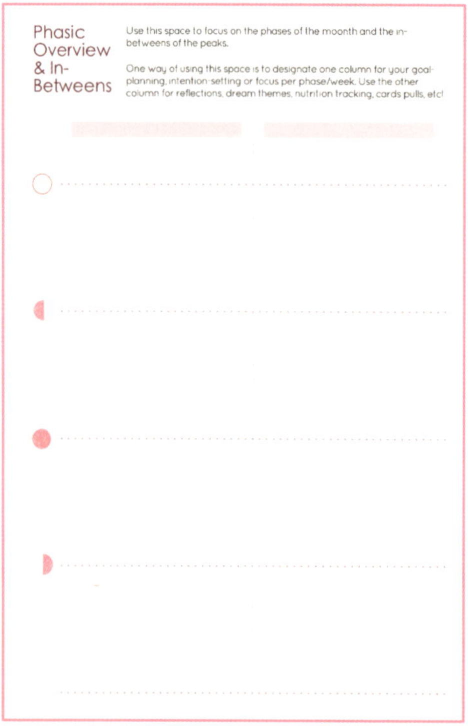

This is an overview to focus on the phases of the moonth and the in-betweens of the peak lunations.

Use this space to add the dates and/or your cycle dates they fall on, and expand into how you'd like to work with this cycle.

One way of using this space is to designate one column for your goal-planning, intention-setting or focus per phase/week.

Use the other column for reflections, dream themes, nutrition tracking, cards pulls, etc!

Practicing Cyclical Mindfulness

By Rachael Amber (they/she) • Intuitive Nature-Centric Channel & Artist • @rachael.amber • @embodiedecosystems • cyclicalroots.com •

Cyclical Mindfulness or Wholistic Cycle Awareness is finding our center of awareness within the ever-changing nature of life.

It's honoring all parts of the whole, through noticing patterns, connections, and intersections.

It's trust within the endless cycles of growth & decay; embodying our true nature. Following instinct & intuition, it is presence in both painful and pleasurable polarities – holding space for the in-betweens.

It is not just of the mind, but of all we perceive, feel and are.

Living within the unknowns, you are a beacon of potential. All you need is to stay anchored in presence so you can release and flow.

This is a practice of presence with patterns.

There are corresponding elemental symbols on the daily pages in this journal for you to use as cues for practices and prompts if you'd like. Or, let them be décor.

PROMPTS:

▽ I am pausing/grounding because…

▽ I notice / feel…

△ I allow / open to…

△ I respond / release…

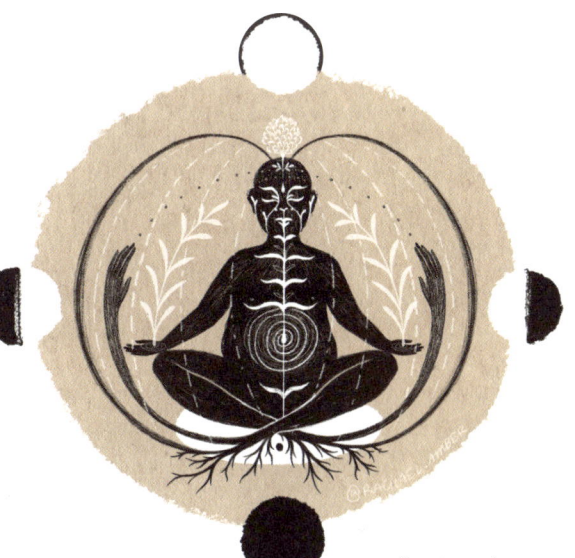

PRACTICE:

▽ **1. Pause • Ground (Earth)**
• take a break • set boundaries • allow space…

▽ **2. Notice • Feel (Water)**
• tune in • observe your experience & senses…

△ **3. Allow • Open (Fire)**
• move • create • self-compassion • find support…

△ **4. Reflect • Release (Air)**
• write • analyze • integrate • rest • respond…

Receive a free meditation →

& the option to go deeper in understanding this methodology…

A letter of devotion to yourself;

Dear _____,
         (your name here)

I honor you. As we embark on this journey in this space, I promise to devote time & energy to getting to know you better. I will learn to say "no" when I need more time with you, and "yes" when it feels nourishing & pleasurable for you.

In this space we will find release & flow. I will love & embrace you openly — I promise to be a better listener.

I strive to create nurturing habits & invigorating rituals that deeply respect your needs & boundaries.

I am here with you through all the pain, doubt, blame, & worry — that is not who you are, but conditions we are working to release and transmute.

I honor the beauty & magic in your natural cycles. I promise to plan my life with you always in mind & to check in with you before making big decisions. I will be more present with you. I trust that you forgive me for any unintentional absence of presence from the past so that we can move forward into better unity & allyship.

I trust in you & your wisdom and messages. I trust in the flow of your cycles & patterns and I will no longer go against or disregard it.

I see you & all of your potential, worthiness, & abundance. I am here to help you embrace it. I am here for you & I love you.

Here & for the rest of this year in Cycles Journal, I devote myself to you.

In this next chapter together, I hope to . . .

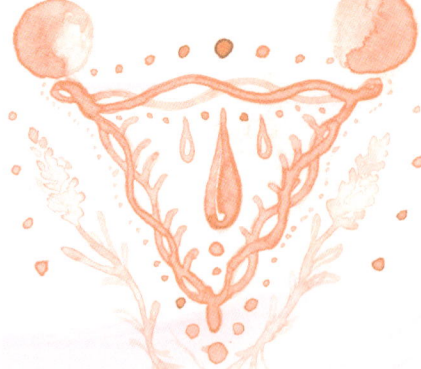

Love,

_____
     (your name here)

Once you've completed adding your own words to this letter,
read it out loud while facing yourself in a mirror & then sign + date at the bottom.

2025 Intentions

Endless growth & potential lives within you, ready . . .

In 2025 I will focus on . . .
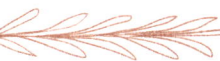

In 2025 I will stop focusing on . . .
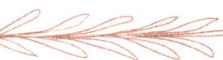

In 2025 I will experience . . .
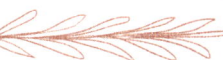

In 2025 I will travel to . . .
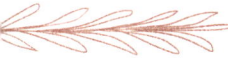

In 2025 I will learn to . . .
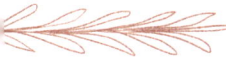

My affirmation going into 2025 is . . .
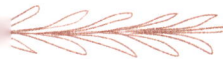

In 2025 . . .
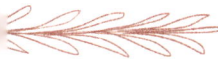

Where are you starting...?

Do you know of any patterns or recurring symptoms within your cycle? (emotional, physical, etc.) (if not, no worries)

Is there anything specific you experience that you're trying to understand the root cause & pattern of?

What do you want to know about your body &/or menstrual cycle?

How do you want to feel about your body &/or menstrual cycle?

How often do you tune into your body & spend time listening & reflecting?

What are your goals in using this journal as a healing tool, record-keeper, & ritual guide?

What is stopping you from making self-care a priority & how can you shift that?

Inquire Within • guidance for when you feel stuck
Prompts for meditation, reflection &/or tarot or oracle card pulls.

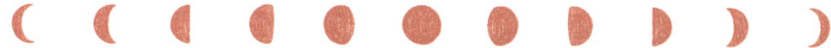

Suggested ritual:

• Ground yourself – take a few deep breaths. Breathe & move until you feel clear, centered and present.

• Hold and connect to your cards. Then pull a card as you focus on each inquiry.

• One at a time, reflect on your card pulls – focus on the imagery of the cards instead of written meanings. How does it make you feel? What is this guidance offering you? Try looking at it from a few perspectives without judgment. Keep what resonates within and leave the rest.

---

1. What energy or feeling is presently blocking me?

2. What is at the root of this?

3. What needs to be released?

4. What area of my life is asking for attention?

5. What (inner) guidance can best support me?

Tracking Key Replacements:

If you'd like to replace & customize the moonthly overview tracking features, you can cut out a column, and tape it to the left edge of page 35 so it can serve as a replacement flap. Video instructions:

PHYSICAL — EMOTIONAL — HABITUAL

PHYSICAL — EMOTIONAL — HABITUAL

PHYSICAL — EMOTIONAL — HABITUAL

Tracking Key Replacement Options:

If you'd like to replace or customize the moonthly overview tracking features, you can cut out a column, and tape it to the left edge of page 35 so it can serve as a replacement flap. Video instructions:

PHYSICAL — EMOTIONAL — HABITUAL

PHYSICAL — EMOTIONAL — HABITUAL

PHYSICAL — EMOTIONAL — HABITUAL

DEC | JAN

☾ 13th Moon Cycle 2024

☼ ♑ → ♒ 1/19

	♑	♑	♒	♒	♒	♓	♓	♓	♈	♈	♉	♉	♊	♊	♋
	M	T	W	T	F	S	S	M	T	W	T	F	S	S
	30	31	1	2	3	4	5	6	7	8	9	10	11	12

PHYSICAL

- Cycle Day #
- Basal Body Temp.
- Cervical Mucus | 🩸
- Cramps
- Bloating
- Fatigue
- Sore | Tender
- Headache
- Aroused
- Sensory Sensitivity
- Energy Level
- Acne | Breakout
- _____
- _____
- _____

EMOTIONAL

- Blissful | Excited
- Centered | Calm
- Sensitive | Tender
- Foggy | Unfocused
- Stressed | Anxious
- Sad | Down
- Irritable | Angry
- Confidence Level
- _____
- _____
- _____

HABITUAL

- Meditation
- Movement | Exercise
- Self-Care
- Intimacy | Pleasure
- Hours of Sleep
- Sleep Quality
- Intense Dreams
- Vitamins | Meds
- Creation | Play
- _____
- _____
- _____

JANUARY

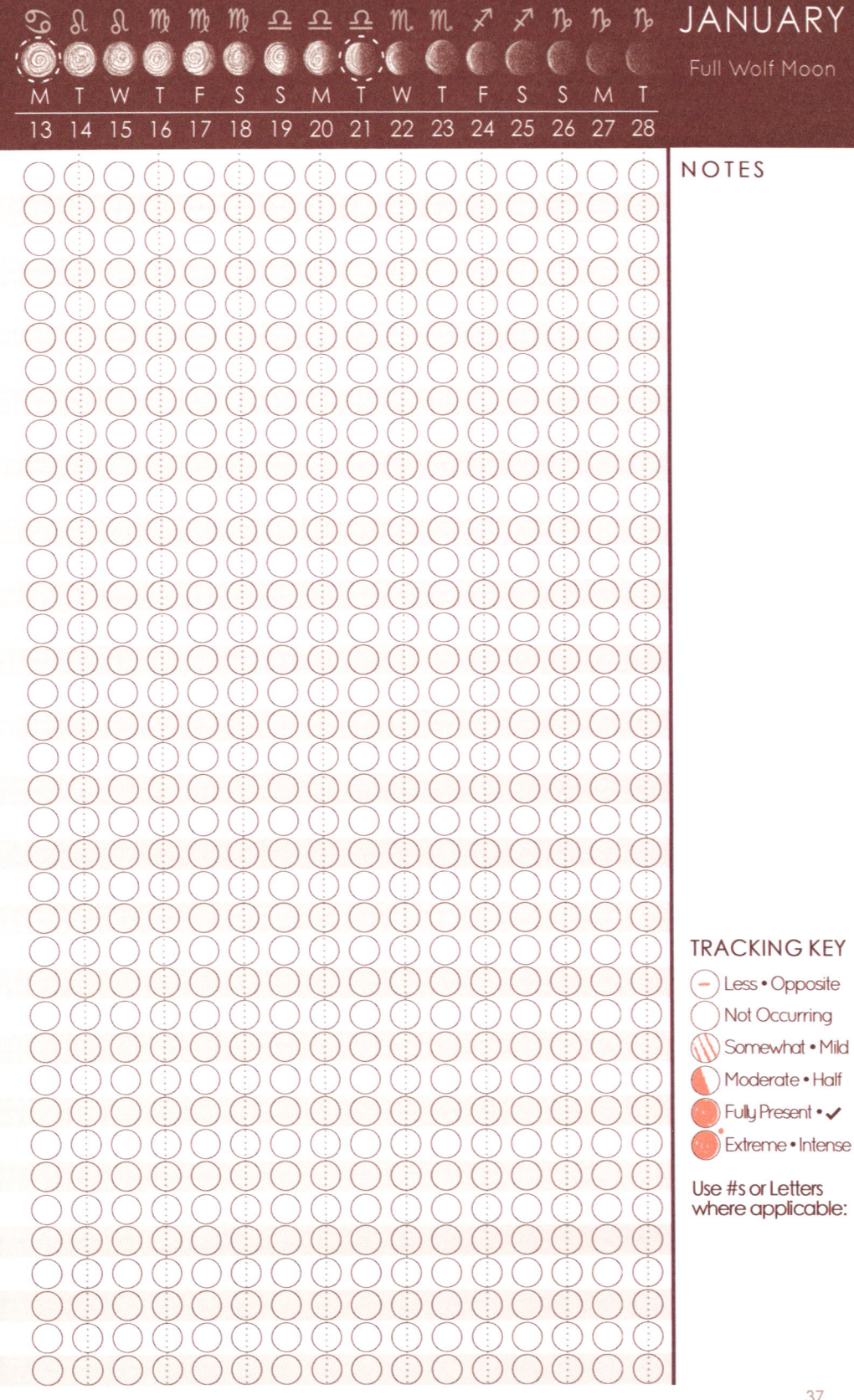

Full Wolf Moon

M	T	W	T	F	S	S	M	T	W	T	F	S	S	M	T
13	14	15	16	17	18	19	20	21	22	23	24	25	26	27	28

NOTES

TRACKING KEY

- ⊖ Less • Opposite
- ○ Not Occurring
- ◐ Somewhat • Mild
- ◑ Moderate • Half
- ● Fully Present • ✓
- ● Extreme • Intense

Use #s or Letters where applicable:

JAN | FEB

☾ 1st Moon Cycle 2025

☀ ♒ → ♓ 2/18

	W 29	T 30	F 31	S 1	S 2	M 3	T 4	W 5	T 6	F 7	S 8	S 9	M 10	T 11
PHYSICAL														
Cycle Day #	○	○	○	○	○	○	○	○	○	○	○	○	○	○
Basal Body Temp.	○	○	○	○	○	○	○	○	○	○	○	○	○	○
Cervical Mucus | 🩸	○	○	○	○	○	○	○	○	○	○	○	○	○	○
Cramps	○	○	○	○	○	○	○	○	○	○	○	○	○	○
Bloating	○	○	○	○	○	○	○	○	○	○	○	○	○	○
Fatigue	○	○	○	○	○	○	○	○	○	○	○	○	○	○
Sore | Tender	○	○	○	○	○	○	○	○	○	○	○	○	○	○
Headache	○	○	○	○	○	○	○	○	○	○	○	○	○	○
Aroused	○	○	○	○	○	○	○	○	○	○	○	○	○	○
Sensory Sensitivity	○	○	○	○	○	○	○	○	○	○	○	○	○	○
Energy Level	○	○	○	○	○	○	○	○	○	○	○	○	○	○
Acne | Breakout	○	○	○	○	○	○	○	○	○	○	○	○	○	○
_____	○	○	○	○	○	○	○	○	○	○	○	○	○	○
_____	○	○	○	○	○	○	○	○	○	○	○	○	○	○
_____	○	○	○	○	○	○	○	○	○	○	○	○	○	○
EMOTIONAL														
Blissful | Excited	○	○	○	○	○	○	○	○	○	○	○	○	○	○
Centered | Calm	○	○	○	○	○	○	○	○	○	○	○	○	○	○
Sensitive | Tender	○	○	○	○	○	○	○	○	○	○	○	○	○	○
Foggy | Unfocused	○	○	○	○	○	○	○	○	○	○	○	○	○	○
Stressed | Anxious	○	○	○	○	○	○	○	○	○	○	○	○	○	○
Sad | Down	○	○	○	○	○	○	○	○	○	○	○	○	○	○
Irritable | Angry	○	○	○	○	○	○	○	○	○	○	○	○	○	○
Confidence Level	○	○	○	○	○	○	○	○	○	○	○	○	○	○
_____	○	○	○	○	○	○	○	○	○	○	○	○	○	○
_____	○	○	○	○	○	○	○	○	○	○	○	○	○	○
_____	○	○	○	○	○	○	○	○	○	○	○	○	○	○
HABITUAL														
Meditation	○	○	○	○	○	○	○	○	○	○	○	○	○	○
Movement | Exercise	○	○	○	○	○	○	○	○	○	○	○	○	○	○
Self-Care	○	○	○	○	○	○	○	○	○	○	○	○	○	○
Intimacy | Pleasure	○	○	○	○	○	○	○	○	○	○	○	○	○	○
Hours of Sleep	○	○	○	○	○	○	○	○	○	○	○	○	○	○
Sleep Quality	○	○	○	○	○	○	○	○	○	○	○	○	○	○
Intense Dreams	○	○	○	○	○	○	○	○	○	○	○	○	○	○
Vitamins | Meds	○	○	○	○	○	○	○	○	○	○	○	○	○	○
Creation | Play	○	○	○	○	○	○	○	○	○	○	○	○	○	○
_____	○	○	○	○	○	○	○	○	○	○	○	○	○	○
_____	○	○	○	○	○	○	○	○	○	○	○	○	○	○
_____	○	○	○	○	○	○	○	○	○	○	○	○	○	○

FEBRUARY
Full Snow Moon

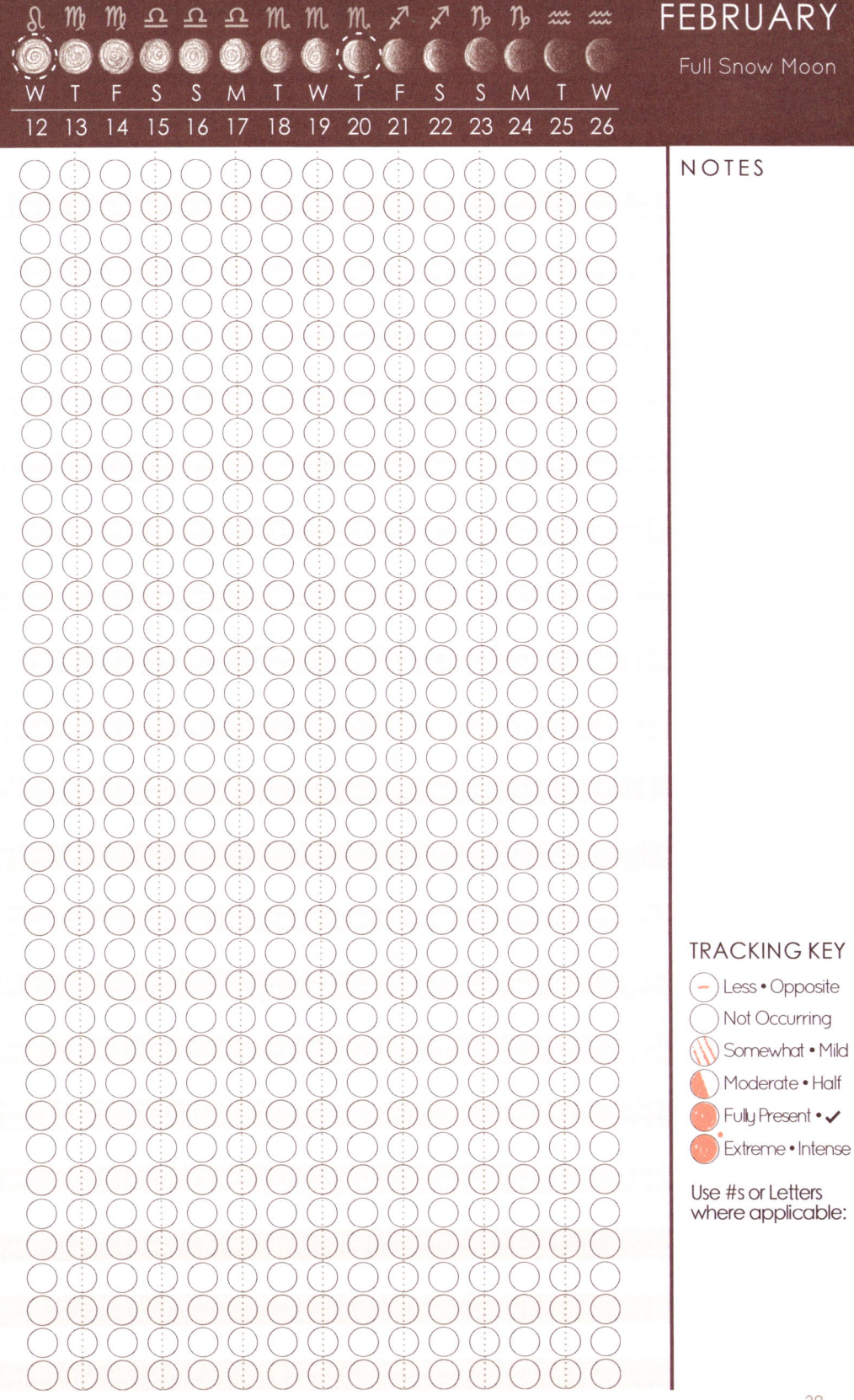

W	T	F	S	S	M	T	W	T	F	S	S	M	T	W
12	13	14	15	16	17	18	19	20	21	22	23	24	25	26

NOTES

TRACKING KEY
- — Less • Opposite
- ○ Not Occurring
- ◐ Somewhat • Mild
- ◐ Moderate • Half
- ● Fully Present • ✓
- ● Extreme • Intense

Use #s or Letters where applicable:

FEB | MAR

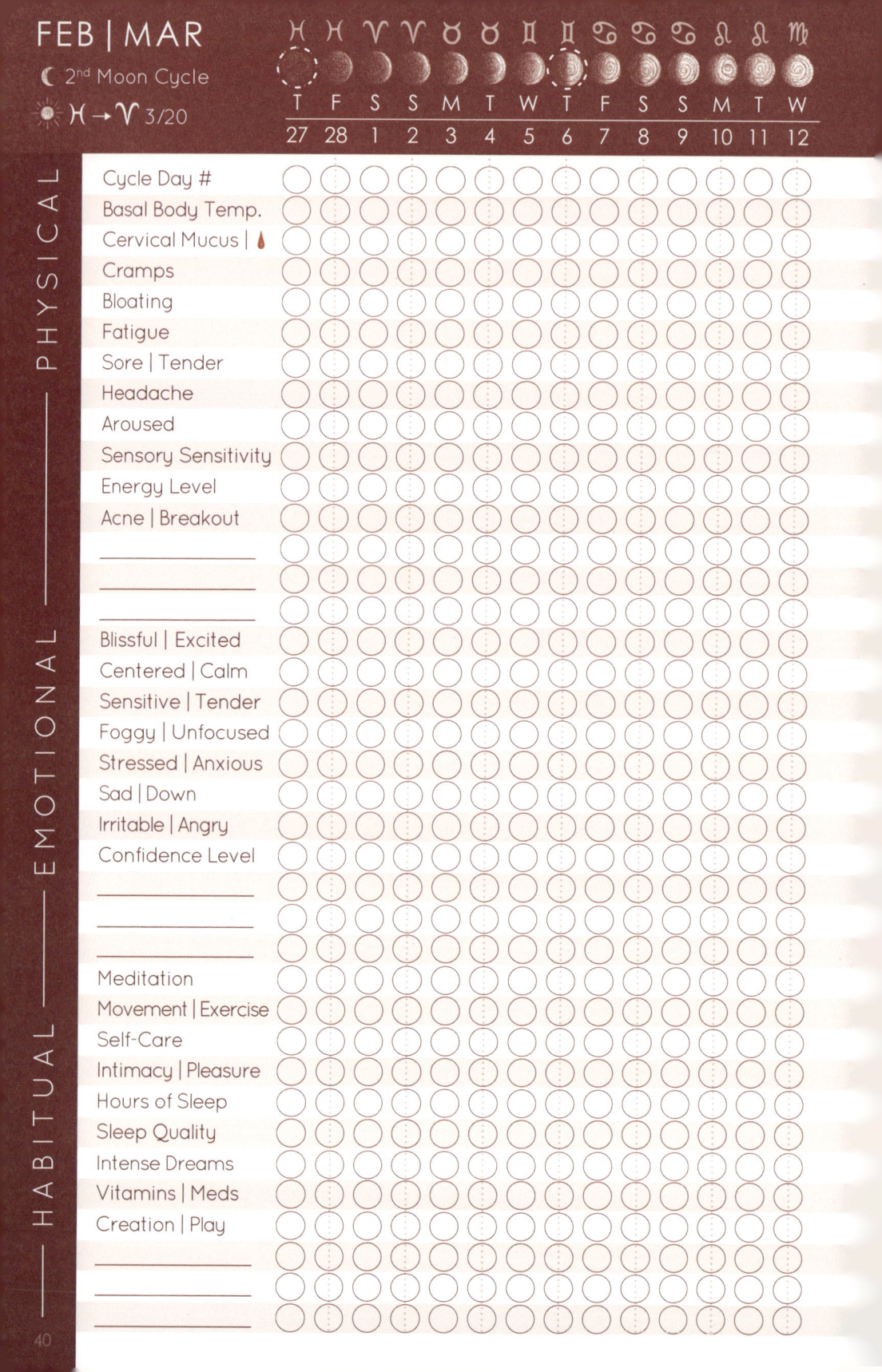

☾ 2nd Moon Cycle

☀ ♓ → ♈ 3/20

	T 27	F 28	S 1	S 2	M 3	T 4	W 5	T 6	F 7	S 8	S 9	M 10	T 11	W 12

PHYSICAL

- Cycle Day #
- Basal Body Temp.
- Cervical Mucus | 🩸
- Cramps
- Bloating
- Fatigue
- Sore | Tender
- Headache
- Aroused
- Sensory Sensitivity
- Energy Level
- Acne | Breakout
- _____
- _____

EMOTIONAL

- Blissful | Excited
- Centered | Calm
- Sensitive | Tender
- Foggy | Unfocused
- Stressed | Anxious
- Sad | Down
- Irritable | Angry
- Confidence Level
- _____
- _____

HABITUAL

- Meditation
- Movement | Exercise
- Self-Care
- Intimacy | Pleasure
- Hours of Sleep
- Sleep Quality
- Intense Dreams
- Vitamins | Meds
- Creation | Play
- _____
- _____
- _____

MARCH

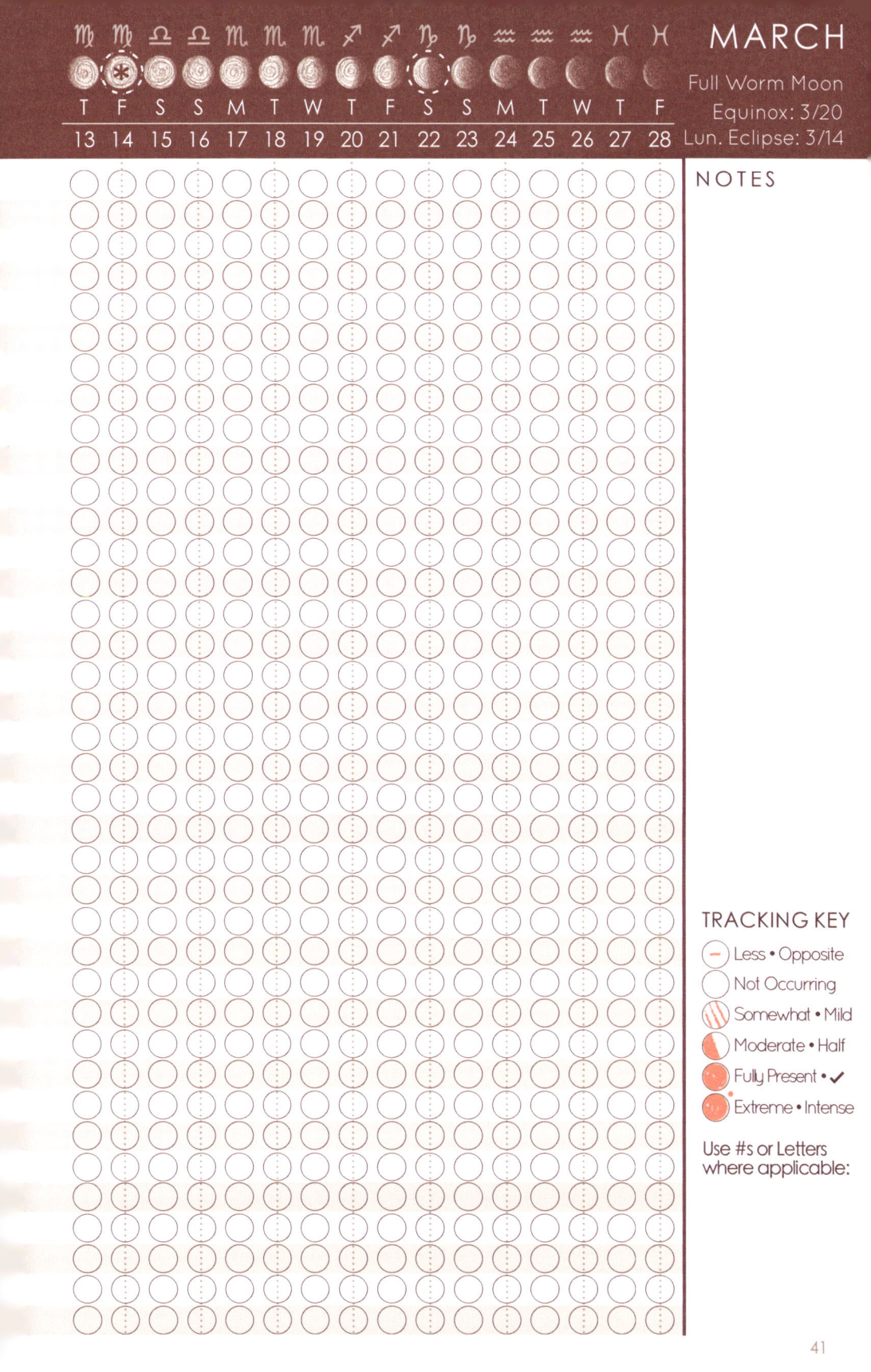

Full Worm Moon
Equinox: 3/20
Lun. Eclipse: 3/14

T	F	S	S	M	T	W	T	F	S	S	M	T	W	T	F
13	14	15	16	17	18	19	20	21	22	23	24	25	26	27	28

NOTES

TRACKING KEY

- Less • Opposite
- Not Occurring
- Somewhat • Mild
- Moderate • Half
- Fully Present • ✓
- Extreme • Intense

Use #s or Letters where applicable:

41

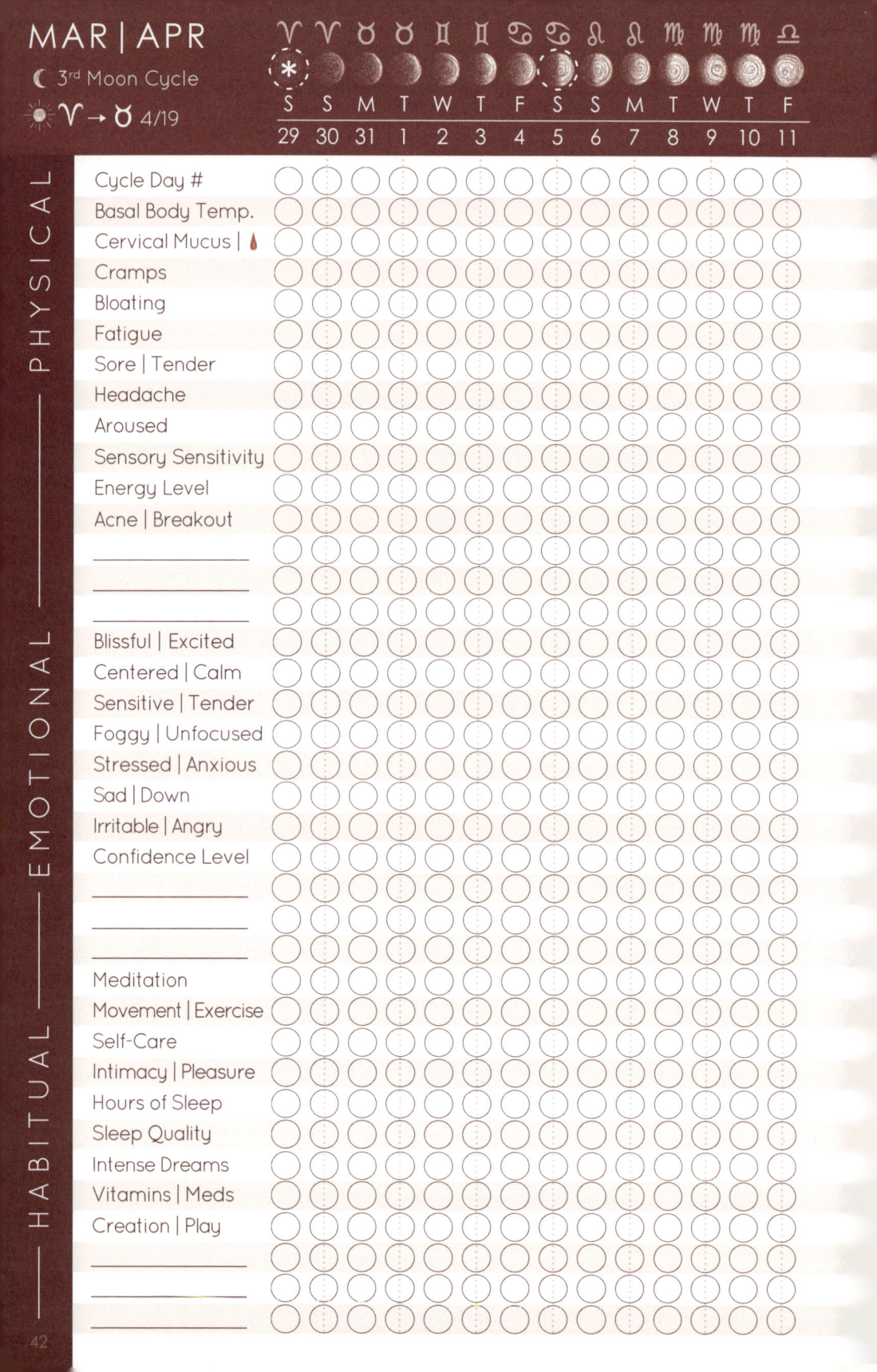

MAR | APR
☾ 3rd Moon Cycle
☀ ♈ → ♉ 4/19

	♈	♈	♉	♉	♊	♊	♋	♋	♌	♌	♍	♍	♏	♎
	S	S	M	T	W	T	F	S	S	M	T	W	T	F
	29	30	31	1	2	3	4	5	6	7	8	9	10	11

PHYSICAL

Cycle Day #	○	○	○	○	○	○	○	○	○	○	○	○	○	○
Basal Body Temp.	○	○	○	○	○	○	○	○	○	○	○	○	○	○
Cervical Mucus | 🩸	○	○	○	○	○	○	○	○	○	○	○	○	○	○
Cramps	○	○	○	○	○	○	○	○	○	○	○	○	○	○
Bloating	○	○	○	○	○	○	○	○	○	○	○	○	○	○
Fatigue	○	○	○	○	○	○	○	○	○	○	○	○	○	○
Sore | Tender	○	○	○	○	○	○	○	○	○	○	○	○	○	○
Headache	○	○	○	○	○	○	○	○	○	○	○	○	○	○
Aroused	○	○	○	○	○	○	○	○	○	○	○	○	○	○
Sensory Sensitivity	○	○	○	○	○	○	○	○	○	○	○	○	○	○
Energy Level	○	○	○	○	○	○	○	○	○	○	○	○	○	○
Acne | Breakout	○	○	○	○	○	○	○	○	○	○	○	○	○	○
_____	○	○	○	○	○	○	○	○	○	○	○	○	○	○
_____	○	○	○	○	○	○	○	○	○	○	○	○	○	○
_____	○	○	○	○	○	○	○	○	○	○	○	○	○	○

EMOTIONAL

Blissful | Excited	○	○	○	○	○	○	○	○	○	○	○	○	○	○
Centered | Calm	○	○	○	○	○	○	○	○	○	○	○	○	○	○
Sensitive | Tender	○	○	○	○	○	○	○	○	○	○	○	○	○	○
Foggy | Unfocused	○	○	○	○	○	○	○	○	○	○	○	○	○	○
Stressed | Anxious	○	○	○	○	○	○	○	○	○	○	○	○	○	○
Sad | Down	○	○	○	○	○	○	○	○	○	○	○	○	○	○
Irritable | Angry	○	○	○	○	○	○	○	○	○	○	○	○	○	○
Confidence Level	○	○	○	○	○	○	○	○	○	○	○	○	○	○
_____	○	○	○	○	○	○	○	○	○	○	○	○	○	○
_____	○	○	○	○	○	○	○	○	○	○	○	○	○	○
_____	○	○	○	○	○	○	○	○	○	○	○	○	○	○

HABITUAL

Meditation	○	○	○	○	○	○	○	○	○	○	○	○	○	○
Movement | Exercise	○	○	○	○	○	○	○	○	○	○	○	○	○	○
Self-Care	○	○	○	○	○	○	○	○	○	○	○	○	○	○
Intimacy | Pleasure	○	○	○	○	○	○	○	○	○	○	○	○	○	○
Hours of Sleep	○	○	○	○	○	○	○	○	○	○	○	○	○	○
Sleep Quality	○	○	○	○	○	○	○	○	○	○	○	○	○	○
Intense Dreams	○	○	○	○	○	○	○	○	○	○	○	○	○	○
Vitamins | Meds	○	○	○	○	○	○	○	○	○	○	○	○	○	○
Creation | Play	○	○	○	○	○	○	○	○	○	○	○	○	○	○
_____	○	○	○	○	○	○	○	○	○	○	○	○	○	○
_____	○	○	○	○	○	○	○	○	○	○	○	○	○	○
_____	○	○	○	○	○	○	○	○	○	○	○	○	○	○

APRIL

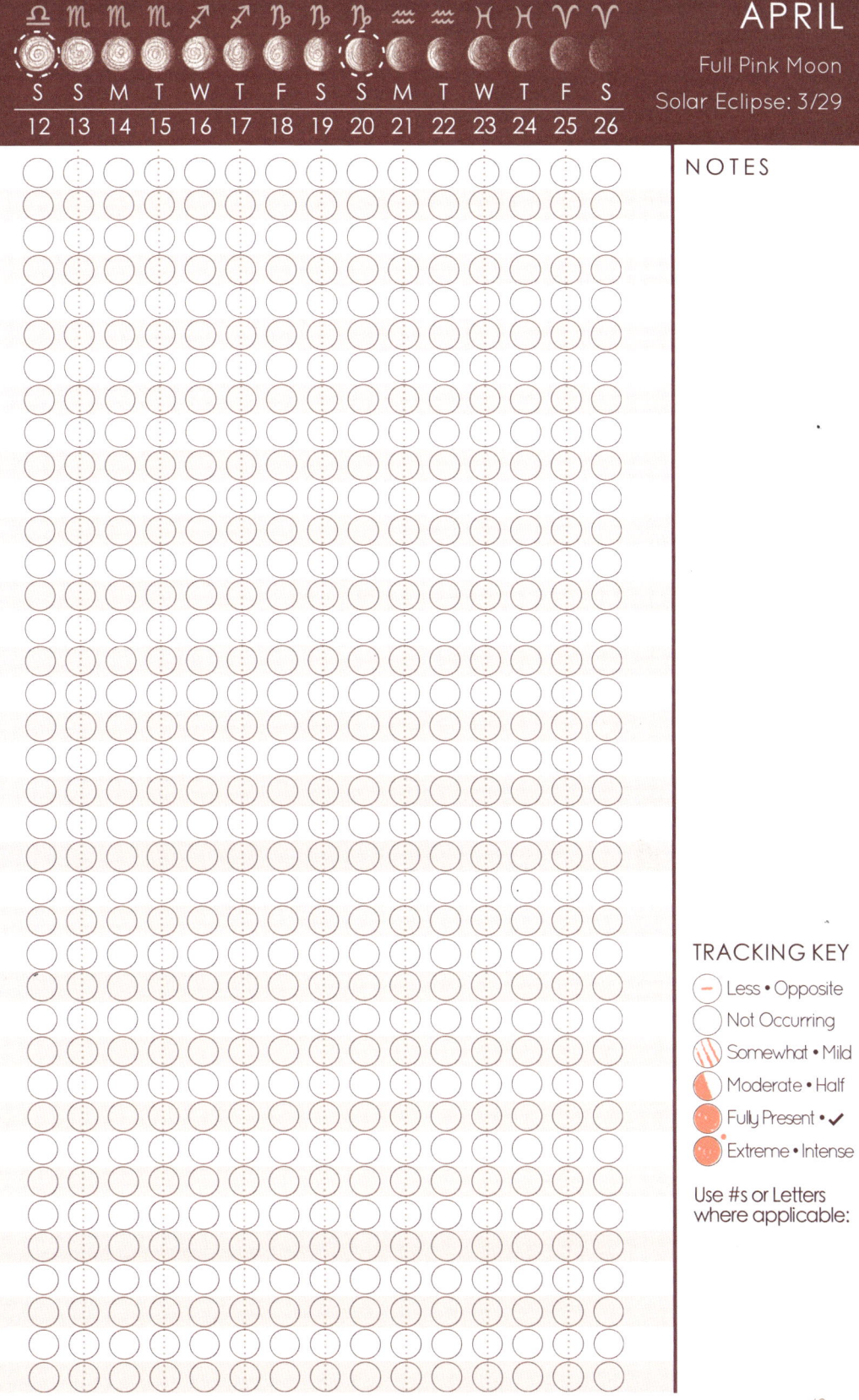

Full Pink Moon
Solar Eclipse: 3/29

S	S	M	T	W	T	F	S	S	M	T	W	T	F	S
12	13	14	15	16	17	18	19	20	21	22	23	24	25	26

NOTES

TRACKING KEY

− Less • Opposite
◯ Not Occurring
▨ Somewhat • Mild
◐ Moderate • Half
● Fully Present • ✓
● Extreme • Intense

Use #s or Letters where applicable:

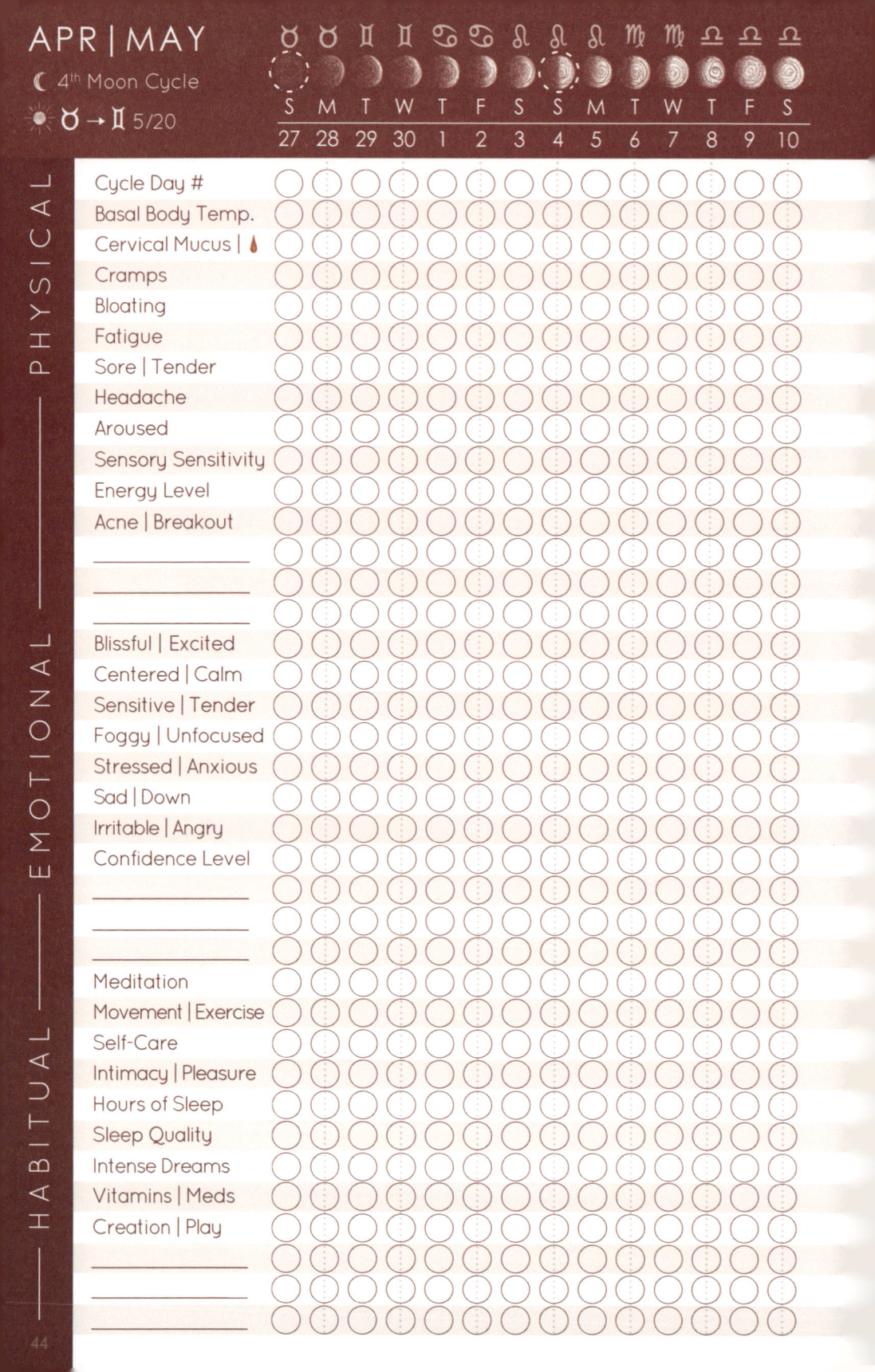

APR | MAY
☾ 4th Moon Cycle
☼ ♉ → ♊ 5/20

	S	M	T	W	T	F	S	S	M	T	W	T	F	S
	27	28	29	30	1	2	3	4	5	6	7	8	9	10

PHYSICAL

- Cycle Day #
- Basal Body Temp.
- Cervical Mucus | 💧
- Cramps
- Bloating
- Fatigue
- Sore | Tender
- Headache
- Aroused
- Sensory Sensitivity
- Energy Level
- Acne | Breakout
- _____
- _____
- _____

EMOTIONAL

- Blissful | Excited
- Centered | Calm
- Sensitive | Tender
- Foggy | Unfocused
- Stressed | Anxious
- Sad | Down
- Irritable | Angry
- Confidence Level
- _____
- _____
- _____

HABITUAL

- Meditation
- Movement | Exercise
- Self-Care
- Intimacy | Pleasure
- Hours of Sleep
- Sleep Quality
- Intense Dreams
- Vitamins | Meds
- Creation | Play
- _____
- _____
- _____

44

MAY
Full Flower Moon

S	M	T	W	T	F	S	S	M	T	W	T	F	S	S
11	12	13	14	15	16	17	18	19	20	21	22	23	24	25

NOTES

TRACKING KEY
- ⊖ Less • Opposite
- ○ Not Occurring
- ◍ Somewhat • Mild
- ◐ Moderate • Half
- ● Fully Present • ✓
- ● Extreme • Intense

Use #s or Letters where applicable:

MAY | JUN

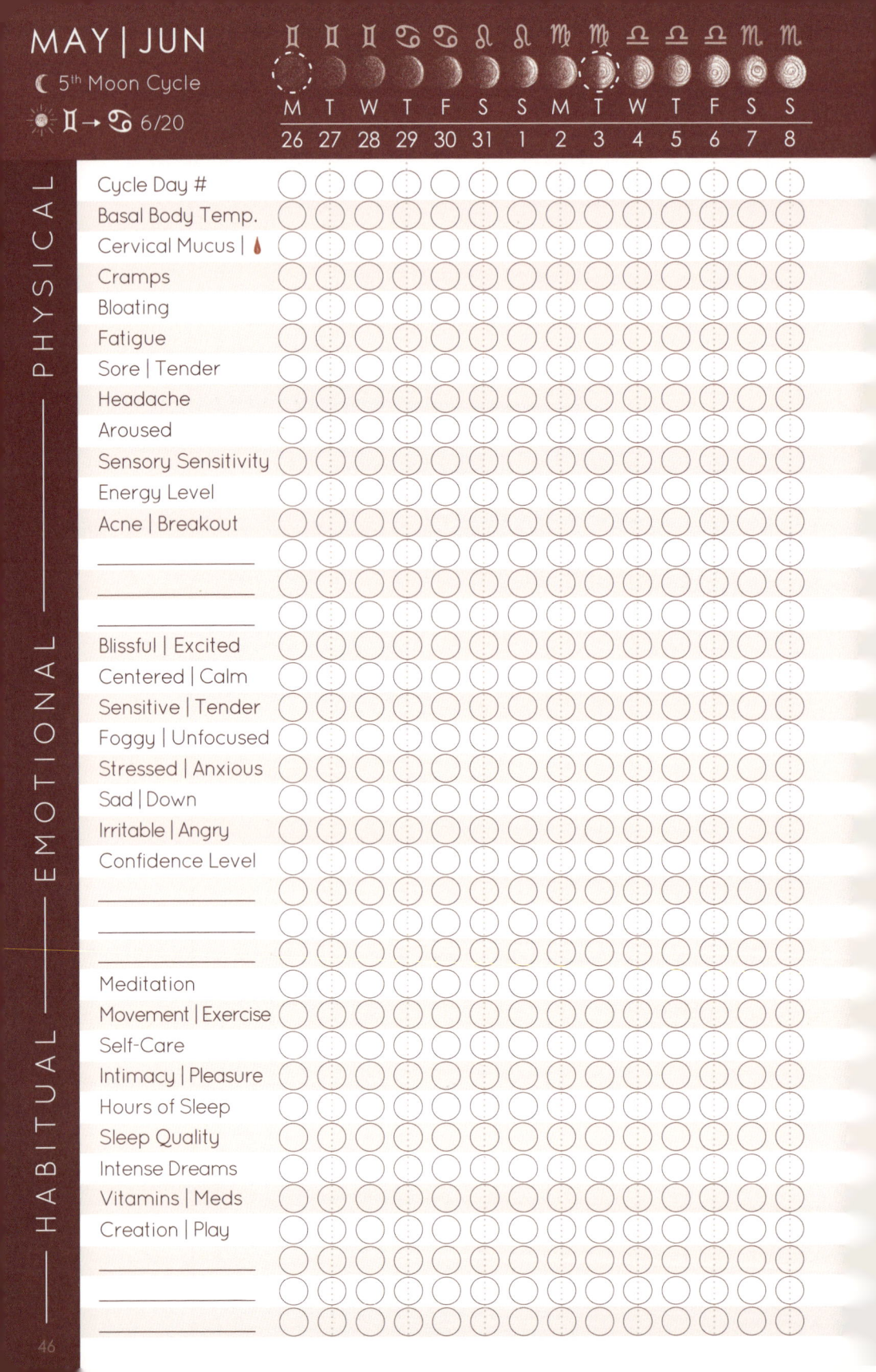

☾ 5th Moon Cycle

☀ ♊ → ♋ 6/20

	♊	♊	♊	♋	♋	♌	♌	♍	♍	♎	♎	♏	♏
	M	T	W	T	F	S	S	M	T	W	T	F	S	S
	26	27	28	29	30	31	1	2	3	4	5	6	7	8

PHYSICAL

Cycle Day #	○	○	○	○	○	○	○	○	○	○	○	○	○	○
Basal Body Temp.	○	○	○	○	○	○	○	○	○	○	○	○	○	○
Cervical Mucus | 🩸	○	○	○	○	○	○	○	○	○	○	○	○	○	○
Cramps	○	○	○	○	○	○	○	○	○	○	○	○	○	○
Bloating	○	○	○	○	○	○	○	○	○	○	○	○	○	○
Fatigue	○	○	○	○	○	○	○	○	○	○	○	○	○	○
Sore | Tender	○	○	○	○	○	○	○	○	○	○	○	○	○	○
Headache	○	○	○	○	○	○	○	○	○	○	○	○	○	○
Aroused	○	○	○	○	○	○	○	○	○	○	○	○	○	○
Sensory Sensitivity	○	○	○	○	○	○	○	○	○	○	○	○	○	○
Energy Level	○	○	○	○	○	○	○	○	○	○	○	○	○	○
Acne | Breakout	○	○	○	○	○	○	○	○	○	○	○	○	○	○
_____	○	○	○	○	○	○	○	○	○	○	○	○	○	○
_____	○	○	○	○	○	○	○	○	○	○	○	○	○	○
_____	○	○	○	○	○	○	○	○	○	○	○	○	○	○

EMOTIONAL

Blissful | Excited	○	○	○	○	○	○	○	○	○	○	○	○	○	○
Centered | Calm	○	○	○	○	○	○	○	○	○	○	○	○	○	○
Sensitive | Tender	○	○	○	○	○	○	○	○	○	○	○	○	○	○
Foggy | Unfocused	○	○	○	○	○	○	○	○	○	○	○	○	○	○
Stressed | Anxious	○	○	○	○	○	○	○	○	○	○	○	○	○	○
Sad | Down	○	○	○	○	○	○	○	○	○	○	○	○	○	○
Irritable | Angry	○	○	○	○	○	○	○	○	○	○	○	○	○	○
Confidence Level	○	○	○	○	○	○	○	○	○	○	○	○	○	○
_____	○	○	○	○	○	○	○	○	○	○	○	○	○	○
_____	○	○	○	○	○	○	○	○	○	○	○	○	○	○

HABITUAL

Meditation	○	○	○	○	○	○	○	○	○	○	○	○	○	○
Movement | Exercise	○	○	○	○	○	○	○	○	○	○	○	○	○	○
Self-Care	○	○	○	○	○	○	○	○	○	○	○	○	○	○
Intimacy | Pleasure	○	○	○	○	○	○	○	○	○	○	○	○	○	○
Hours of Sleep	○	○	○	○	○	○	○	○	○	○	○	○	○	○
Sleep Quality	○	○	○	○	○	○	○	○	○	○	○	○	○	○
Intense Dreams	○	○	○	○	○	○	○	○	○	○	○	○	○	○
Vitamins | Meds	○	○	○	○	○	○	○	○	○	○	○	○	○	○
Creation | Play	○	○	○	○	○	○	○	○	○	○	○	○	○	○
_____	○	○	○	○	○	○	○	○	○	○	○	○	○	○
_____	○	○	○	○	○	○	○	○	○	○	○	○	○	○

JUNE

Strawberry Moon

Solstice: 6/20

M	T	W	T	F	S	S	M	T	W	T	F	S	S	M	T
9	10	11	12	13	14	15	16	17	18	19	20	21	22	23	24

NOTES

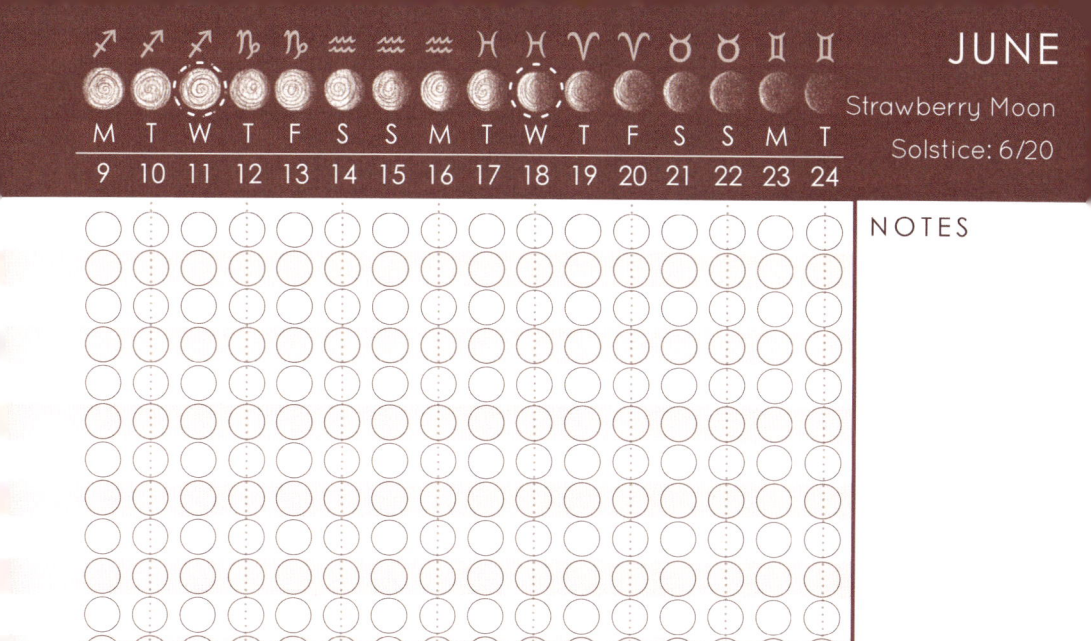

TRACKING KEY

- — Less • Opposite
- ○ Not Occurring
- ◔ Somewhat • Mild
- ◑ Moderate • Half
- ● Fully Present • ✓
- ● Extreme • Intense

Use #s or Letters where applicable:

JUN | JUL

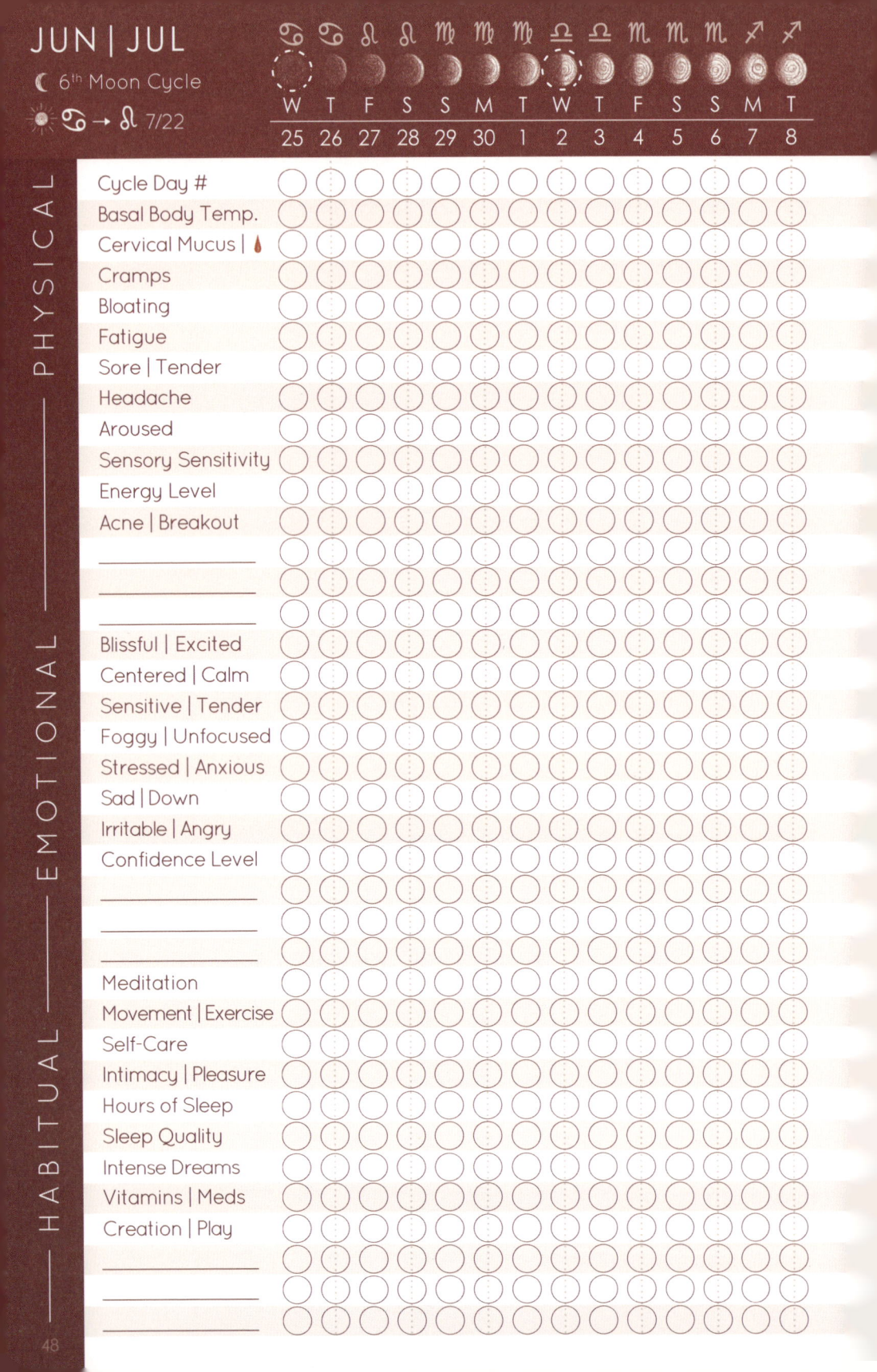

☾ 6th Moon Cycle

☀ ♋ → ♌ 7/22

	♋	♋	♌	♌	♍	♍	♍	♎	♎	♏	♏	♏	♐	♐
	W	T	F	S	S	M	T	W	T	F	S	S	M	T
	25	26	27	28	29	30	1	2	3	4	5	6	7	8

PHYSICAL

- Cycle Day #
- Basal Body Temp.
- Cervical Mucus | 💧
- Cramps
- Bloating
- Fatigue
- Sore | Tender
- Headache
- Aroused
- Sensory Sensitivity
- Energy Level
- Acne | Breakout
- _____
- _____
- _____

EMOTIONAL

- Blissful | Excited
- Centered | Calm
- Sensitive | Tender
- Foggy | Unfocused
- Stressed | Anxious
- Sad | Down
- Irritable | Angry
- Confidence Level
- _____
- _____

HABITUAL

- Meditation
- Movement | Exercise
- Self-Care
- Intimacy | Pleasure
- Hours of Sleep
- Sleep Quality
- Intense Dreams
- Vitamins | Meds
- Creation | Play
- _____
- _____

JULY
Full Buck Moon

W	T	F	S	S	M	T	W	T	F	S	S	M	T	W
9	10	11	12	13	14	15	16	17	18	19	20	21	22	23

NOTES

TRACKING KEY
- Less • Opposite
- Not Occurring
- Somewhat • Mild
- Moderate • Half
- Fully Present • ✓
- Extreme • Intense

Use #'s or Letters where applicable:

49

JUL | AUG

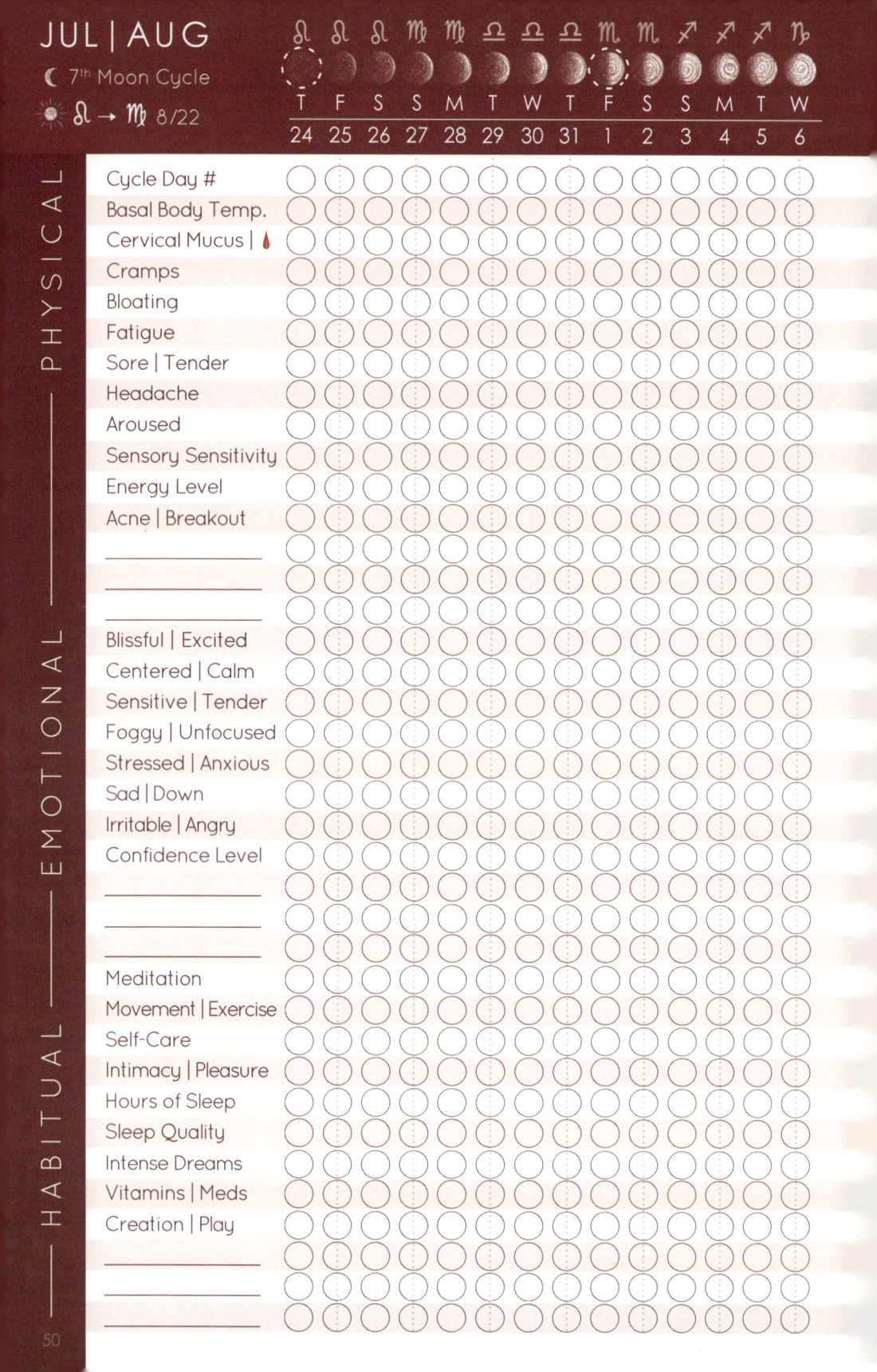

☾ 7th Moon Cycle

☀ ♌ → ♍ 8/22

	♌	♌	♍	♍	♎	♎	♎	♏	♏	♐	♐	♐	♑
	T	F	S	S	M	T	W	T	F	S	S	M	T	W
	24	25	26	27	28	29	30	31	1	2	3	4	5	6

PHYSICAL

- Cycle Day #
- Basal Body Temp.
- Cervical Mucus | 🩸
- Cramps
- Bloating
- Fatigue
- Sore | Tender
- Headache
- Aroused
- Sensory Sensitivity
- Energy Level
- Acne | Breakout
- _____
- _____
- _____

EMOTIONAL

- Blissful | Excited
- Centered | Calm
- Sensitive | Tender
- Foggy | Unfocused
- Stressed | Anxious
- Sad | Down
- Irritable | Angry
- Confidence Level
- _____
- _____
- _____

HABITUAL

- Meditation
- Movement | Exercise
- Self-Care
- Intimacy | Pleasure
- Hours of Sleep
- Sleep Quality
- Intense Dreams
- Vitamins | Meds
- Creation | Play
- _____
- _____
- _____

AUGUST

Full Sturgeon Moon

T	F	S	S	M	T	W	T	F	S	S	M	T	W	T	F
7	8	9	10	11	12	13	14	15	16	17	18	19	20	21	22

NOTES

TRACKING KEY

- – Less • Opposite
- ◯ Not Occurring
- Somewhat • Mild
- Moderate • Half
- Fully Present • ✓
- Extreme • Intense

Use #s or Letters where applicable:

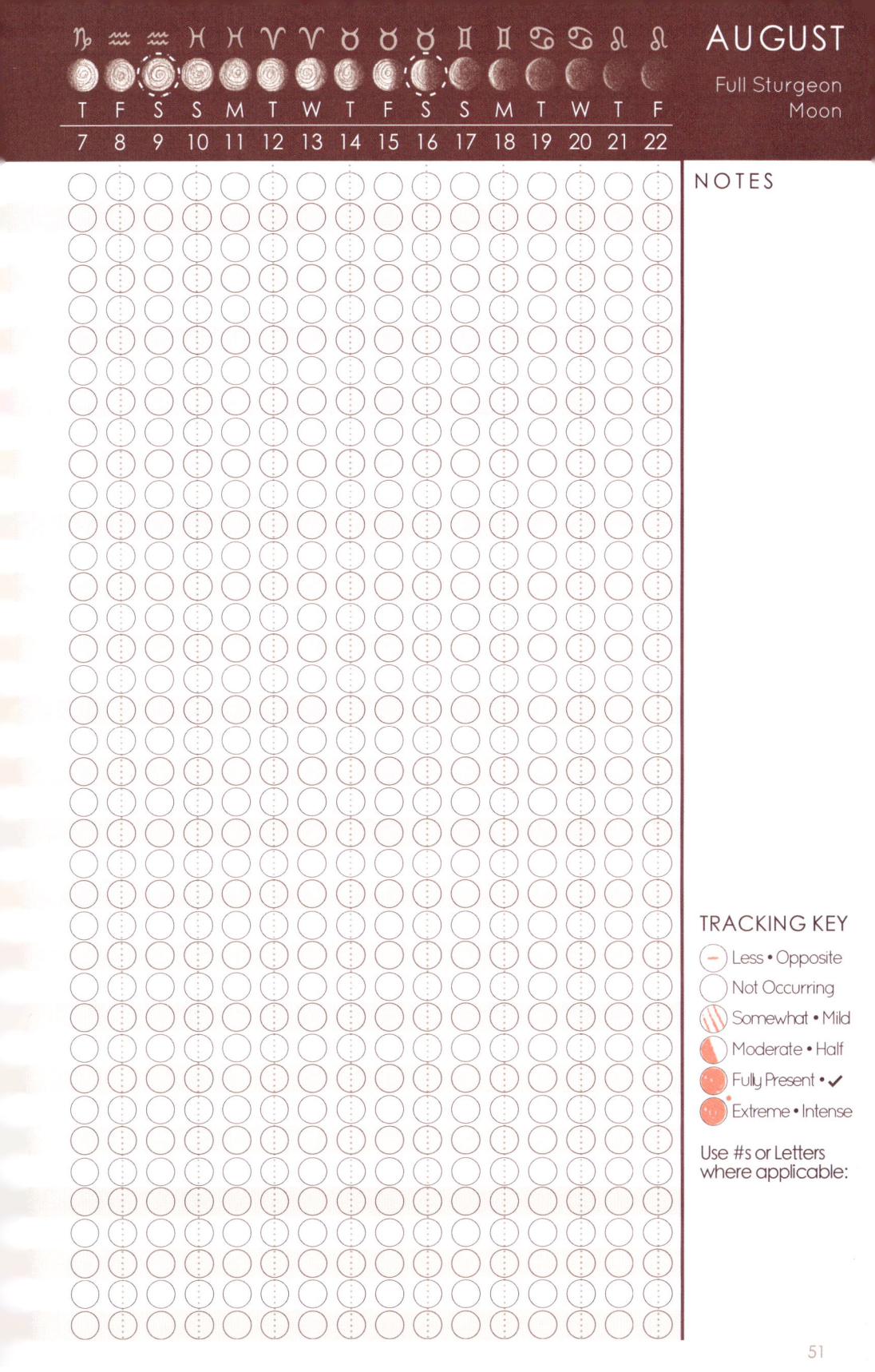

AUG | SEP

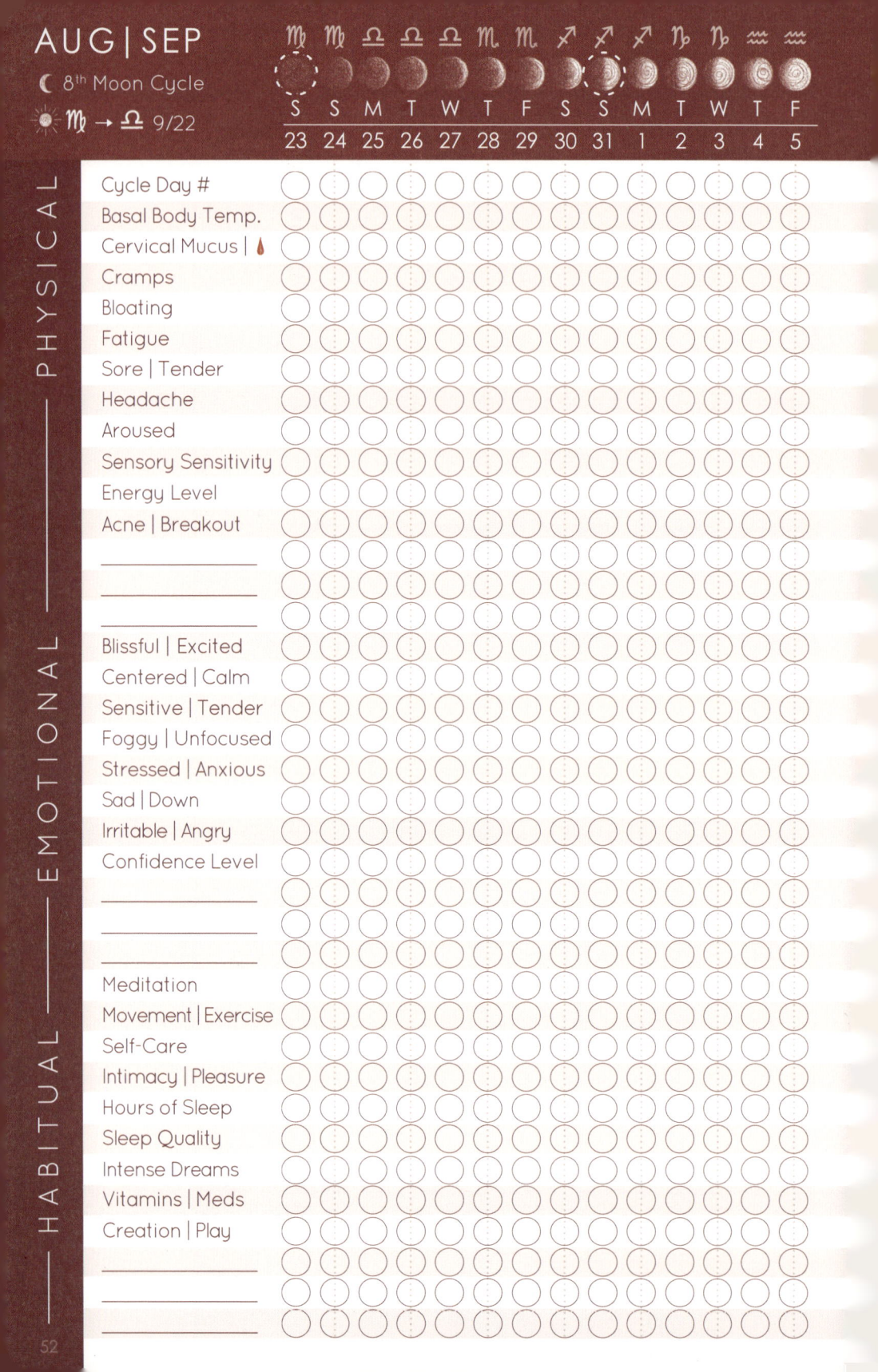

☾ 8th Moon Cycle

☀ ♏ → ♎ 9/22

	♏	♏	♎	♎	♏	♏	♐	♐	♐	♑	♑	♒	♒
	S	S	M	T	W	T	F	S	S	M	T	W	T	F
	23	24	25	26	27	28	29	30	31	1	2	3	4	5

PHYSICAL

Cycle Day #	○	○	○	○	○	○	○	○	○	○	○	○	○	○
Basal Body Temp.	○	○	○	○	○	○	○	○	○	○	○	○	○	○
Cervical Mucus | 🩸	○	○	○	○	○	○	○	○	○	○	○	○	○	○
Cramps	○	○	○	○	○	○	○	○	○	○	○	○	○	○
Bloating	○	○	○	○	○	○	○	○	○	○	○	○	○	○
Fatigue	○	○	○	○	○	○	○	○	○	○	○	○	○	○
Sore | Tender	○	○	○	○	○	○	○	○	○	○	○	○	○	○
Headache	○	○	○	○	○	○	○	○	○	○	○	○	○	○
Aroused	○	○	○	○	○	○	○	○	○	○	○	○	○	○
Sensory Sensitivity	○	○	○	○	○	○	○	○	○	○	○	○	○	○
Energy Level	○	○	○	○	○	○	○	○	○	○	○	○	○	○
Acne | Breakout	○	○	○	○	○	○	○	○	○	○	○	○	○	○
_____	○	○	○	○	○	○	○	○	○	○	○	○	○	○
_____	○	○	○	○	○	○	○	○	○	○	○	○	○	○

EMOTIONAL

Blissful | Excited	○	○	○	○	○	○	○	○	○	○	○	○	○	○
Centered | Calm	○	○	○	○	○	○	○	○	○	○	○	○	○	○
Sensitive | Tender	○	○	○	○	○	○	○	○	○	○	○	○	○	○
Foggy | Unfocused	○	○	○	○	○	○	○	○	○	○	○	○	○	○
Stressed | Anxious	○	○	○	○	○	○	○	○	○	○	○	○	○	○
Sad | Down	○	○	○	○	○	○	○	○	○	○	○	○	○	○
Irritable | Angry	○	○	○	○	○	○	○	○	○	○	○	○	○	○
Confidence Level	○	○	○	○	○	○	○	○	○	○	○	○	○	○
_____	○	○	○	○	○	○	○	○	○	○	○	○	○	○
_____	○	○	○	○	○	○	○	○	○	○	○	○	○	○

HABITUAL

Meditation	○	○	○	○	○	○	○	○	○	○	○	○	○	○
Movement | Exercise	○	○	○	○	○	○	○	○	○	○	○	○	○	○
Self-Care	○	○	○	○	○	○	○	○	○	○	○	○	○	○
Intimacy | Pleasure	○	○	○	○	○	○	○	○	○	○	○	○	○	○
Hours of Sleep	○	○	○	○	○	○	○	○	○	○	○	○	○	○
Sleep Quality	○	○	○	○	○	○	○	○	○	○	○	○	○	○
Intense Dreams	○	○	○	○	○	○	○	○	○	○	○	○	○	○
Vitamins | Meds	○	○	○	○	○	○	○	○	○	○	○	○	○	○
Creation | Play	○	○	○	○	○	○	○	○	○	○	○	○	○	○
_____	○	○	○	○	○	○	○	○	○	○	○	○	○	○
_____	○	○	○	○	○	○	○	○	○	○	○	○	○	○
_____	○	○	○	○	○	○	○	○	○	○	○	○	○	○

SEPTEMBER

Harvest Moon
Lun. Eclipse: 9/7
Equinox: 9/22

S	S	M	T	W	T	F	S	S	M	T	W	T	F	S
6	7	8	9	10	11	12	13	14	15	16	17	18	19	20

NOTES

TRACKING KEY

- Less • Opposite
- Not Occurring
- Somewhat • Mild
- Moderate • Half
- Fully Present • ✓
- Extreme • Intense

Use #s or Letters where applicable:

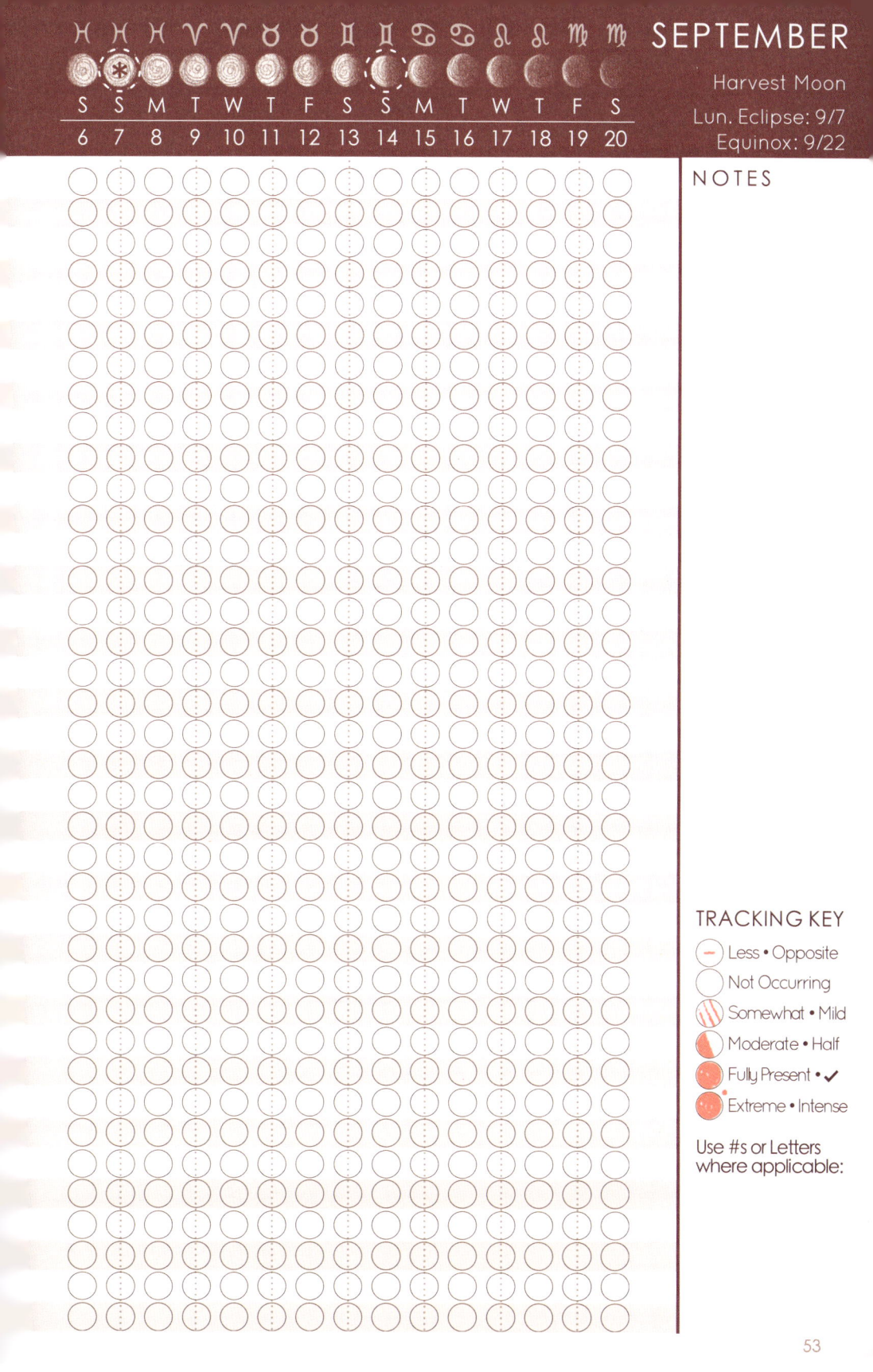

53

SEP | OCT

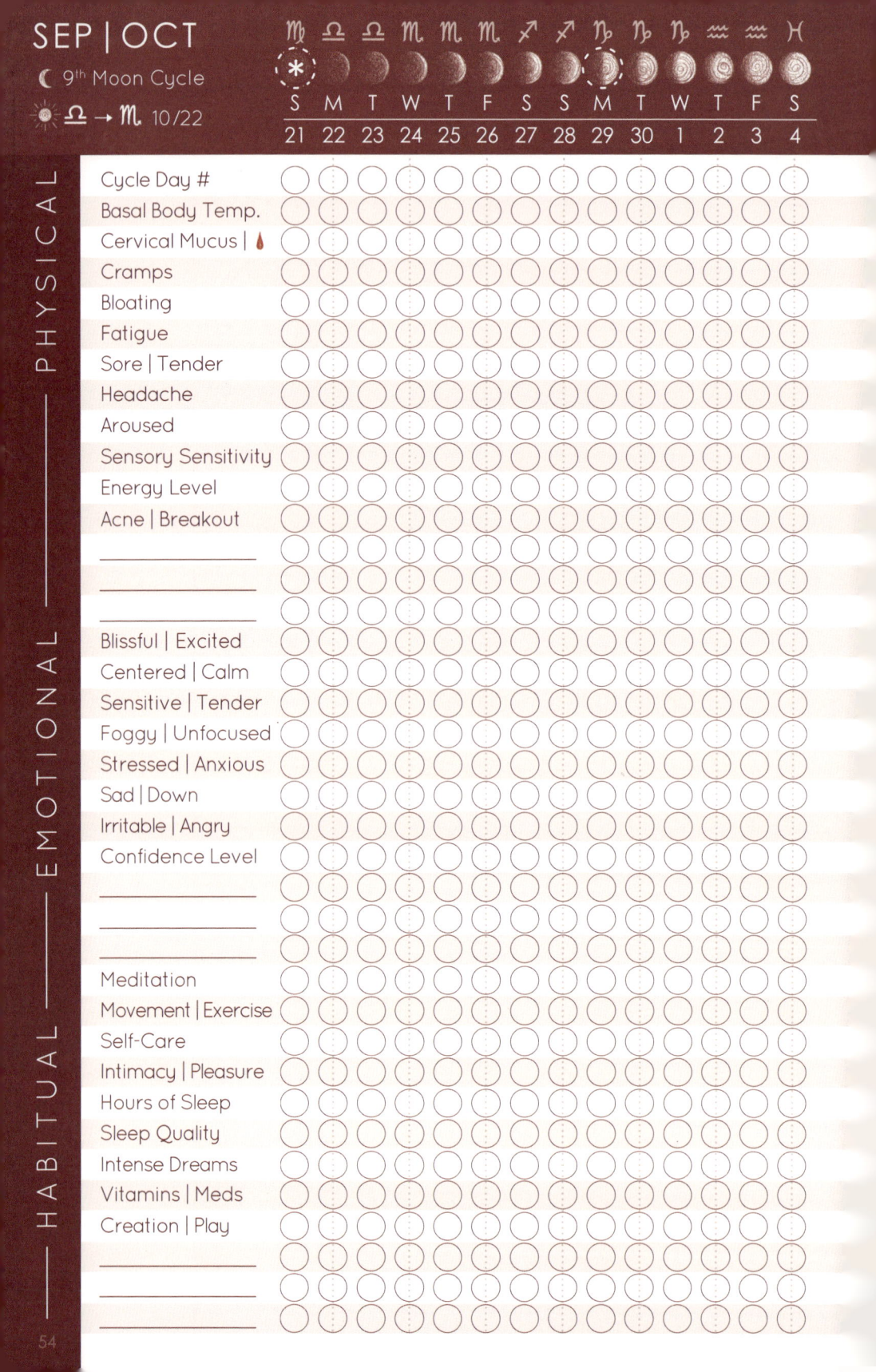

☾ 9th Moon Cycle

☀ ♎ → ♏ 10/22

	♍	♎	♎	♏	♏	♏	♐	♐	♑	♑	♑	♒	♒	♓
	S	M	T	W	T	F	S	S	M	T	W	T	F	S
	21	22	23	24	25	26	27	28	29	30	1	2	3	4

PHYSICAL

- Cycle Day #
- Basal Body Temp.
- Cervical Mucus | 🩸
- Cramps
- Bloating
- Fatigue
- Sore | Tender
- Headache
- Aroused
- Sensory Sensitivity
- Energy Level
- Acne | Breakout
- _____
- _____
- _____

EMOTIONAL

- Blissful | Excited
- Centered | Calm
- Sensitive | Tender
- Foggy | Unfocused
- Stressed | Anxious
- Sad | Down
- Irritable | Angry
- Confidence Level
- _____
- _____
- _____

HABITUAL

- Meditation
- Movement | Exercise
- Self-Care
- Intimacy | Pleasure
- Hours of Sleep
- Sleep Quality
- Intense Dreams
- Vitamins | Meds
- Creation | Play
- _____
- _____
- _____

54

OCTOBER

Full Hunter's Moon
Sol. Eclipse: 9/21

S	M	T	W	T	F	S	S	M	T	W	T	F	S	S	M
5	6	7	8	9	10	11	12	13	14	15	16	17	18	19	20

NOTES

TRACKING KEY

- ⊖ Less • Opposite
- ◯ Not Occurring
- ◐ Somewhat • Mild
- ◑ Moderate • Half
- ● Fully Present • ✓
- ⬤ Extreme • Intense

Use #s or Letters where applicable:

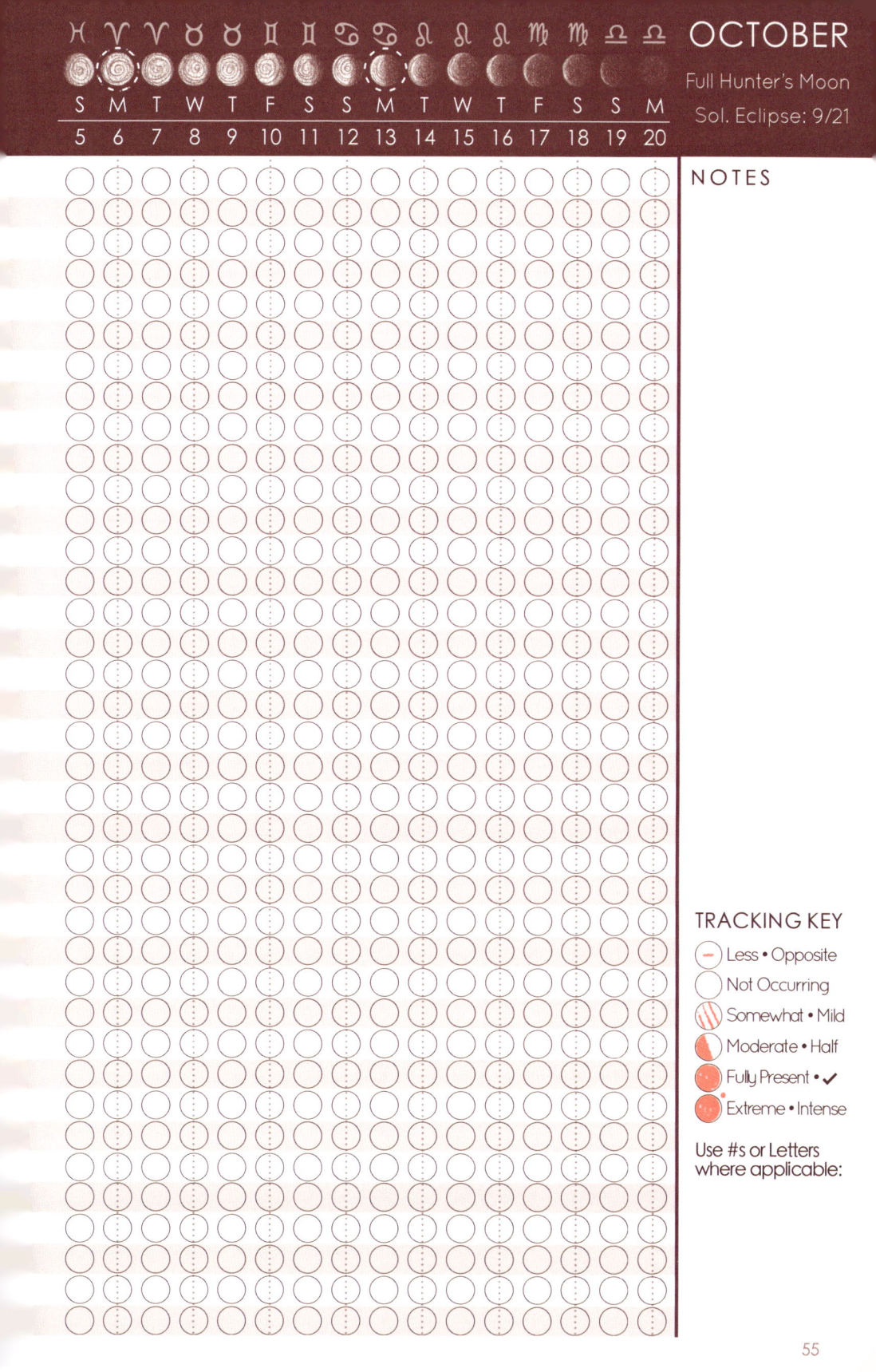

55

OCT | NOV

☾ 10th Moon Cycle

☀ ♏ → ♐ 11/21

	♏	♏	♏	♐	♐	♐	♑	♑	♒	♒	♓	♓	♈	♈
	T	W	T	F	S	S	M	T	W	T	F	S	S	M
	21	22	23	24	25	26	27	28	29	30	31	1	2	3

PHYSICAL

Cycle Day #	○	○	○	○	○	○	○	○	○	○	○	○	○	○
Basal Body Temp.	○	○	○	○	○	○	○	○	○	○	○	○	○	○
Cervical Mucus | 🩸	○	○	○	○	○	○	○	○	○	○	○	○	○	○
Cramps	○	○	○	○	○	○	○	○	○	○	○	○	○	○
Bloating	○	○	○	○	○	○	○	○	○	○	○	○	○	○
Fatigue	○	○	○	○	○	○	○	○	○	○	○	○	○	○
Sore | Tender	○	○	○	○	○	○	○	○	○	○	○	○	○	○
Headache	○	○	○	○	○	○	○	○	○	○	○	○	○	○
Aroused	○	○	○	○	○	○	○	○	○	○	○	○	○	○
Sensory Sensitivity	○	○	○	○	○	○	○	○	○	○	○	○	○	○
Energy Level	○	○	○	○	○	○	○	○	○	○	○	○	○	○
Acne | Breakout	○	○	○	○	○	○	○	○	○	○	○	○	○	○
_____	○	○	○	○	○	○	○	○	○	○	○	○	○	○
_____	○	○	○	○	○	○	○	○	○	○	○	○	○	○
_____	○	○	○	○	○	○	○	○	○	○	○	○	○	○

EMOTIONAL

Blissful | Excited	○	○	○	○	○	○	○	○	○	○	○	○	○	○
Centered | Calm	○	○	○	○	○	○	○	○	○	○	○	○	○	○
Sensitive | Tender	○	○	○	○	○	○	○	○	○	○	○	○	○	○
Foggy | Unfocused	○	○	○	○	○	○	○	○	○	○	○	○	○	○
Stressed | Anxious	○	○	○	○	○	○	○	○	○	○	○	○	○	○
Sad | Down	○	○	○	○	○	○	○	○	○	○	○	○	○	○
Irritable | Angry	○	○	○	○	○	○	○	○	○	○	○	○	○	○
Confidence Level	○	○	○	○	○	○	○	○	○	○	○	○	○	○
_____	○	○	○	○	○	○	○	○	○	○	○	○	○	○
_____	○	○	○	○	○	○	○	○	○	○	○	○	○	○
_____	○	○	○	○	○	○	○	○	○	○	○	○	○	○

HABITUAL

Meditation	○	○	○	○	○	○	○	○	○	○	○	○	○	○
Movement | Exercise	○	○	○	○	○	○	○	○	○	○	○	○	○	○
Self-Care	○	○	○	○	○	○	○	○	○	○	○	○	○	○
Intimacy | Pleasure	○	○	○	○	○	○	○	○	○	○	○	○	○	○
Hours of Sleep	○	○	○	○	○	○	○	○	○	○	○	○	○	○
Sleep Quality	○	○	○	○	○	○	○	○	○	○	○	○	○	○
Intense Dreams	○	○	○	○	○	○	○	○	○	○	○	○	○	○
Vitamins | Meds	○	○	○	○	○	○	○	○	○	○	○	○	○	○
Creation | Play	○	○	○	○	○	○	○	○	○	○	○	○	○	○
_____	○	○	○	○	○	○	○	○	○	○	○	○	○	○
_____	○	○	○	○	○	○	○	○	○	○	○	○	○	○
_____	○	○	○	○	○	○	○	○	○	○	○	○	○	○

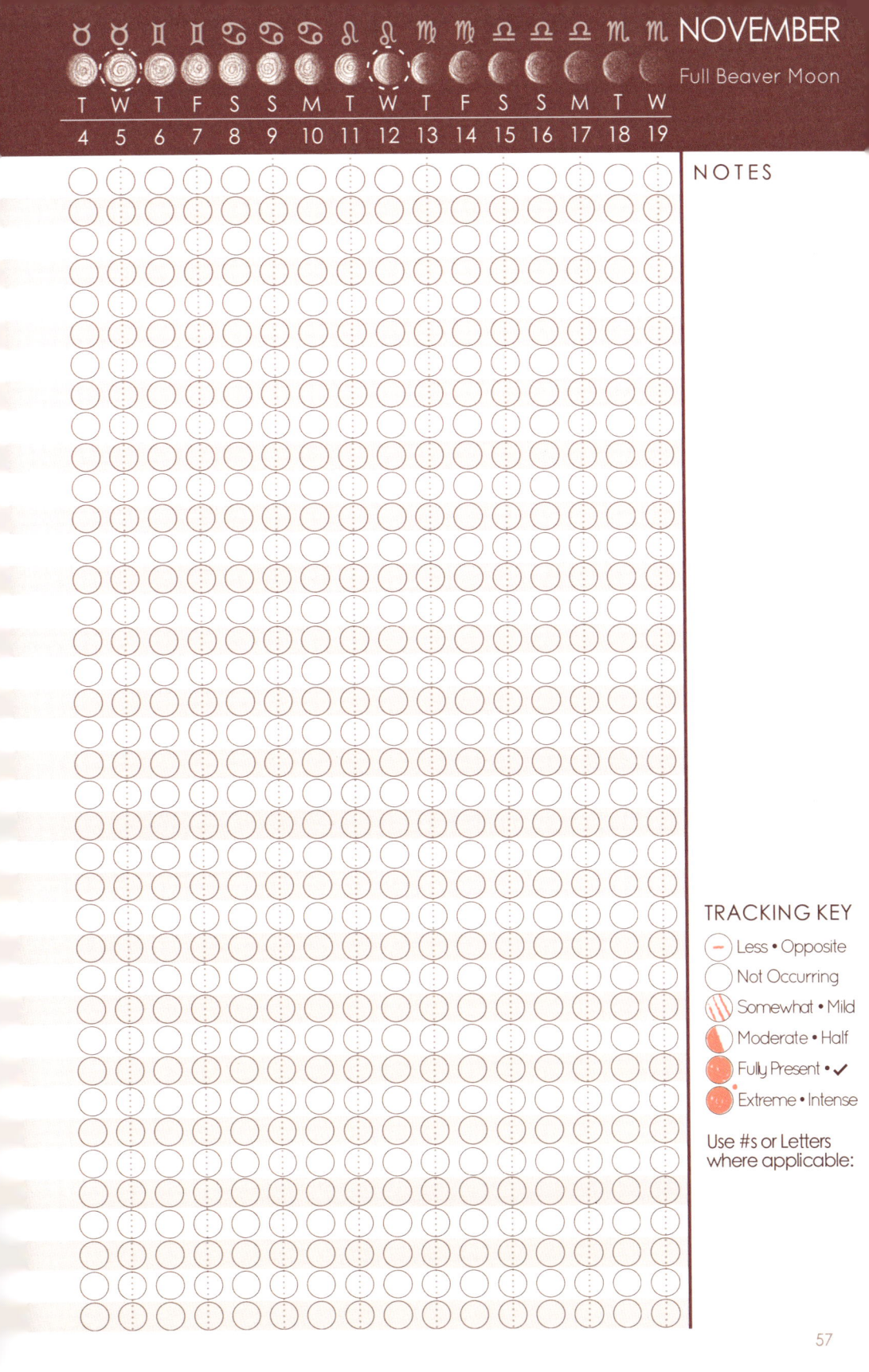

NOVEMBER
Full Beaver Moon

T	W	T	F	S	S	M	T	W	T	F	S	S	M	T	W
4	5	6	7	8	9	10	11	12	13	14	15	16	17	18	19

NOTES

TRACKING KEY
⊖ Less • Opposite
○ Not Occurring
◐ Somewhat • Mild
◑ Moderate • Half
● Fully Present • ✓
● Extreme • Intense

Use #s or Letters where applicable:

57

NOV | DEC
🌙 11th Moon Cycle

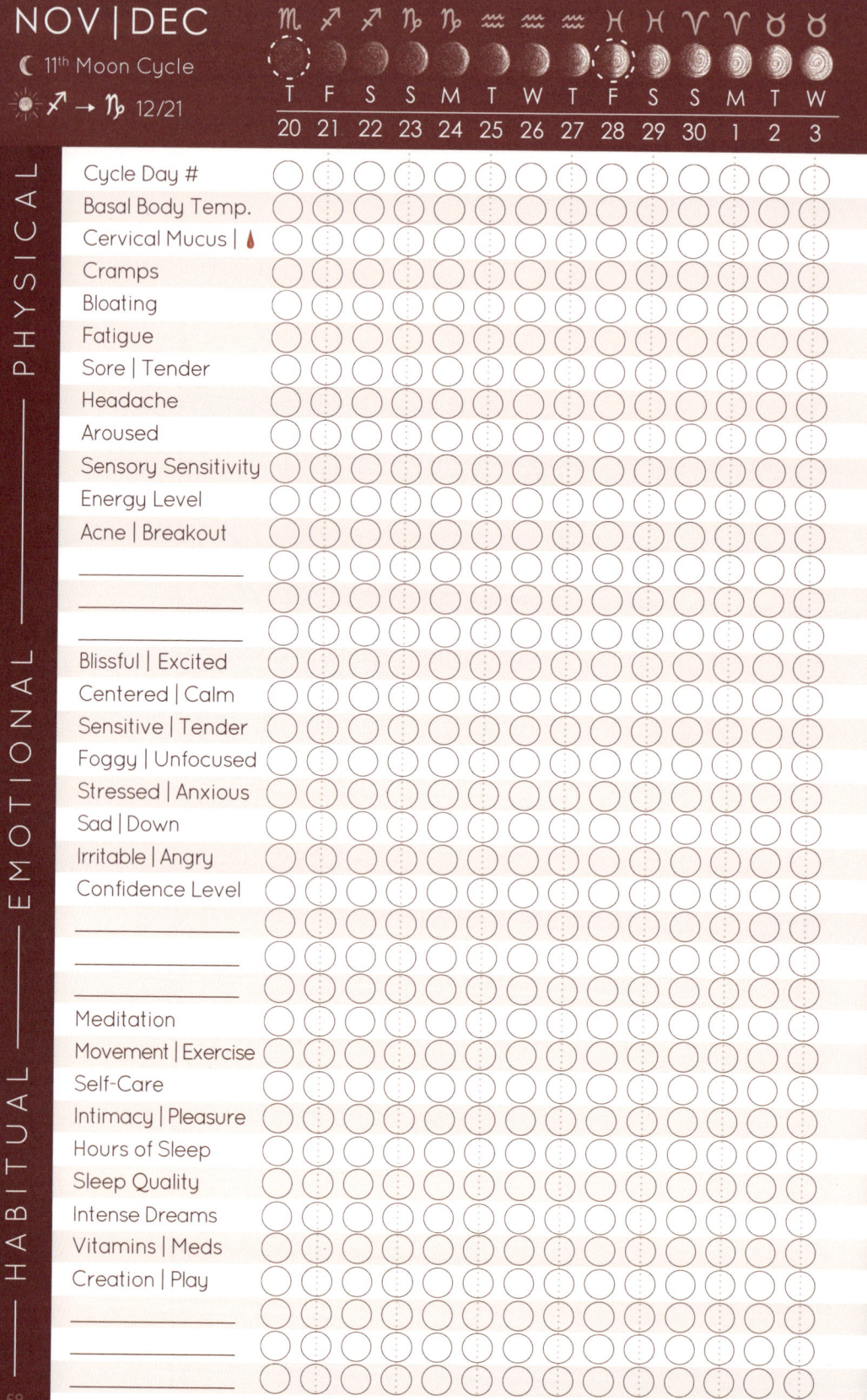

☀ ♐ → ♑ 12/21

	T 20	F 21	S 22	S 23	M 24	T 25	W 26	T 27	F 28	S 29	S 30	M 1	T 2	W 3

PHYSICAL

- Cycle Day #
- Basal Body Temp.
- Cervical Mucus | 🩸
- Cramps
- Bloating
- Fatigue
- Sore | Tender
- Headache
- Aroused
- Sensory Sensitivity
- Energy Level
- Acne | Breakout
- _____
- _____
- _____

EMOTIONAL

- Blissful | Excited
- Centered | Calm
- Sensitive | Tender
- Foggy | Unfocused
- Stressed | Anxious
- Sad | Down
- Irritable | Angry
- Confidence Level
- _____
- _____
- _____

HABITUAL

- Meditation
- Movement | Exercise
- Self-Care
- Intimacy | Pleasure
- Hours of Sleep
- Sleep Quality
- Intense Dreams
- Vitamins | Meds
- Creation | Play
- _____
- _____
- _____

DECEMBER

Full Cold Moon
Solstice: 12/21

T	F	S	S	M	T	W	T	F	S	S	M	T	W	T
4	5	6	7	8	9	10	11	12	13	14	15	16	17	18

NOTES

TRACKING KEY

- ⊖ Less • Opposite
- ◯ Not Occurring
- ◐ Somewhat • Mild
- ◑ Moderate • Half
- ● Fully Present • ✓
- ✸ Extreme • Intense

Use #s or Letters where applicable:

59

DEC | JAN '26
☾ 12th Moon Cycle

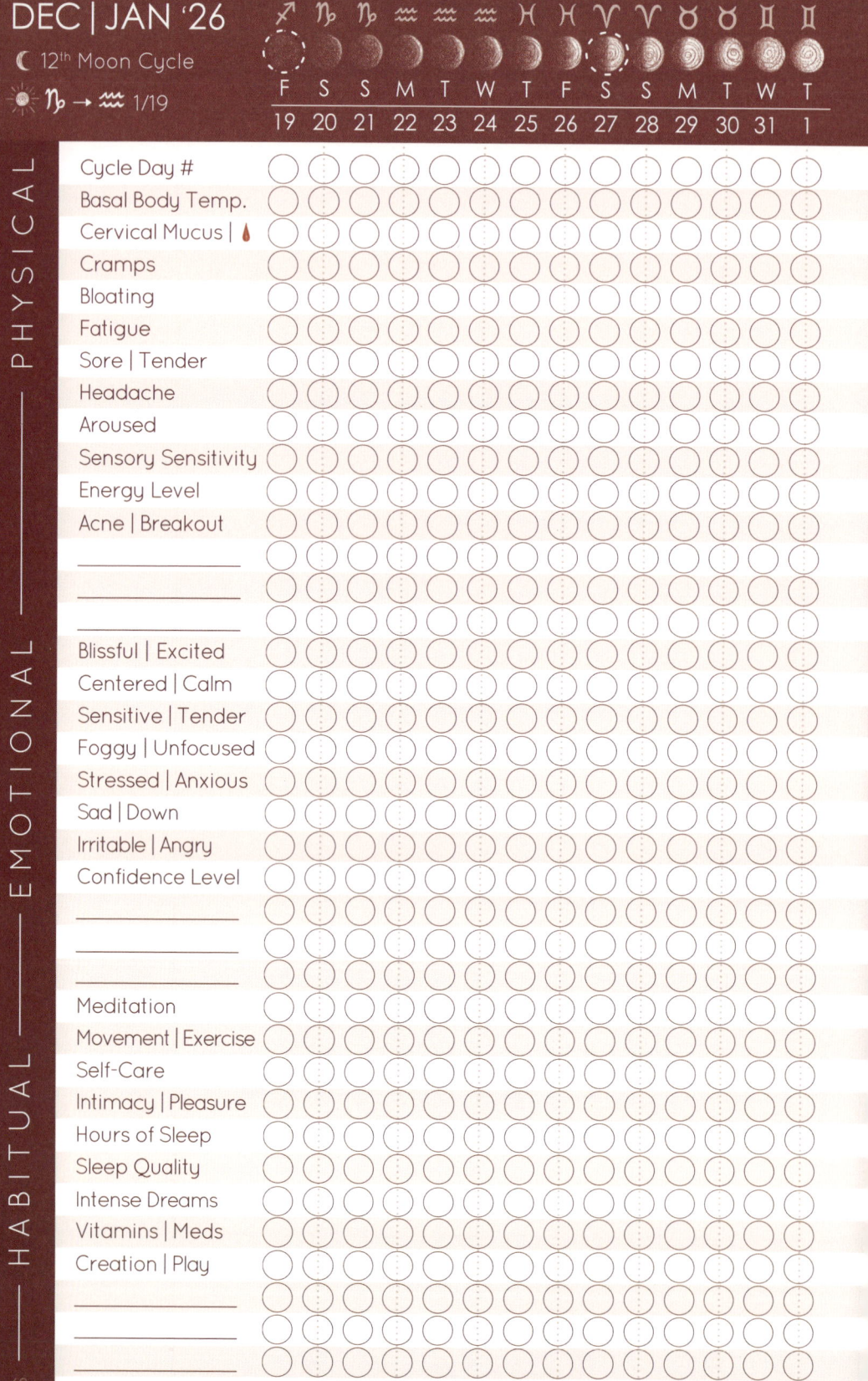

☀ ♑ → ♒ 1/19

	F 19	S 20	S 21	M 22	T 23	W 24	T 25	F 26	S 27	S 28	M 29	T 30	W 31	T 1
PHYSICAL														
Cycle Day #														
Basal Body Temp.														
Cervical Mucus | 🩸														
Cramps														
Bloating														
Fatigue														
Sore | Tender														
Headache														
Aroused														
Sensory Sensitivity														
Energy Level														
Acne | Breakout														
_____														
_____														
_____														
EMOTIONAL														
Blissful | Excited														
Centered | Calm														
Sensitive | Tender														
Foggy | Unfocused														
Stressed | Anxious														
Sad | Down														
Irritable | Angry														
Confidence Level														
_____														
_____														
HABITUAL														
Meditation														
Movement | Exercise														
Self-Care														
Intimacy | Pleasure														
Hours of Sleep														
Sleep Quality														
Intense Dreams														
Vitamins | Meds														
Creation | Play														
_____														
_____														
_____														

M • DEC 30

Day #: _____ | _____°

Phase | Season:

○ Breathe & drop in
○ Moonthly tracking
○ Gratitude practice
○ Celebrate yourself!

Physical State
Flow | Fluids

Emotional &
Mental State

Self-Care
Sleep | Dreams

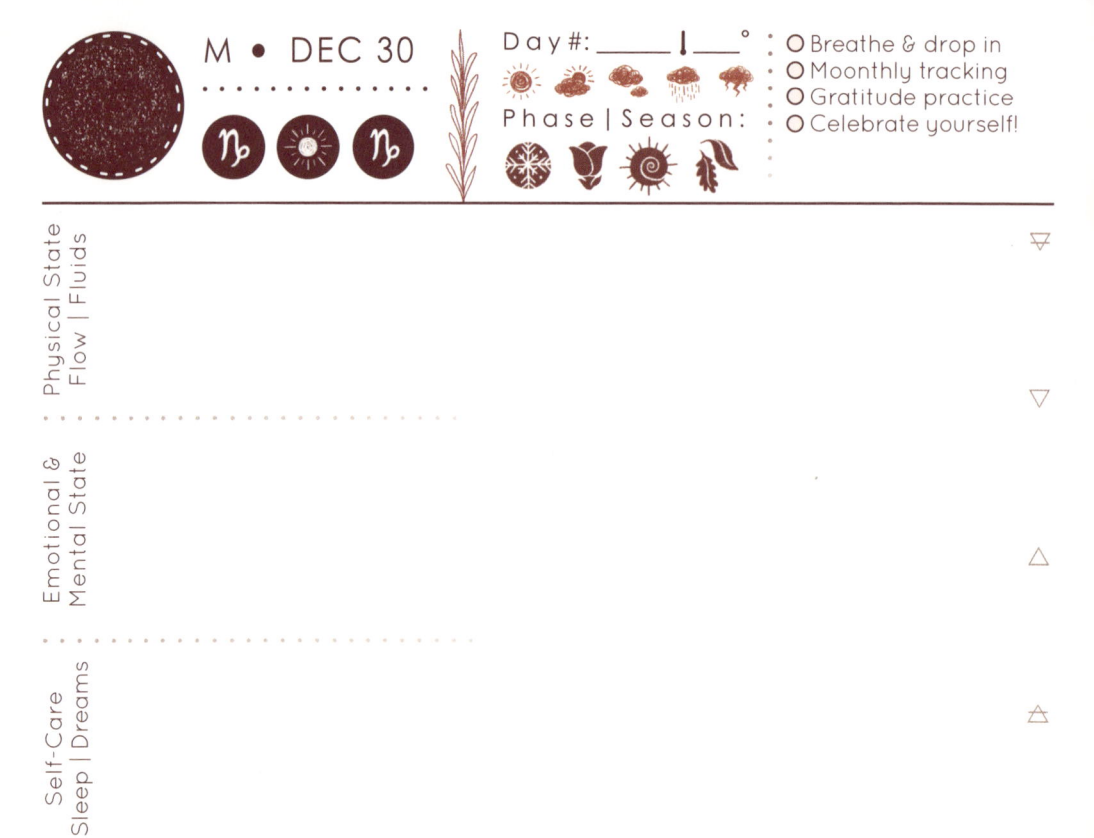

NEW MOON IN CAPRICORN

Initiating new roots to strengthen & deepen desired structures

What do I want to grow & focus on during this lunar cycle?

How will I hold space for this?

T • DEC 31

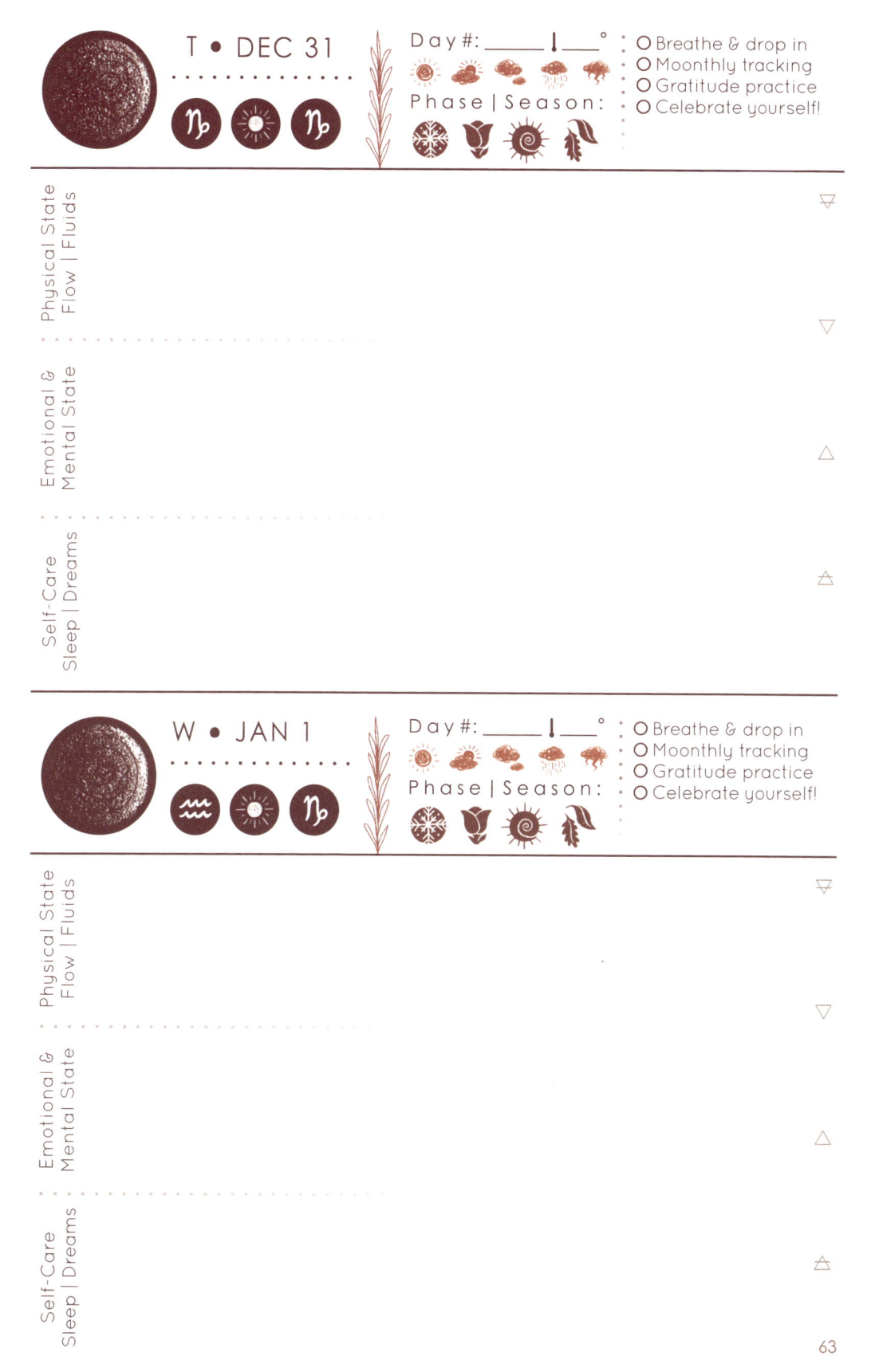

Day #: _____ | _____°

Phase | Season:

- ○ Breathe & drop in
- ○ Moonthly tracking
- ○ Gratitude practice
- ○ Celebrate yourself!

Physical State / Flow | Fluids

Emotional & Mental State

Self-Care / Sleep | Dreams

W • JAN 1

Day #: _____ | _____°

Phase | Season:

- ○ Breathe & drop in
- ○ Moonthly tracking
- ○ Gratitude practice
- ○ Celebrate yourself!

Physical State / Flow | Fluids

Emotional & Mental State

Self-Care / Sleep | Dreams

TH • JAN 2

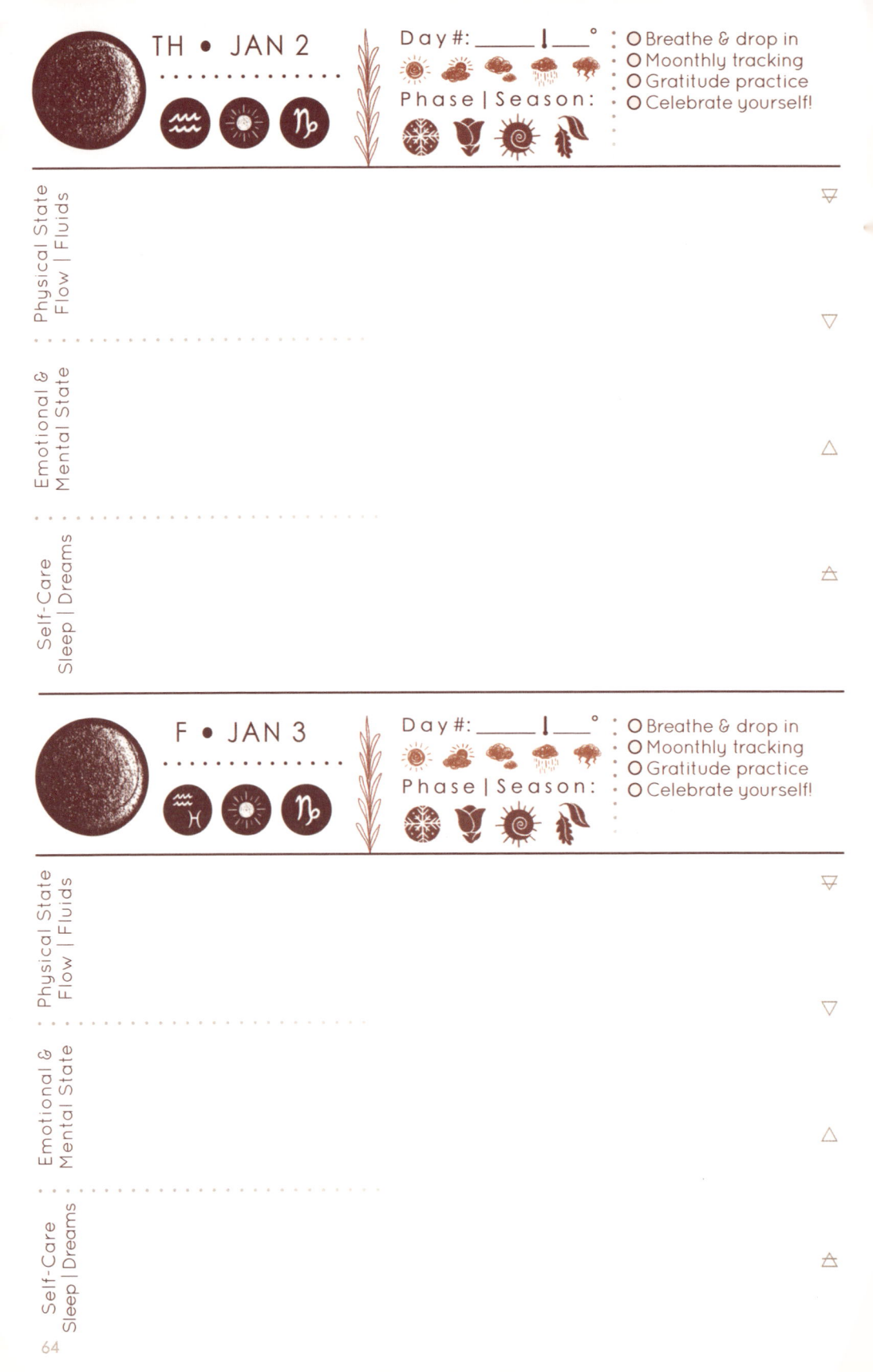

Day #: _____ | _____°

Phase | Season:

- Breathe & drop in
- Moonthly tracking
- Gratitude practice
- Celebrate yourself!

Physical State
Flow | Fluids

Emotional &
Mental State

Self-Care
Sleep | Dreams

F • JAN 3

Day #: _____ | _____°

Phase | Season:

- Breathe & drop in
- Moonthly tracking
- Gratitude practice
- Celebrate yourself!

Physical State
Flow | Fluids

Emotional &
Mental State

Self-Care
Sleep | Dreams

S • JAN 4

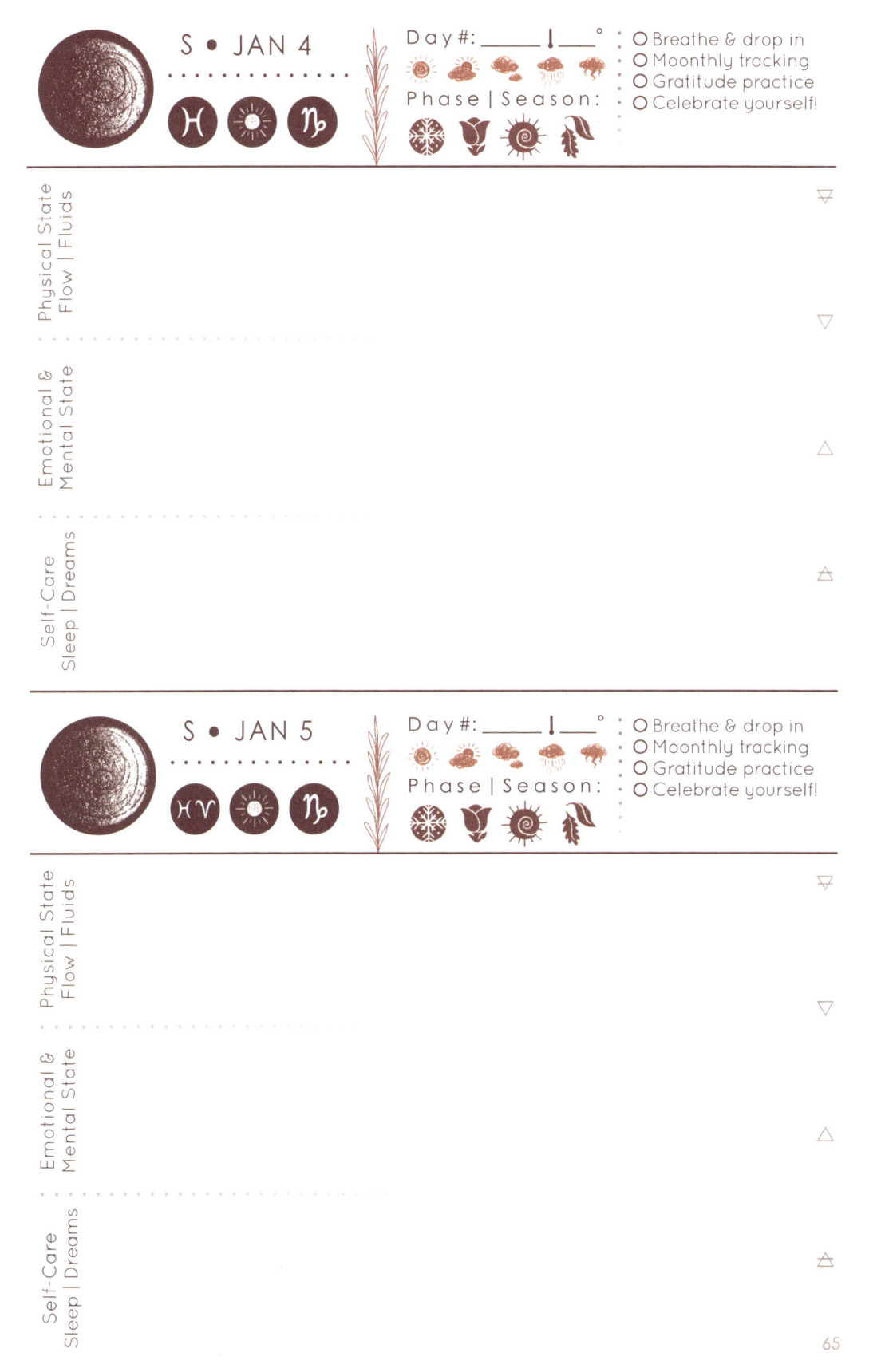

♓ ☀ ♑

Day #: _____ | ___°

Phase | Season:

- ○ Breathe & drop in
- ○ Moonthly tracking
- ○ Gratitude practice
- ○ Celebrate yourself!

Physical State / Flow | Fluids

Emotional & Mental State

Self-Care / Sleep | Dreams

S • JAN 5

♓♈ ☀ ♑

Day #: _____ | ___°

Phase | Season:

- ○ Breathe & drop in
- ○ Moonthly tracking
- ○ Gratitude practice
- ○ Celebrate yourself!

Physical State / Flow | Fluids

Emotional & Mental State

Self-Care / Sleep | Dreams

M • JAN 6

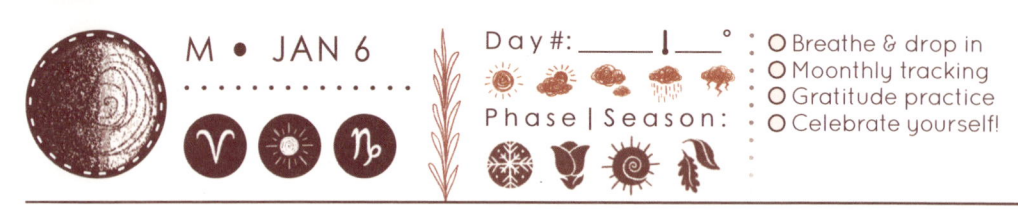

Day #: ____ | ___°
Phase | Season:

- ○ Breathe & drop in
- ○ Moonthly tracking
- ○ Gratitude practice
- ○ Celebrate yourself!

Physical State
Flow | Fluids

Emotional & Mental State

Self-Care
Sleep | Dreams

FIRST QUARTER IN ARIES

Expanding into possibilities led by self-trust

What is sprouting & coming into awareness?

What can I release to make space for further growth & grounding?

66

T • JAN 7

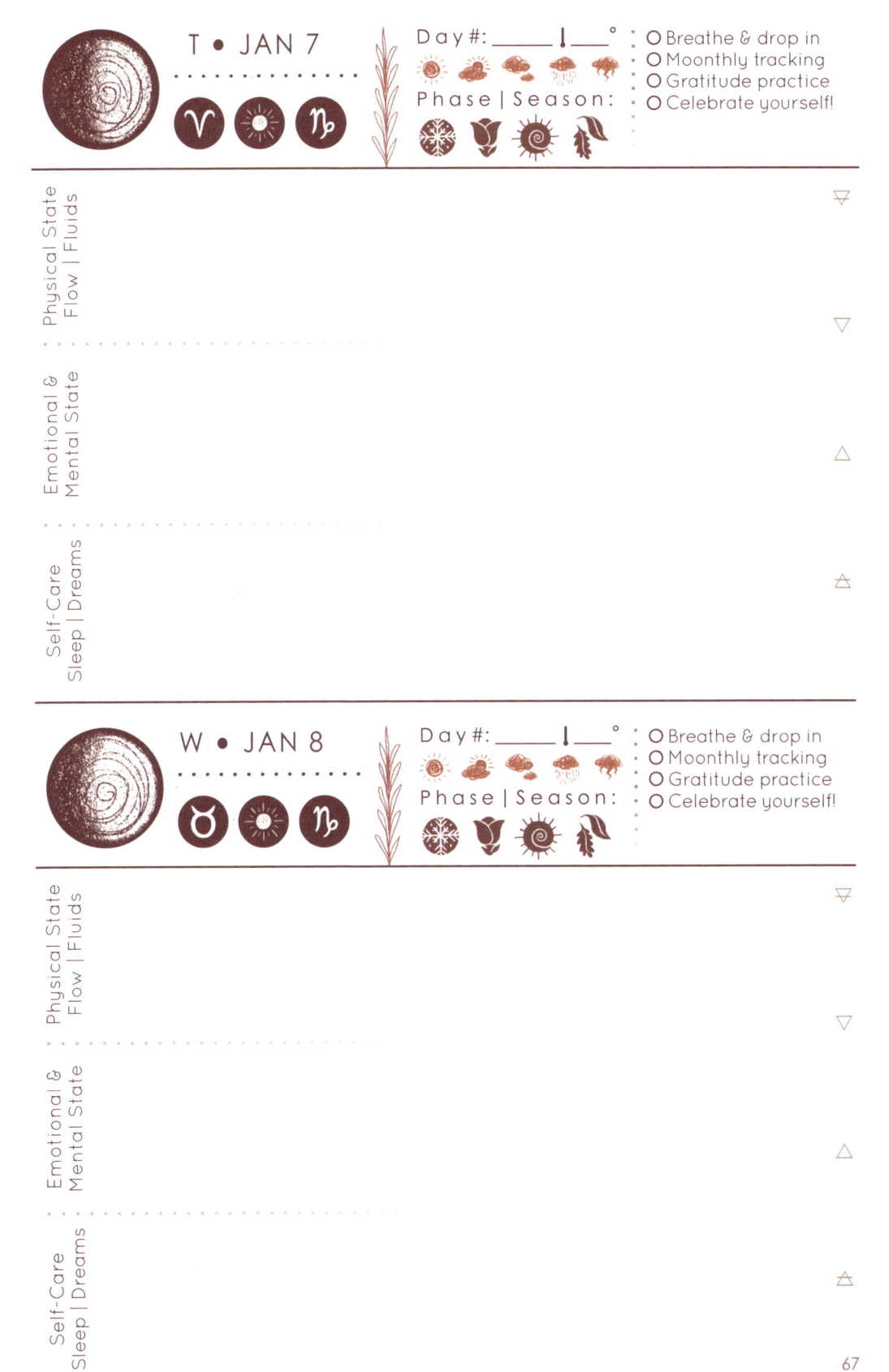

Day #: _____ | _____°

Phase | Season:

- ○ Breathe & drop in
- ○ Moonthly tracking
- ○ Gratitude practice
- ○ Celebrate yourself!

Physical State / Flow | Fluids

Emotional & Mental State

Self-Care / Sleep | Dreams

W • JAN 8

Day #: _____ | _____°

Phase | Season:

- ○ Breathe & drop in
- ○ Moonthly tracking
- ○ Gratitude practice
- ○ Celebrate yourself!

Physical State / Flow | Fluids

Emotional & Mental State

Self-Care / Sleep | Dreams

TH • JAN 9

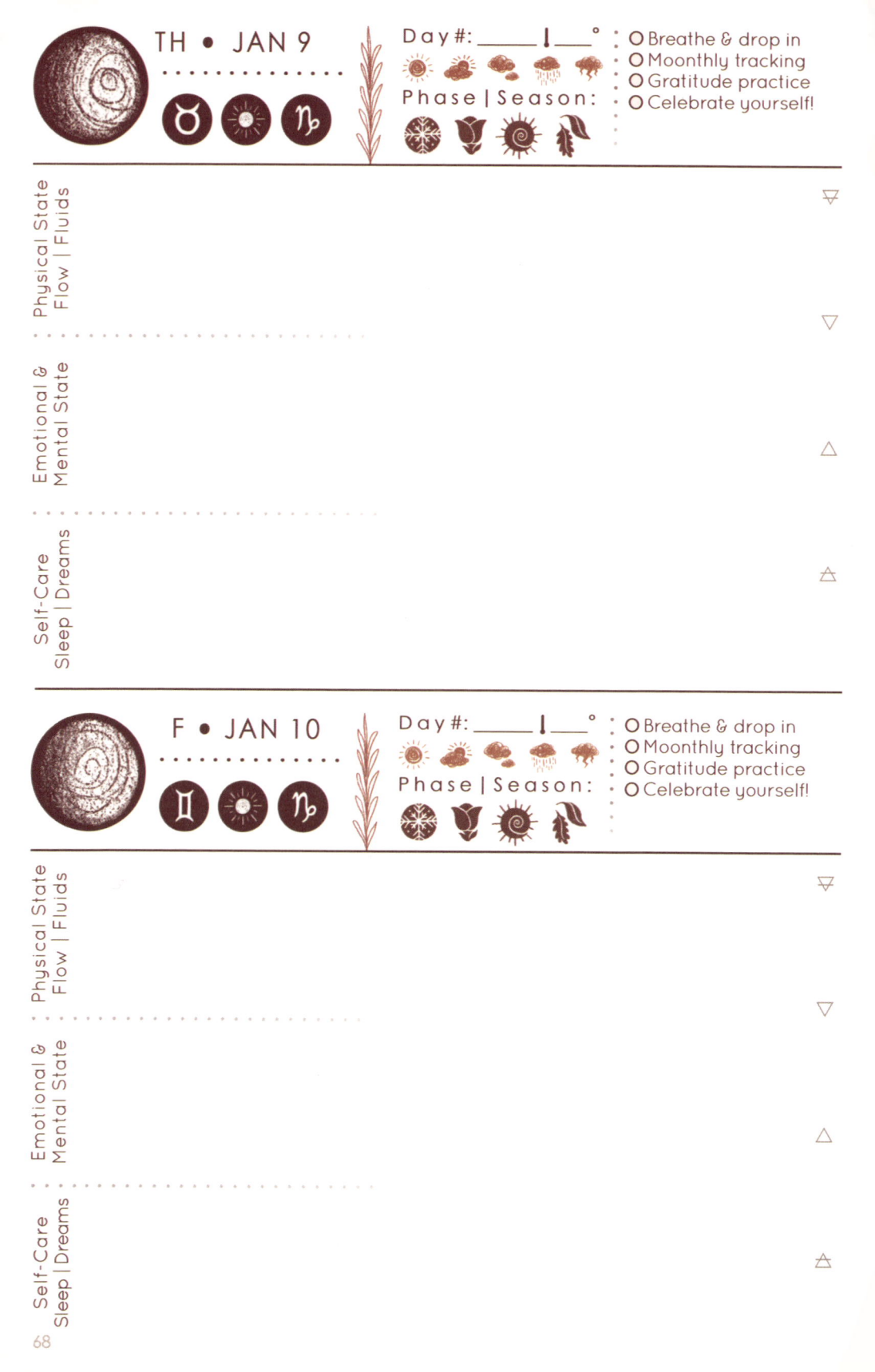

♉ ☼ ♑

Day #: _____ | _____°

Phase | Season:

- ○ Breathe & drop in
- ○ Moonthly tracking
- ○ Gratitude practice
- ○ Celebrate yourself!

Physical State / Flow | Fluids

Emotional & Mental State

Self-Care / Sleep | Dreams

F • JAN 10

♊ ☼ ♑

Day #: _____ | _____°

Phase | Season:

- ○ Breathe & drop in
- ○ Moonthly tracking
- ○ Gratitude practice
- ○ Celebrate yourself!

Physical State / Flow | Fluids

Emotional & Mental State

Self-Care / Sleep | Dreams

S • JAN 11

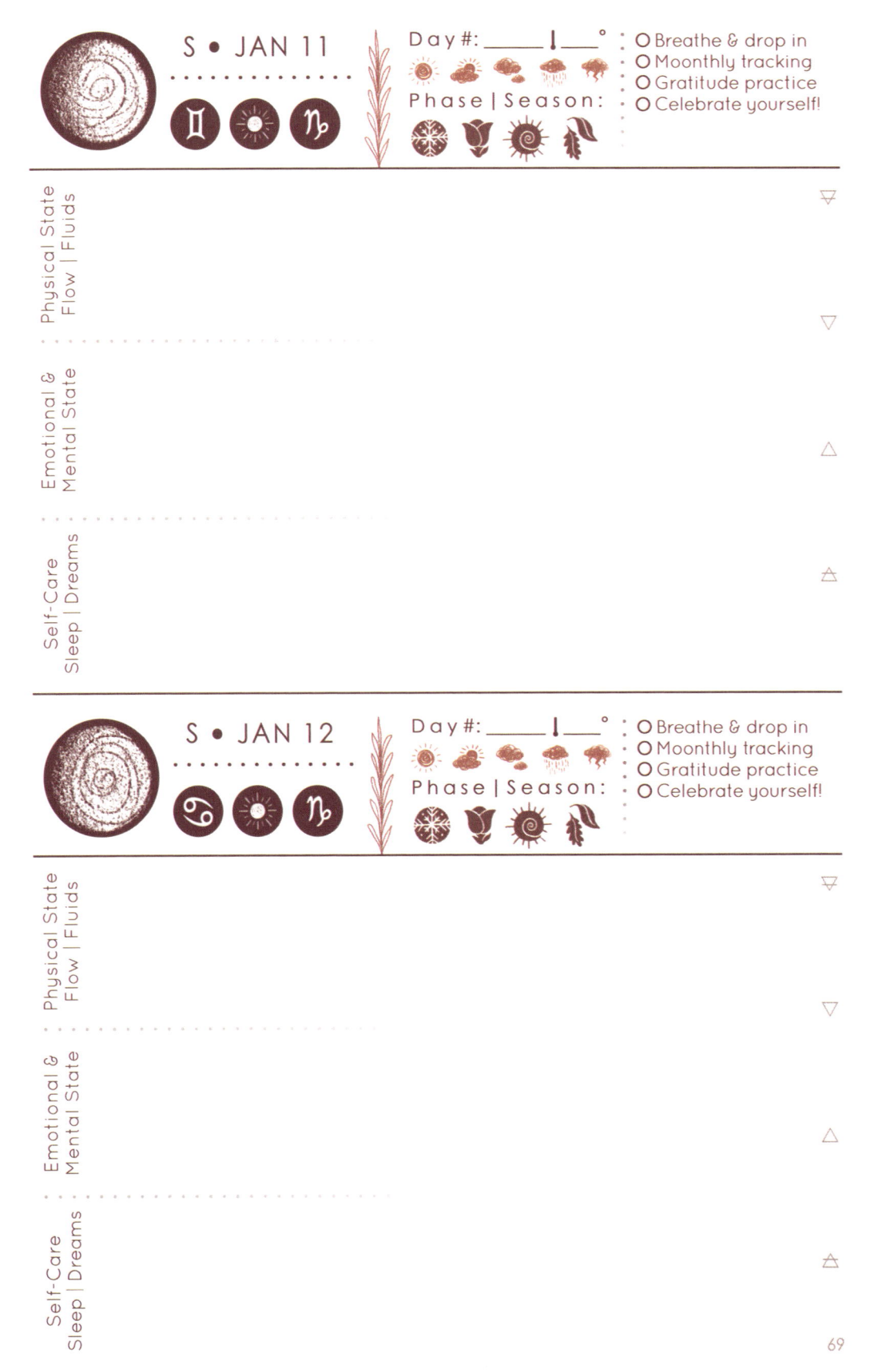

Day #: _____ | _____°

Phase | Season:

○ Breathe & drop in
○ Moonthly tracking
○ Gratitude practice
○ Celebrate yourself!

Physical State
Flow | Fluids

Emotional & Mental State

Self-Care
Sleep | Dreams

S • JAN 12

Day #: _____ | _____°

Phase | Season:

○ Breathe & drop in
○ Moonthly tracking
○ Gratitude practice
○ Celebrate yourself!

Physical State
Flow | Fluids

Emotional & Mental State

Self-Care
Sleep | Dreams

M • JAN 13

Day #: _____ | _____°

Phase | Season:

- Breathe & drop in
- Moonthly tracking
- Gratitude practice
- Celebrate yourself!

Physical State / Flow | Fluids

Emotional & Mental State

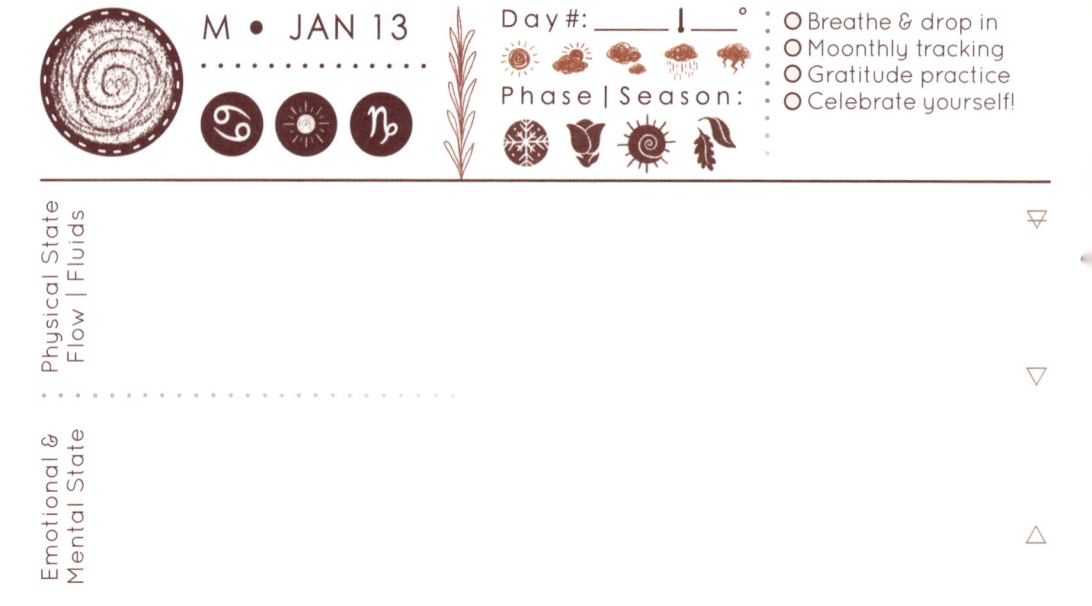

Self-Care / Sleep | Dreams

FULL MOON IN CANCER

Finding present awareness in all forms of feelings

What is being illuminated?

I give gratitude for what is & what is becoming:

T • JAN 14

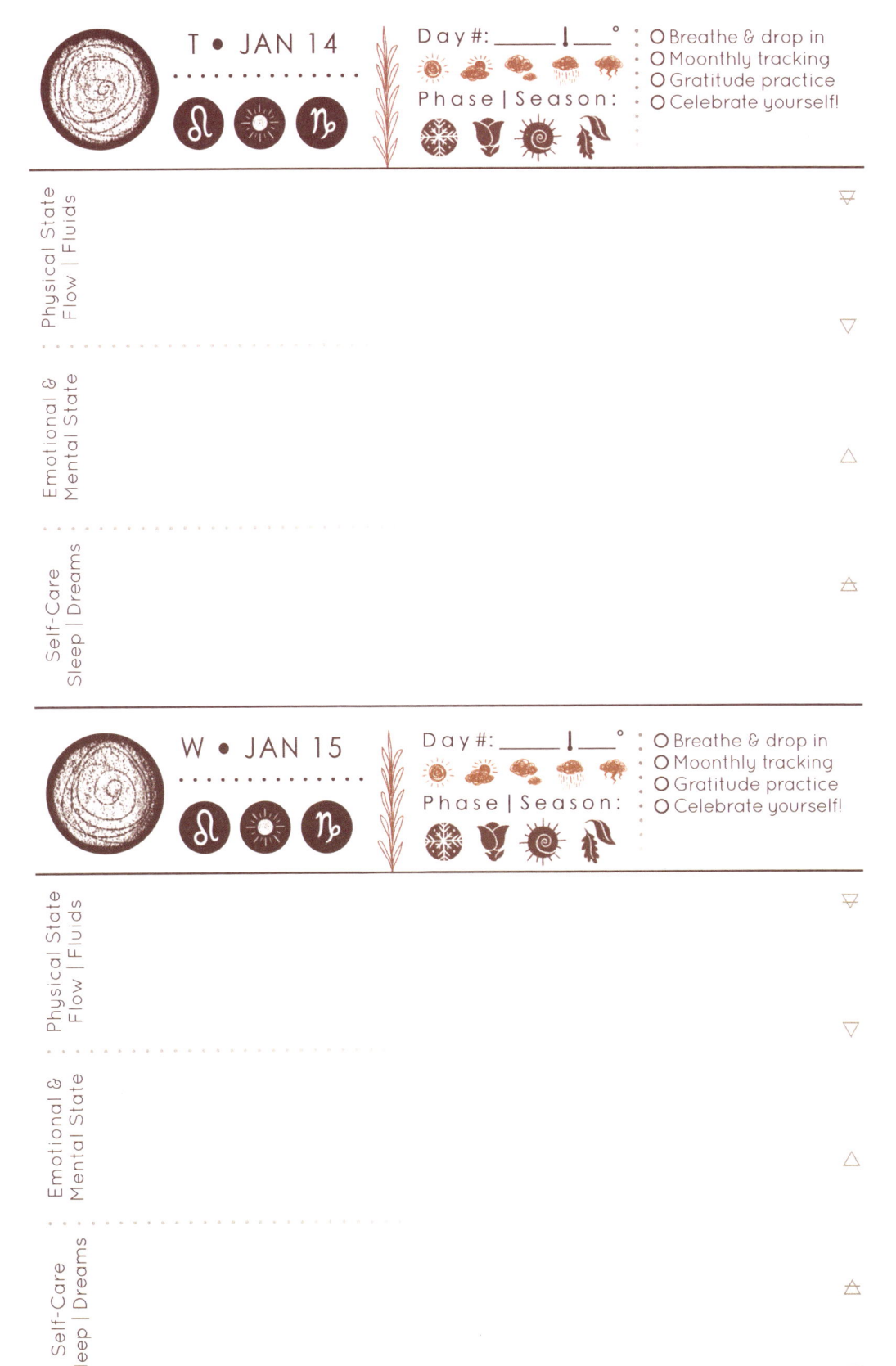

♌ ☀ ♑

Day #: _____ | _____°

Phase | Season:

- Breathe & drop in
- Moonthly tracking
- Gratitude practice
- Celebrate yourself!

Physical State
Flow | Fluids

Emotional &
Mental State

Self-Care
Sleep | Dreams

W • JAN 15

♌ ☀ ♑

Day #: _____ | _____°

Phase | Season:

- Breathe & drop in
- Moonthly tracking
- Gratitude practice
- Celebrate yourself!

Physical State
Flow | Fluids

Emotional &
Mental State

Self-Care
Sleep | Dreams

TH • JAN 16

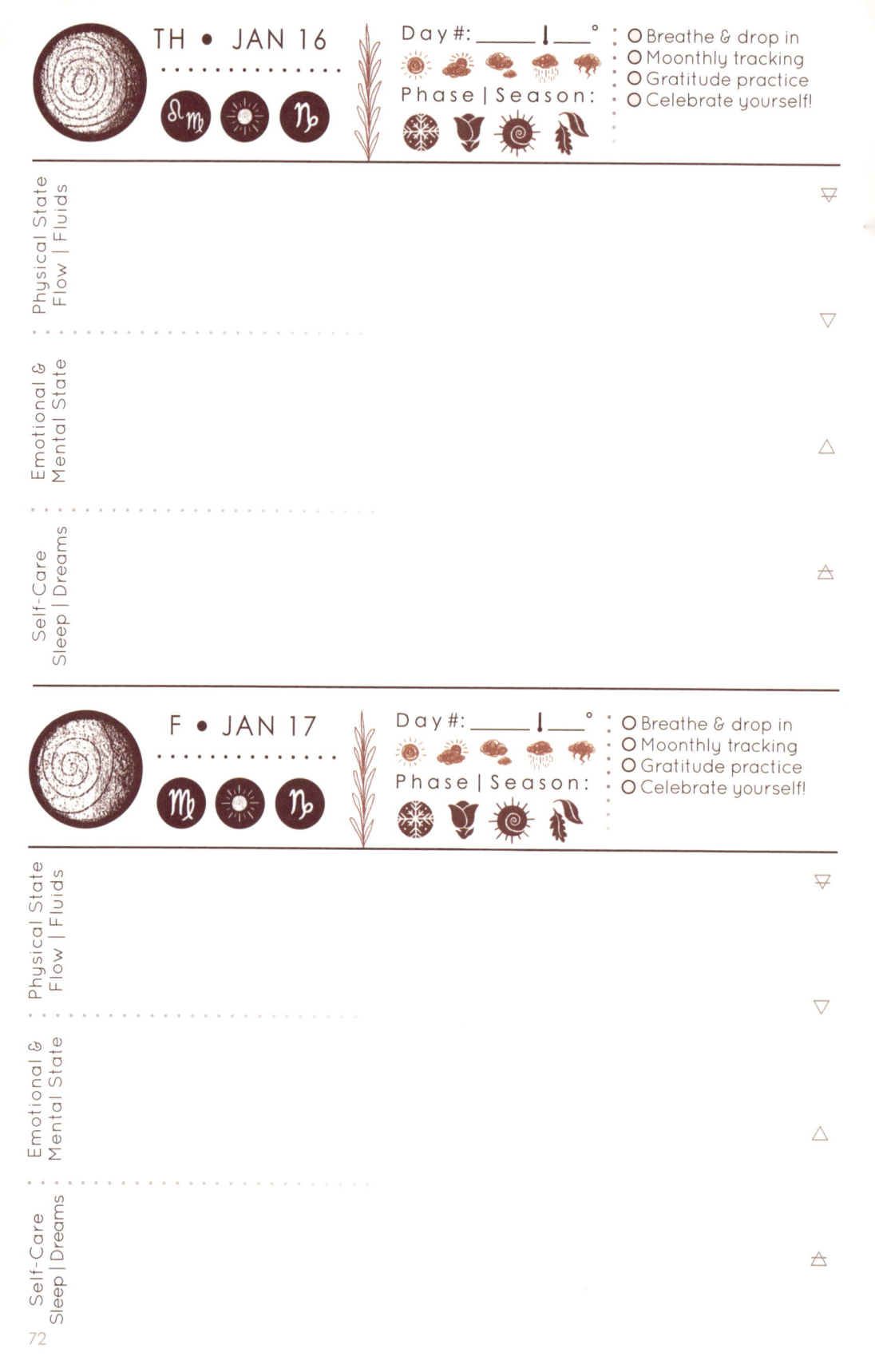

Day #: _____ | _____°

Phase | Season:

- ○ Breathe & drop in
- ○ Moonthly tracking
- ○ Gratitude practice
- ○ Celebrate yourself!

Physical State
Flow | Fluids

Emotional & Mental State

Self-Care
Sleep | Dreams

F • JAN 17

Day #: _____ | _____°

Phase | Season:

- ○ Breathe & drop in
- ○ Moonthly tracking
- ○ Gratitude practice
- ○ Celebrate yourself!

Physical State
Flow | Fluids

Emotional & Mental State

Self-Care
Sleep | Dreams

S • JAN 18

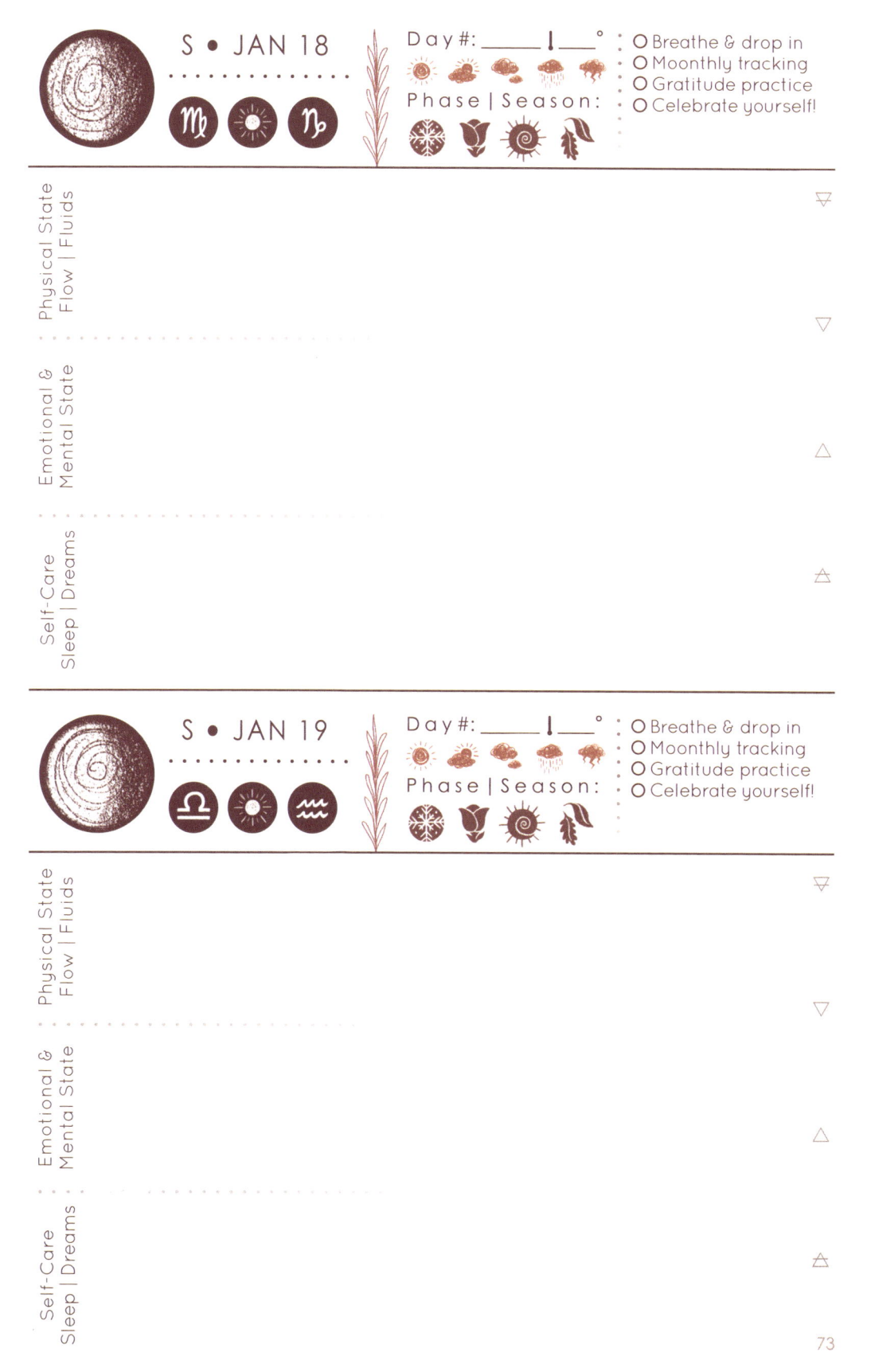

♍ ☀ ♑

Day #: _____ | _____°

Phase | Season:

○ Breathe & drop in
○ Moonthly tracking
○ Gratitude practice
○ Celebrate yourself!

Physical State
Flow | Fluids

Emotional &
Mental State

Self-Care
Sleep | Dreams

S • JAN 19

♎ ☀ ♒

Day #: _____ | _____°

Phase | Season:

○ Breathe & drop in
○ Moonthly tracking
○ Gratitude practice
○ Celebrate yourself!

Physical State
Flow | Fluids

Emotional &
Mental State

Self-Care
Sleep | Dreams

M • JAN 20

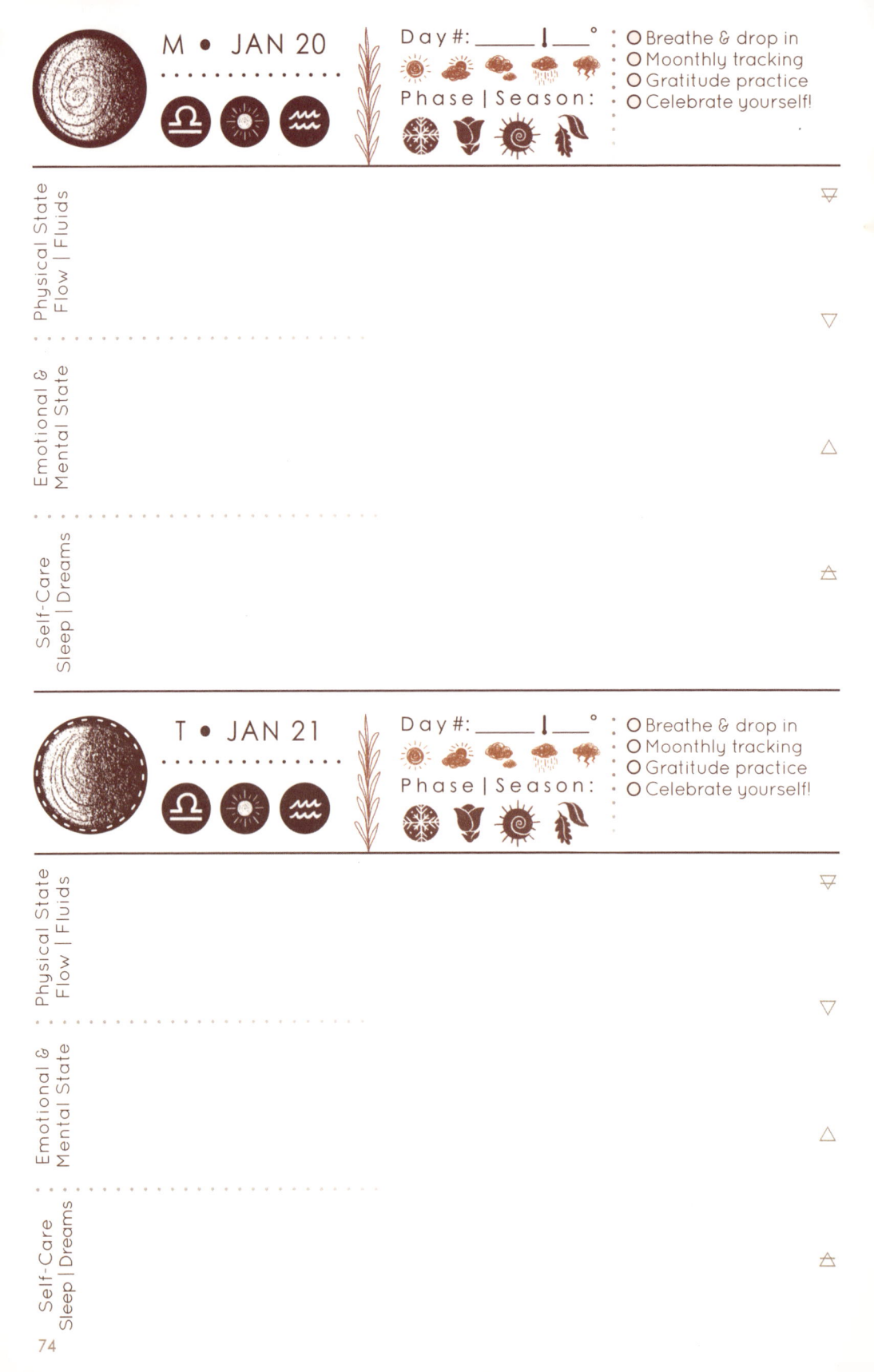

Day #: _____ | ____°

Phase | Season:

○ Breathe & drop in
○ Moonthly tracking
○ Gratitude practice
○ Celebrate yourself!

Physical State
Flow | Fluids

Emotional &
Mental State

Self-Care
Sleep | Dreams

T • JAN 21

Day #: _____ | ____°

Phase | Season:

○ Breathe & drop in
○ Moonthly tracking
○ Gratitude practice
○ Celebrate yourself!

Physical State
Flow | Fluids

Emotional &
Mental State

Self-Care
Sleep | Dreams

LAST QUARTER IN LIBRA

A deep surrender towards finding peace in non-polarity

What am I leaving behind this lunar cycle?

Where can I make more space for reflection &/or integration?

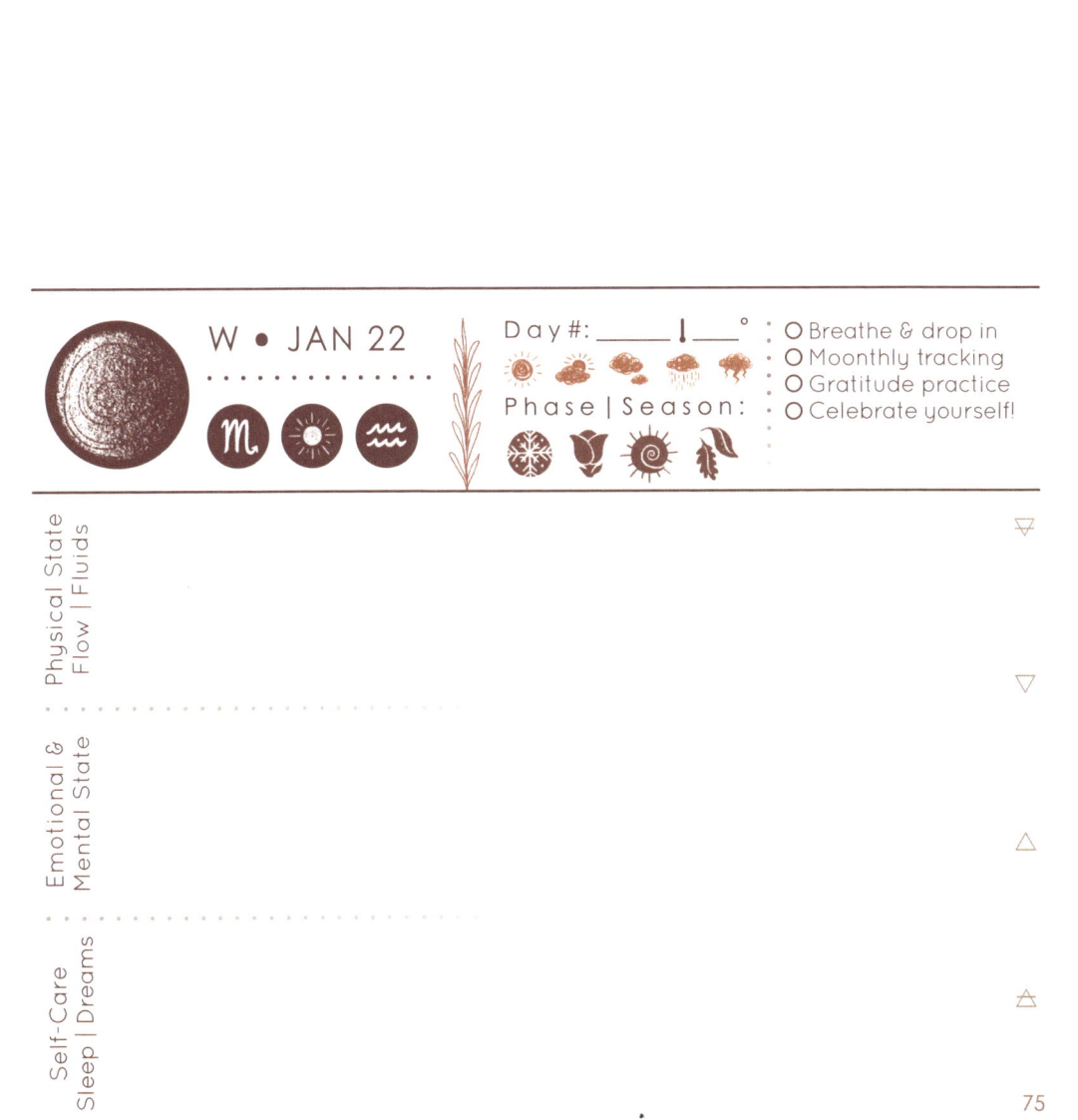

W • JAN 22

Day #: _____ | _____°

Phase | Season:

- ○ Breathe & drop in
- ○ Moonthly tracking
- ○ Gratitude practice
- ○ Celebrate yourself!

Physical State
Flow | Fluids

Emotional &
Mental State

Self-Care
Sleep | Dreams

TH • JAN 23

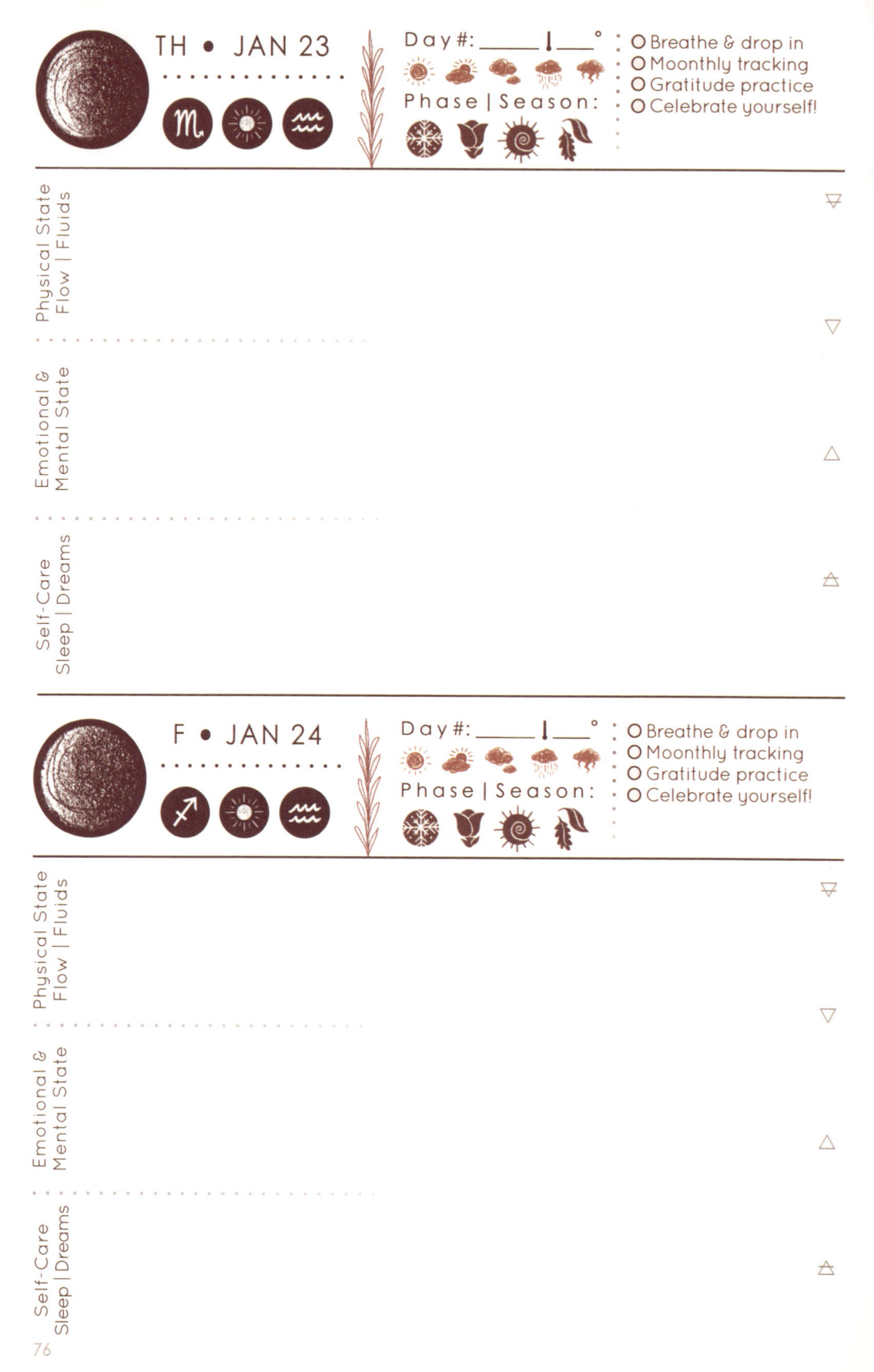

Day #: _____ | _____°

Phase | Season:

- ○ Breathe & drop in
- ○ Moonthly tracking
- ○ Gratitude practice
- ○ Celebrate yourself!

Physical State / Flow | Fluids

Emotional & Mental State

Self-Care / Sleep | Dreams

F • JAN 24

Day #: _____ | _____°

Phase | Season:

- ○ Breathe & drop in
- ○ Moonthly tracking
- ○ Gratitude practice
- ○ Celebrate yourself!

Physical State / Flow | Fluids

Emotional & Mental State

Self-Care / Sleep | Dreams

S • JAN 25

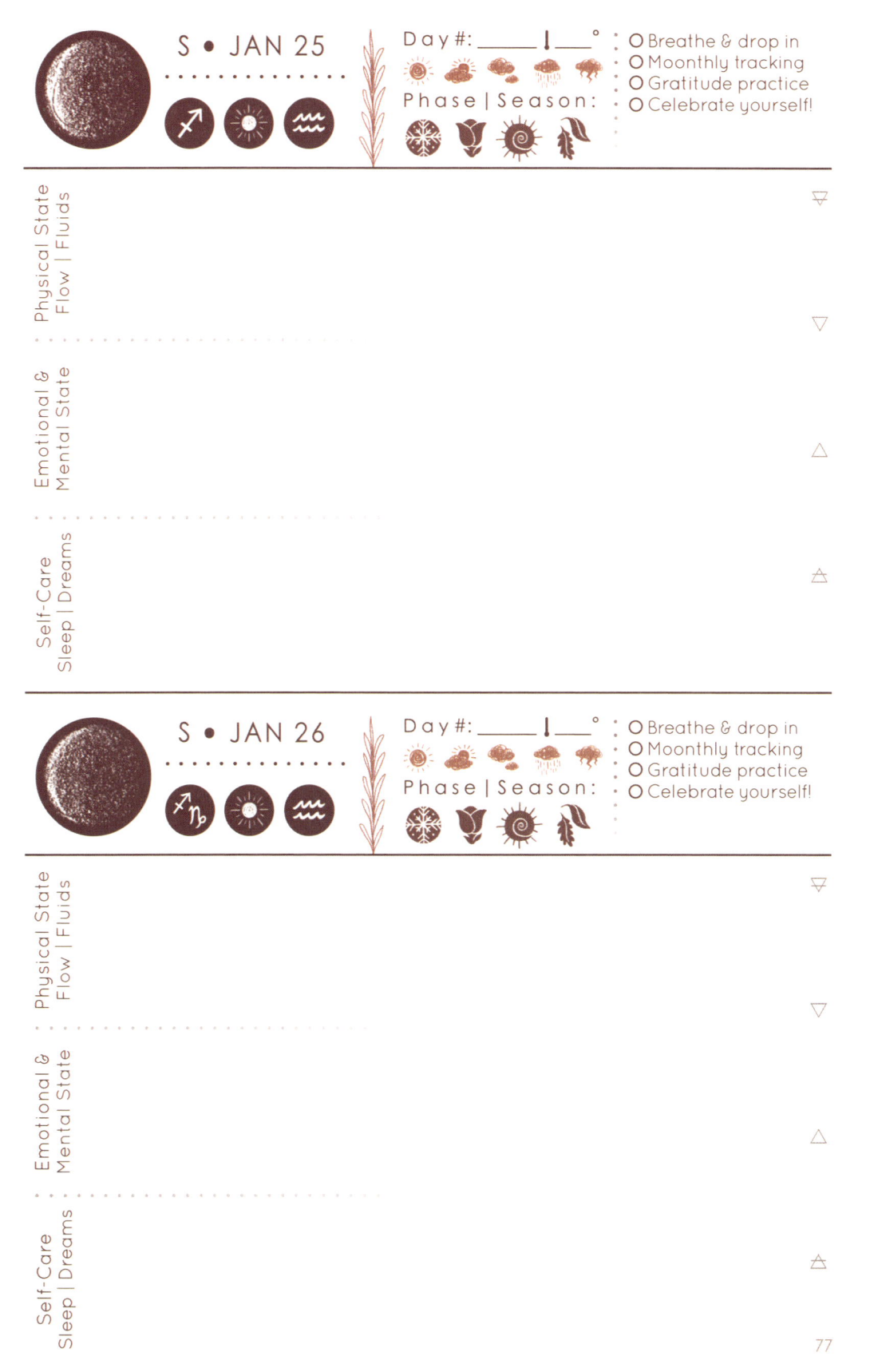

Day #: _____ | ___°

Phase | Season:

- ○ Breathe & drop in
- ○ Moonthly tracking
- ○ Gratitude practice
- ○ Celebrate yourself!

Physical State
Flow | Fluids

Emotional & Mental State

Self-Care
Sleep | Dreams

S • JAN 26

Day #: _____ | ___°

Phase | Season:

- ○ Breathe & drop in
- ○ Moonthly tracking
- ○ Gratitude practice
- ○ Celebrate yourself!

Physical State
Flow | Fluids

Emotional & Mental State

Self-Care
Sleep | Dreams

☾ 13th
12 | 30
01 | 28

CHECK IN & REFLECT

Last Cycle Day 1: _____

Last Cycle Length: _____

Use this space to reflect on your experiences & findings from this ending lunar cycle or your last menstrual cycle. Use cycle day #s if you bleed, or moon phases if you don't.

Circle the phase you bled near:

○ ☾ ☾ ☾ ☽ ● ● ● ● ☾ ☾ ☾ ○

Caution Days: (days I needed space)   **Bliss Days:** (days I felt great)

DAYS TO NOTE — Which cycle days stood out?

OBSERVATIONS — Notice any changes or patterns?

SELF-CARE — What was helpful & nourishing?

PLAN & PREPARE

Next Predicted Cycle:
🩸 ☾ _____

CHECKLIST

Add the following to any other planners or calendars for your next cycle, then check it off.

- ☐ Predicted "days to note" _____
- ☐ Days to slow down (pre-bleed) _____
- ☐ Rest day(s) (next bleed) _____
- ☐ Date with yourself _____
- ☐ _____

- ☐ Self chest/breast exam
- ☐ Meal plan with cycle
- ☐ _____
- ☐ _____
- ☐ _____

OPEN SPACE

Use this space how you wish, or print out one of our free templates to paste here for BBT charting, dream tracking, or something else:

Navigating Life's Phases: The Wisdom of Planetary Cycles

by Julia Simms (she/her) of Child of the Divine Tarot • Tarot Reader & Astrologer • @childofthedivinetarot • childofthedivinetarot.square.site

We can learn to live in alignment with the cyclical rhythms of the universe. One powerful tool for achieving this harmony is the Celestial Guidance Tarot Spread, which integrates the influence of planetary energies into our daily routines.

Shuffle and Cleanse the Deck:
Begin by shuffling your tarot deck while focusing on the day ahead. This process clears any residual energies and prepares the cards to receive guidance from the cosmos.

Find the Card of the Day: Locate the tarot card corresponding to the planetary influence ruling that day. Place the card in front of it in position 1, the day's card in the middle position, and the card behind it in position 3. of the tarot spread below.

1 — **Card in front of daily pull:** Represents your current energy & sets the tone for your day.

2 — **Card of the day:** Reflects the energy of the day, aligned with the corresponding planet's influence.

3 — **Card behind daily pull:** Indicates potential outcomes or energies to embrace as you navigate your day.

Planetary Influences:

Monday - The High Priestess: Trust your intuition and inner wisdom, especially in relation to lunar influences.

Tuesday - The Emperor: Channel the assertive energy of Mars to take decisive action and establish boundaries.

Wednesday - The Magician: Harness the communicative and adaptable energy of Mercury to utilize your skills and resources effectively.

Thursday - Wheel of Fortune: Embrace the expansive energy of Jupiter and trust in the natural cycles of change and abundance.

Friday - The Empress: Cultivate love, beauty, and pleasure in all aspects of your life, aligning with the harmonious energy of Venus.

Saturday - The World: Celebrate accomplishments and milestones while remaining disciplined and grounded under the structured influence of Saturn.

Sunday - The Sun: Radiate optimism, vitality, and joy as you embrace opportunities for growth and self-expression, basking in the illuminating energy of the Sun.

Consciously aligning our actions with planetary energies, we optimize daily cyclical planning.

Phasic Overview & In-Betweens

Use this space to focus on the phases of the moonth and the in-betweens of the peak lunations.

One way of using this space is to designate one column for your goal-planning, intention-setting or focus per phase/week. Use the other column for reflections, dream themes, nutrition tracking, cards pulls, etc!

M • JAN 27

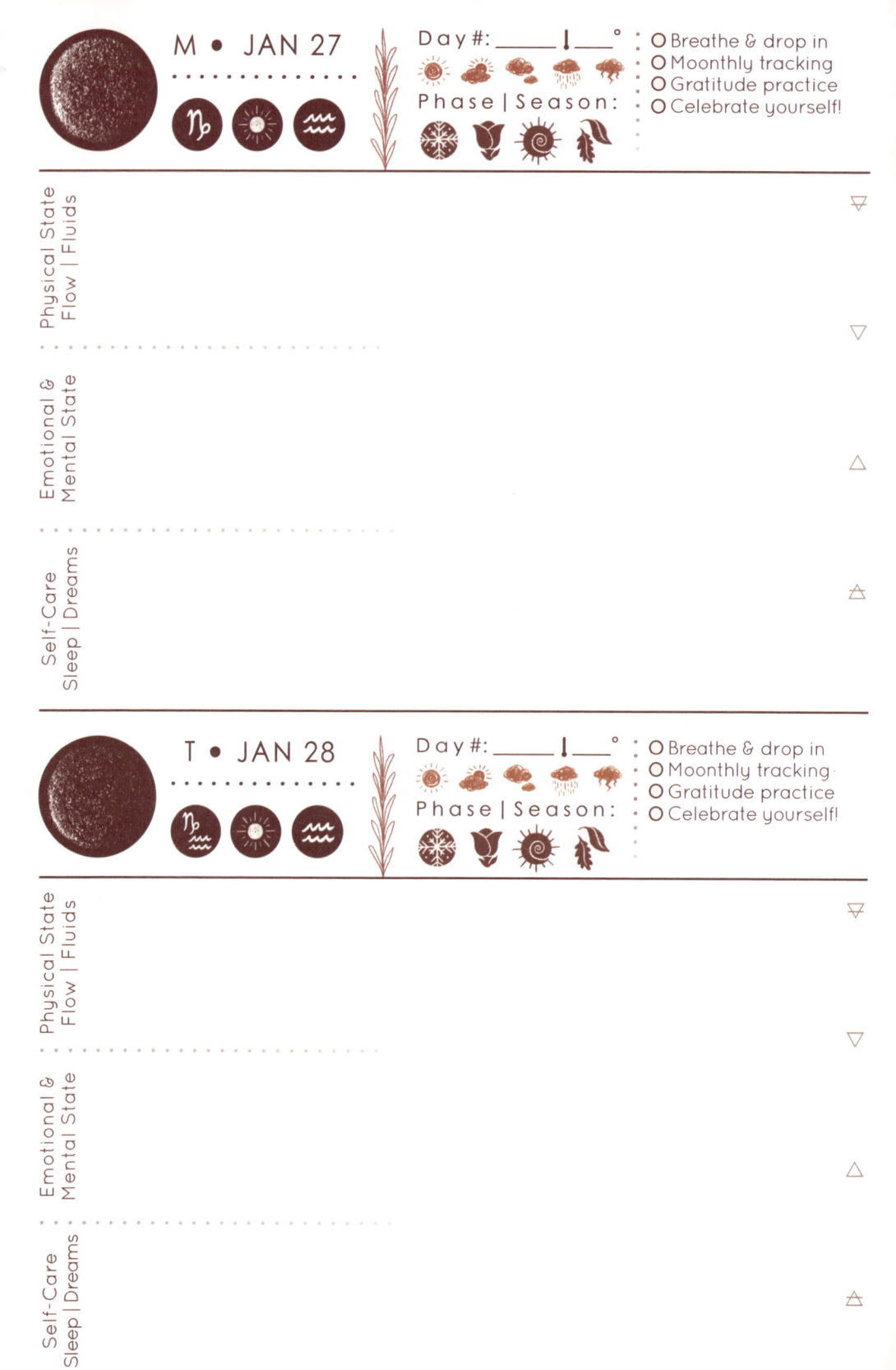

Day #: _____ | _____°

Phase | Season:

- ○ Breathe & drop in
- ○ Moonthly tracking
- ○ Gratitude practice
- ○ Celebrate yourself!

Physical State
Flow | Fluids

Emotional & Mental State

Self-Care
Sleep | Dreams

T • JAN 28

Day #: _____ | _____°

Phase | Season:

- ○ Breathe & drop in
- ○ Moonthly tracking
- ○ Gratitude practice
- ○ Celebrate yourself!

Physical State
Flow | Fluids

Emotional & Mental State

Self-Care
Sleep | Dreams

W • JAN 29

Day #: _____ | ___°

Phase | Season:

- ○ Breathe & drop in
- ○ Moonthly tracking
- ○ Gratitude practice
- ○ Celebrate yourself!

Physical State
Flow | Fluids

Emotional &
Mental State

Self-Care
Sleep | Dreams

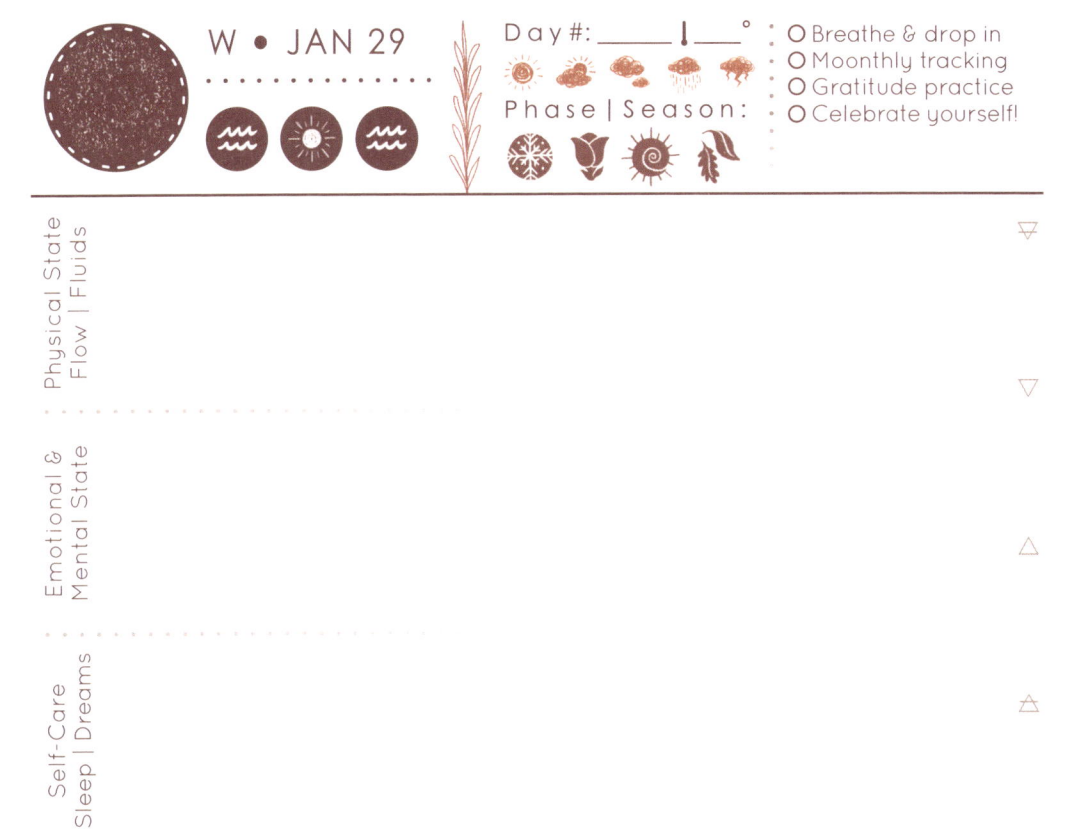

NEW MOON IN AQUARIUS

Initiating new collaborative energy & advocacy for the collective

What do I want to grow & focus on during this lunar cycle?

How will I hold space for this?

TH • JAN 30

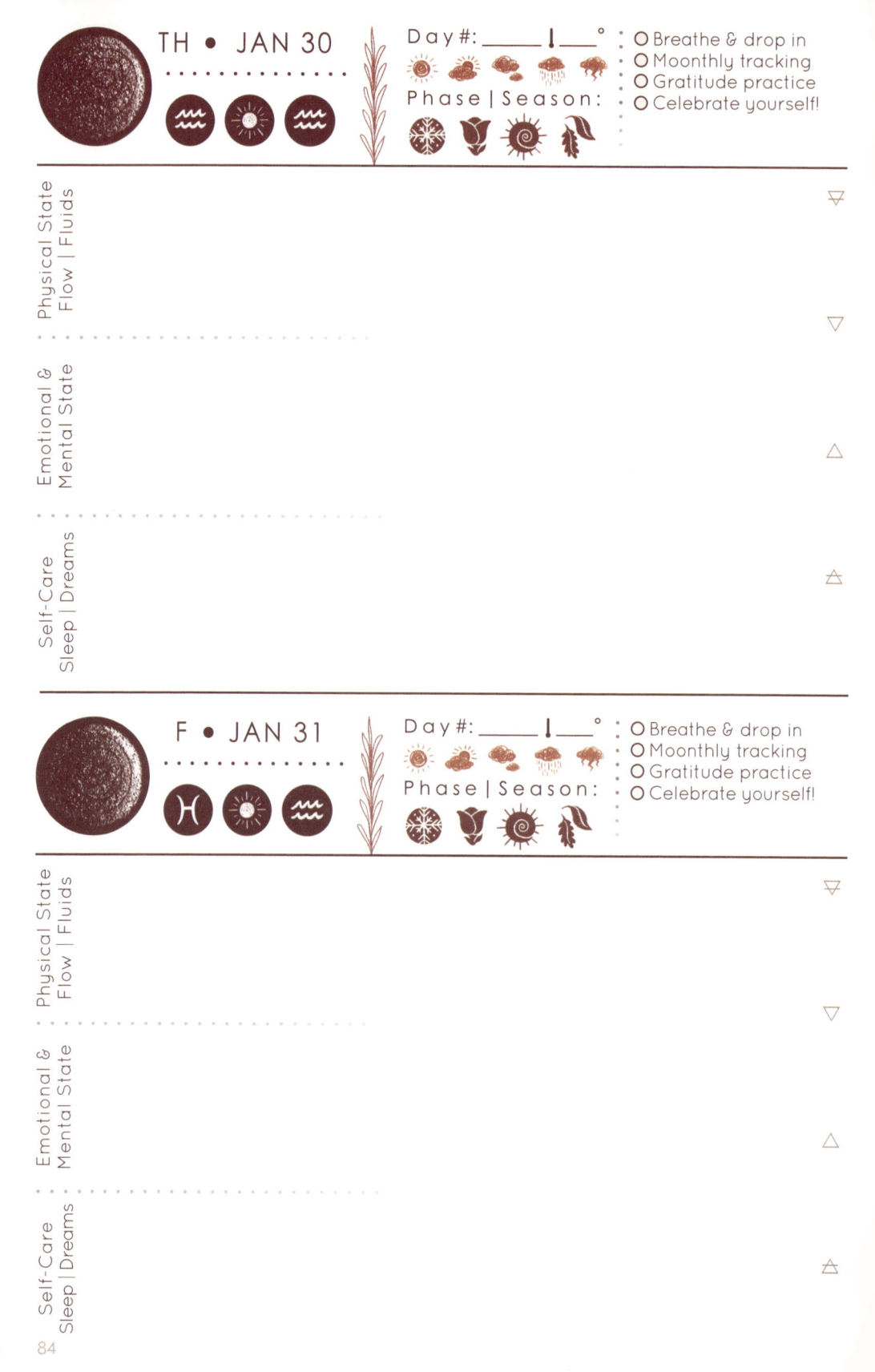

Day #: _____ | _____°

Phase | Season:

- ○ Breathe & drop in
- ○ Moonthly tracking
- ○ Gratitude practice
- ○ Celebrate yourself!

Physical State
Flow | Fluids

Emotional & Mental State

Self-Care
Sleep | Dreams

F • JAN 31

Day #: _____ | _____°

Phase | Season:

- ○ Breathe & drop in
- ○ Moonthly tracking
- ○ Gratitude practice
- ○ Celebrate yourself!

Physical State
Flow | Fluids

Emotional & Mental State

Self-Care
Sleep | Dreams

S • FEB 1

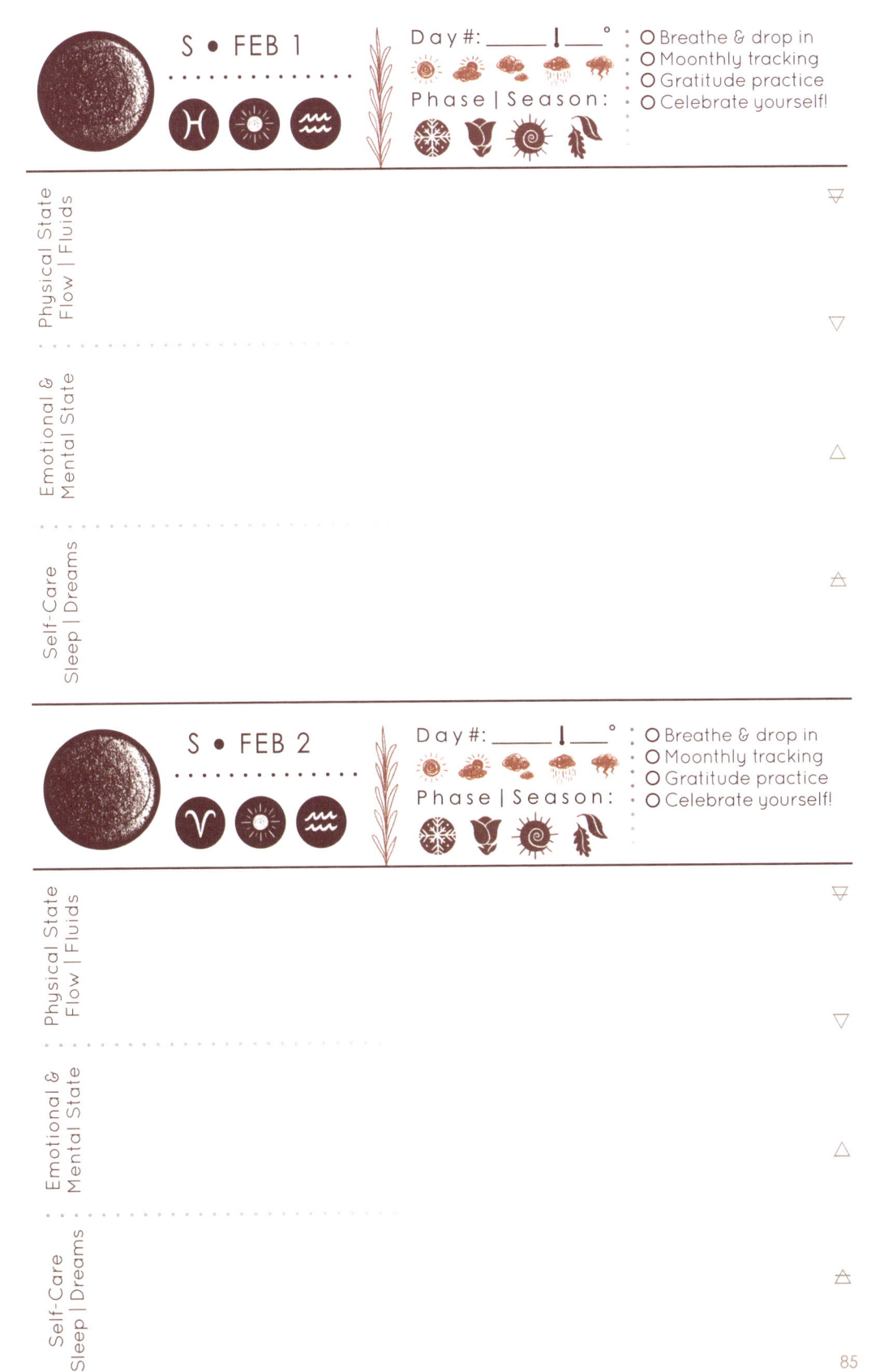

Day #: _____ | ____°

Phase | Season:

- ○ Breathe & drop in
- ○ Moonthly tracking
- ○ Gratitude practice
- ○ Celebrate yourself!

Physical State
Flow | Fluids

Emotional &
Mental State

Self-Care
Sleep | Dreams

S • FEB 2

Day #: _____ | ____°

Phase | Season:

- ○ Breathe & drop in
- ○ Moonthly tracking
- ○ Gratitude practice
- ○ Celebrate yourself!

Physical State
Flow | Fluids

Emotional &
Mental State

Self-Care
Sleep | Dreams

M • FEB 3

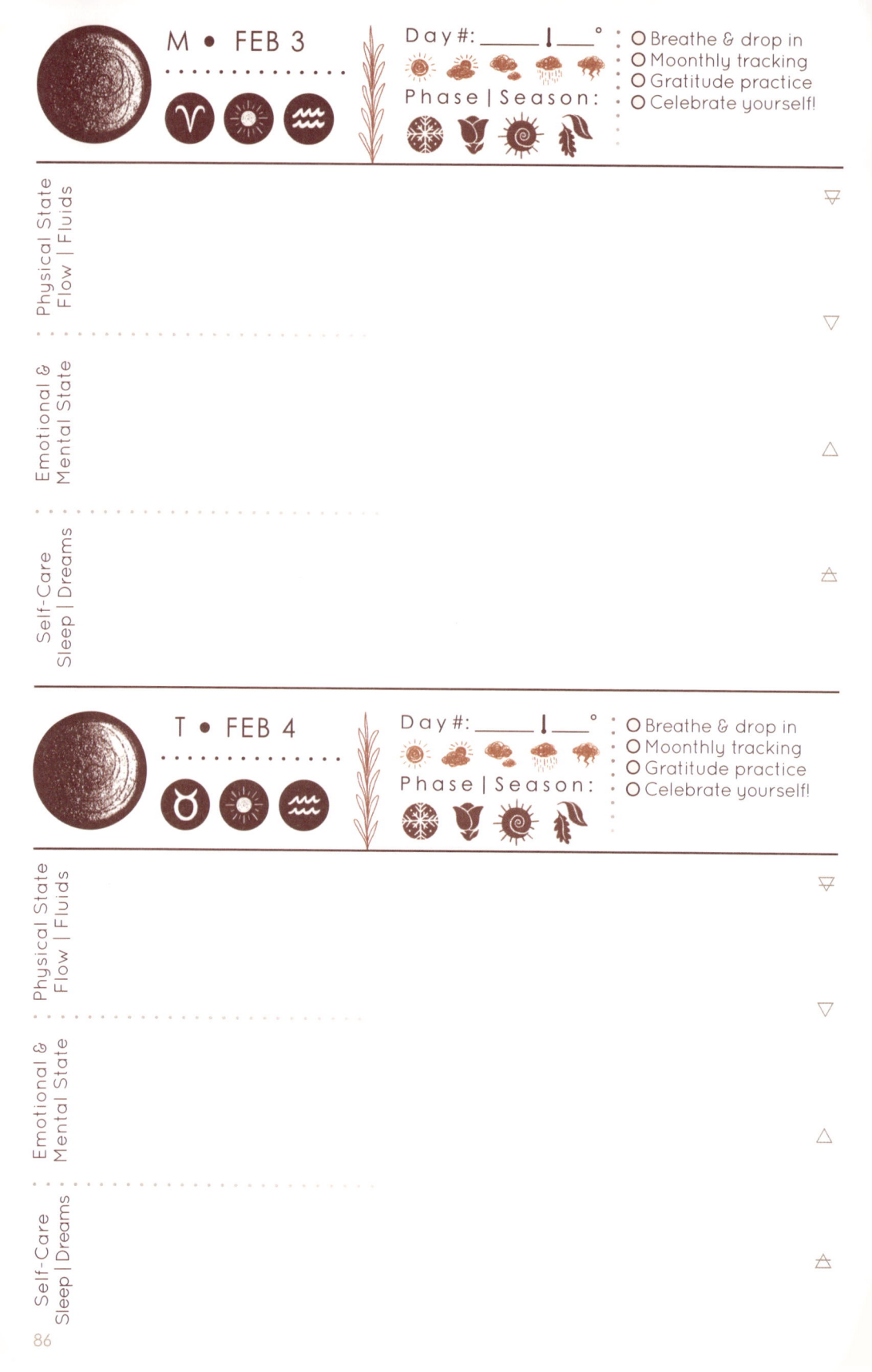

Day #: ____ | ____°
Phase | Season:

- Breathe & drop in
- Moonthly tracking
- Gratitude practice
- Celebrate yourself!

Physical State
Flow | Fluids

Emotional &
Mental State

Self-Care
Sleep | Dreams

T • FEB 4

Day #: ____ | ____°
Phase | Season:

- Breathe & drop in
- Moonthly tracking
- Gratitude practice
- Celebrate yourself!

Physical State
Flow | Fluids

Emotional &
Mental State

Self-Care
Sleep | Dreams

W • FEB 5

Day #: _____ | _____°

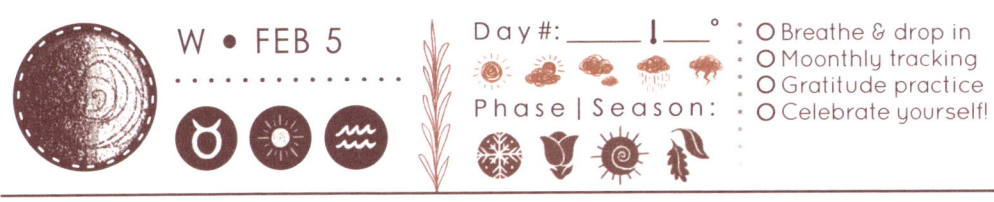

Phase | Season:

- ○ Breathe & drop in
- ○ Moonthly tracking
- ○ Gratitude practice
- ○ Celebrate yourself!

Physical State / Flow | Fluids

Emotional & Mental State

Self-Care / Sleep | Dreams

FIRST QUARTER IN TAURUS

A growing awareness of aligned values & sources of stability

What is sprouting & coming into awareness?

What can I release to make space for further growth & grounding?

TH • FEB 6

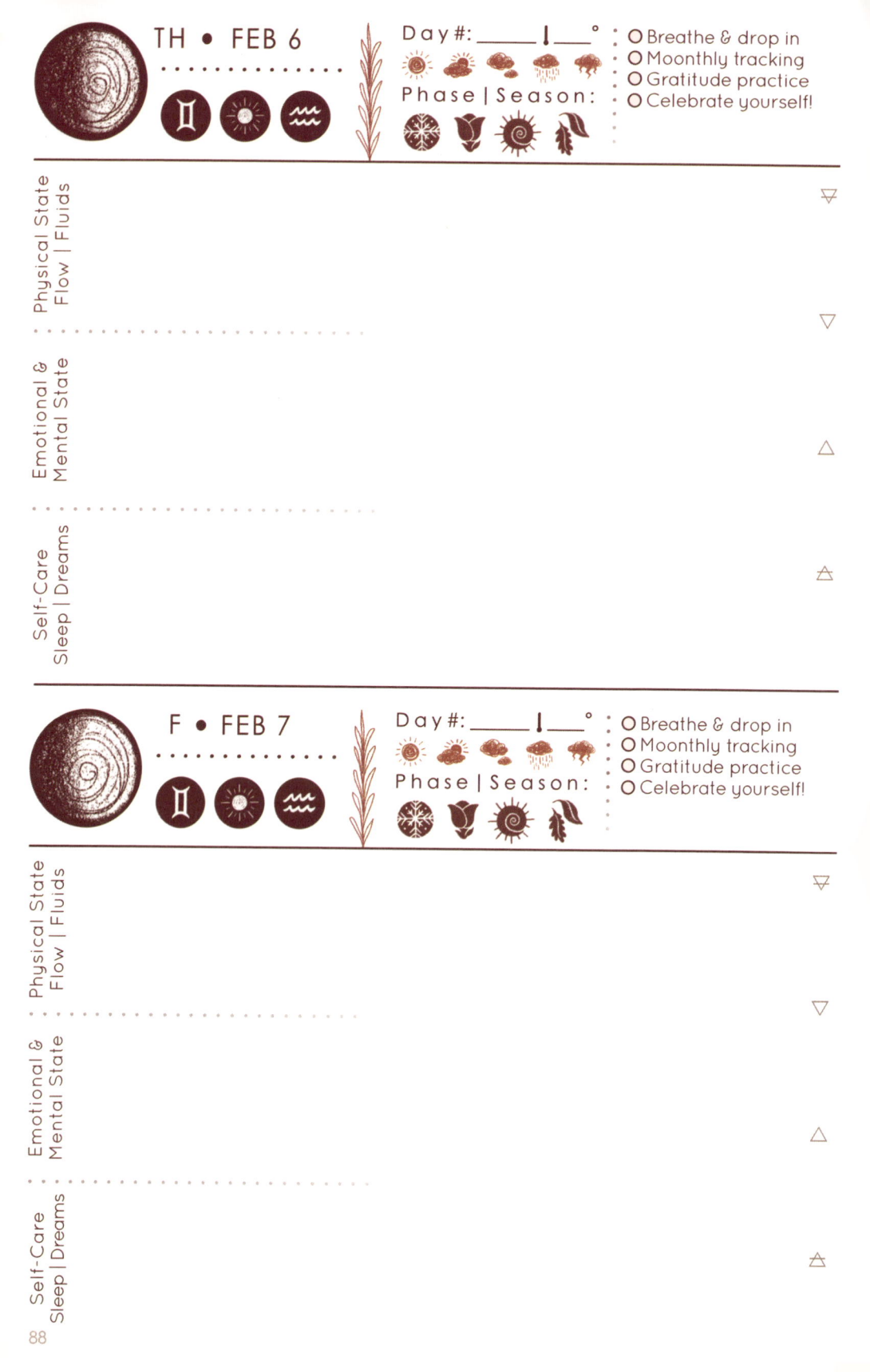

Day #: _____ | _____°

Phase | Season:

- ○ Breathe & drop in
- ○ Moonthly tracking
- ○ Gratitude practice
- ○ Celebrate yourself!

Physical State / Flow | Fluids

Emotional & Mental State

Self-Care / Sleep | Dreams

F • FEB 7

Day #: _____ | _____°

Phase | Season:

- ○ Breathe & drop in
- ○ Moonthly tracking
- ○ Gratitude practice
- ○ Celebrate yourself!

Physical State / Flow | Fluids

Emotional & Mental State

Self-Care / Sleep | Dreams

S • FEB 8

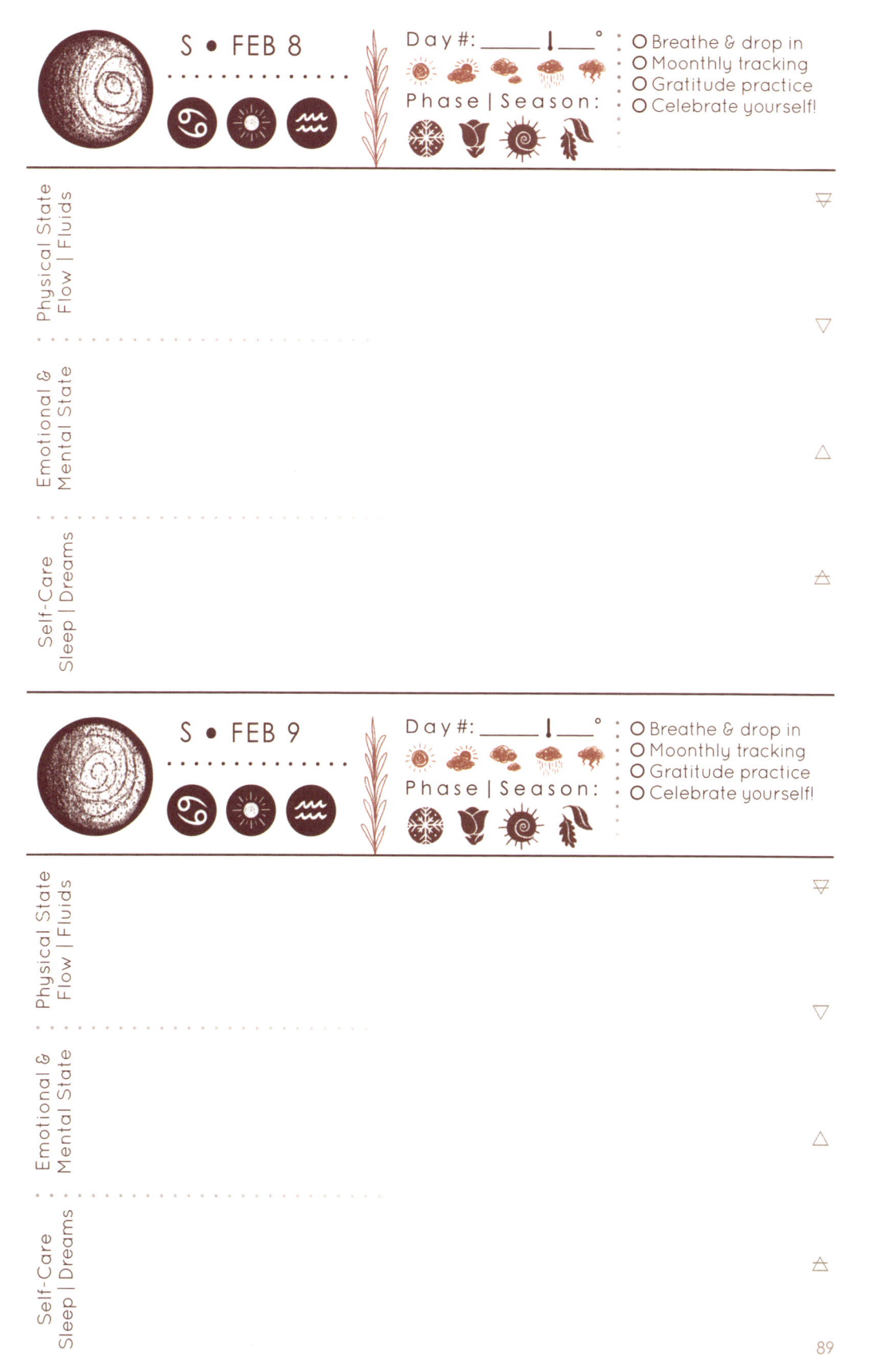

Day #: _____ | _____°

Phase | Season:

- ○ Breathe & drop in
- ○ Moonthly tracking
- ○ Gratitude practice
- ○ Celebrate yourself!

Physical State / Flow | Fluids

Emotional & Mental State

Self-Care / Sleep | Dreams

S • FEB 9

Day #: _____ | _____°

Phase | Season:

- ○ Breathe & drop in
- ○ Moonthly tracking
- ○ Gratitude practice
- ○ Celebrate yourself!

Physical State / Flow | Fluids

Emotional & Mental State

Self-Care / Sleep | Dreams

M • FEB 10

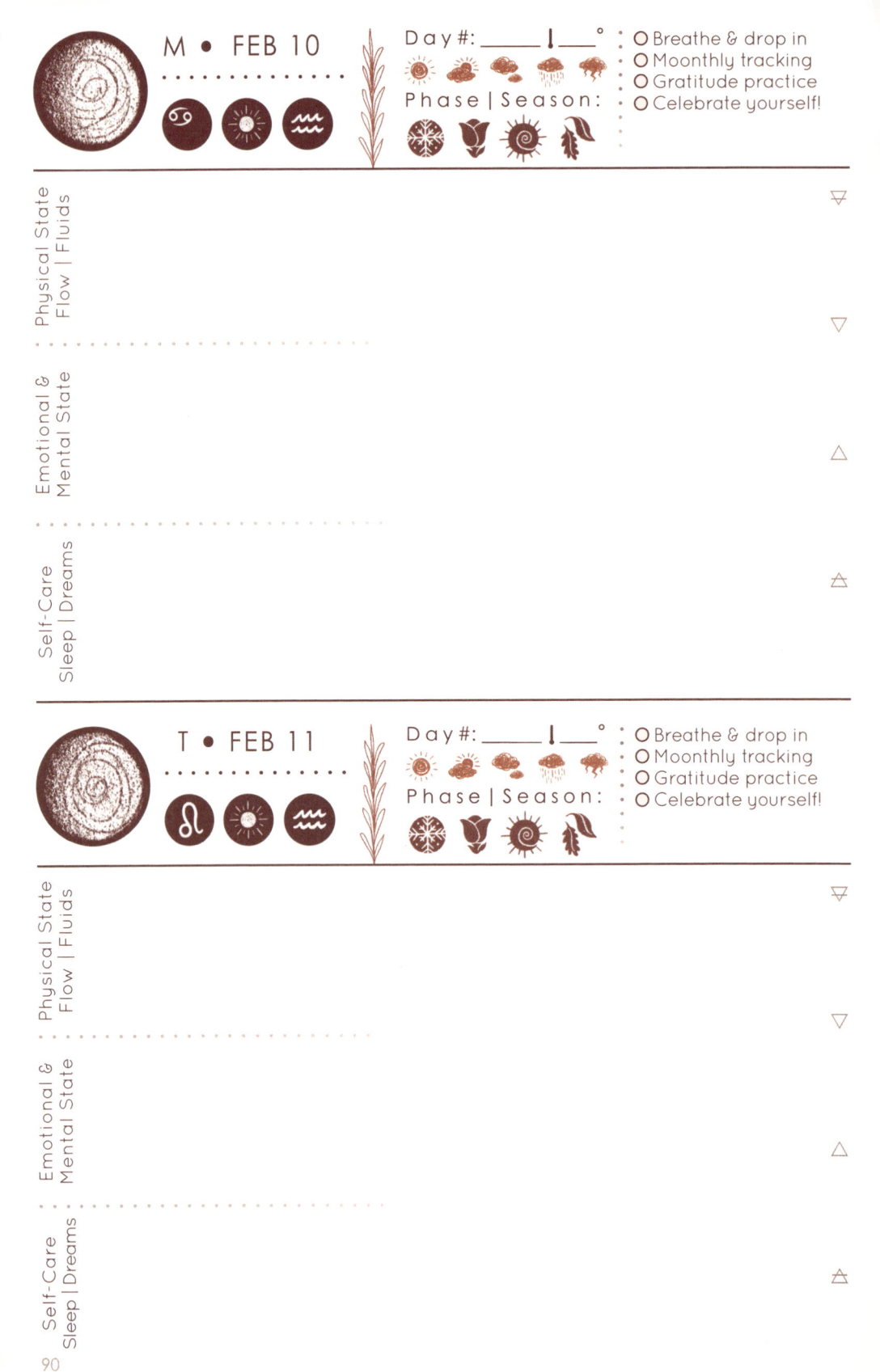

Day #: _____ | _____°

Phase | Season:

- ○ Breathe & drop in
- ○ Moonthly tracking
- ○ Gratitude practice
- ○ Celebrate yourself!

Physical State / Flow | Fluids

Emotional & Mental State

Self-Care / Sleep | Dreams

T • FEB 11

Day #: _____ | _____°

Phase | Season:

- ○ Breathe & drop in
- ○ Moonthly tracking
- ○ Gratitude practice
- ○ Celebrate yourself!

Physical State / Flow | Fluids

Emotional & Mental State

Self-Care / Sleep | Dreams

W • FEB 12

Day #: _____ | ____°

Phase | Season:

- Breathe & drop in
- Moonthly tracking
- Gratitude practice
- Celebrate yourself!

Physical State
Flow | Fluids

Emotional &
Mental State

Self-Care
Sleep | Dreams

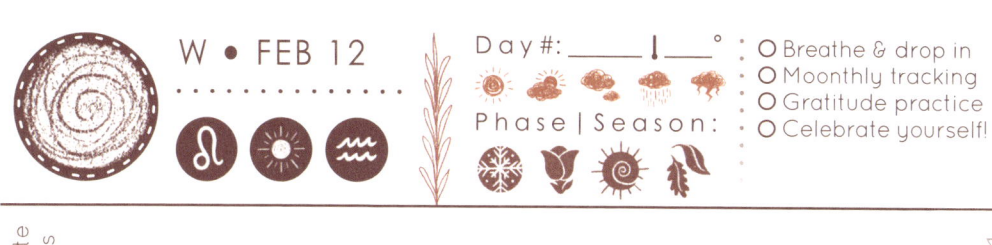

FULL MOON IN LEO

An expansion of creative potential that embraces self-worth

What is being illuminated?

I give gratitude for what is & what is becoming:

TH • FEB 13

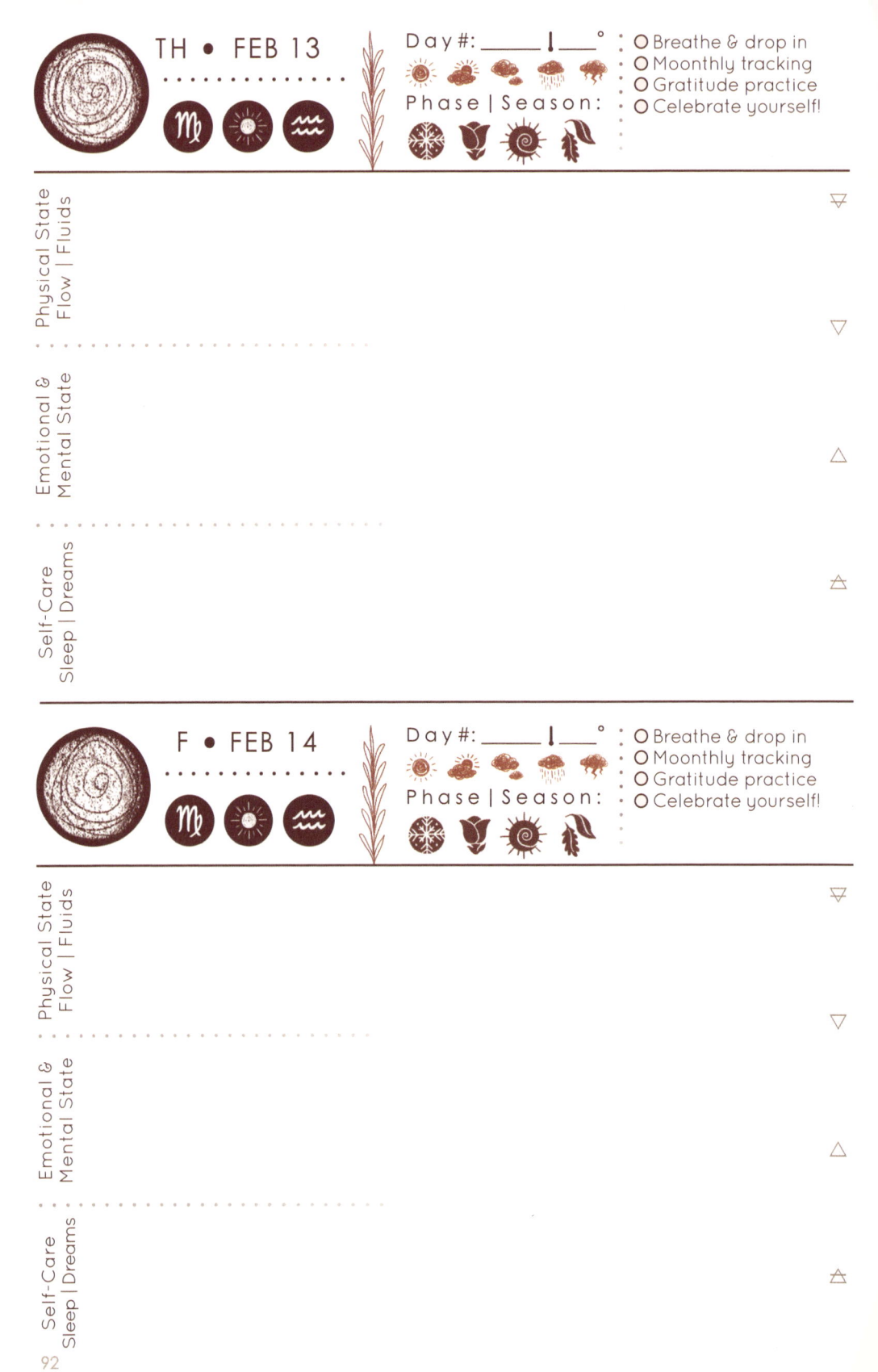

Day #: _____ | _____°

Phase | Season:

- ○ Breathe & drop in
- ○ Moonthly tracking
- ○ Gratitude practice
- ○ Celebrate yourself!

Physical State
Flow | Fluids

Emotional & Mental State

Self-Care
Sleep | Dreams

F • FEB 14

Day #: _____ | _____°

Phase | Season:

- ○ Breathe & drop in
- ○ Moonthly tracking
- ○ Gratitude practice
- ○ Celebrate yourself!

Physical State
Flow | Fluids

Emotional & Mental State

Self-Care
Sleep | Dreams

S • FEB 15

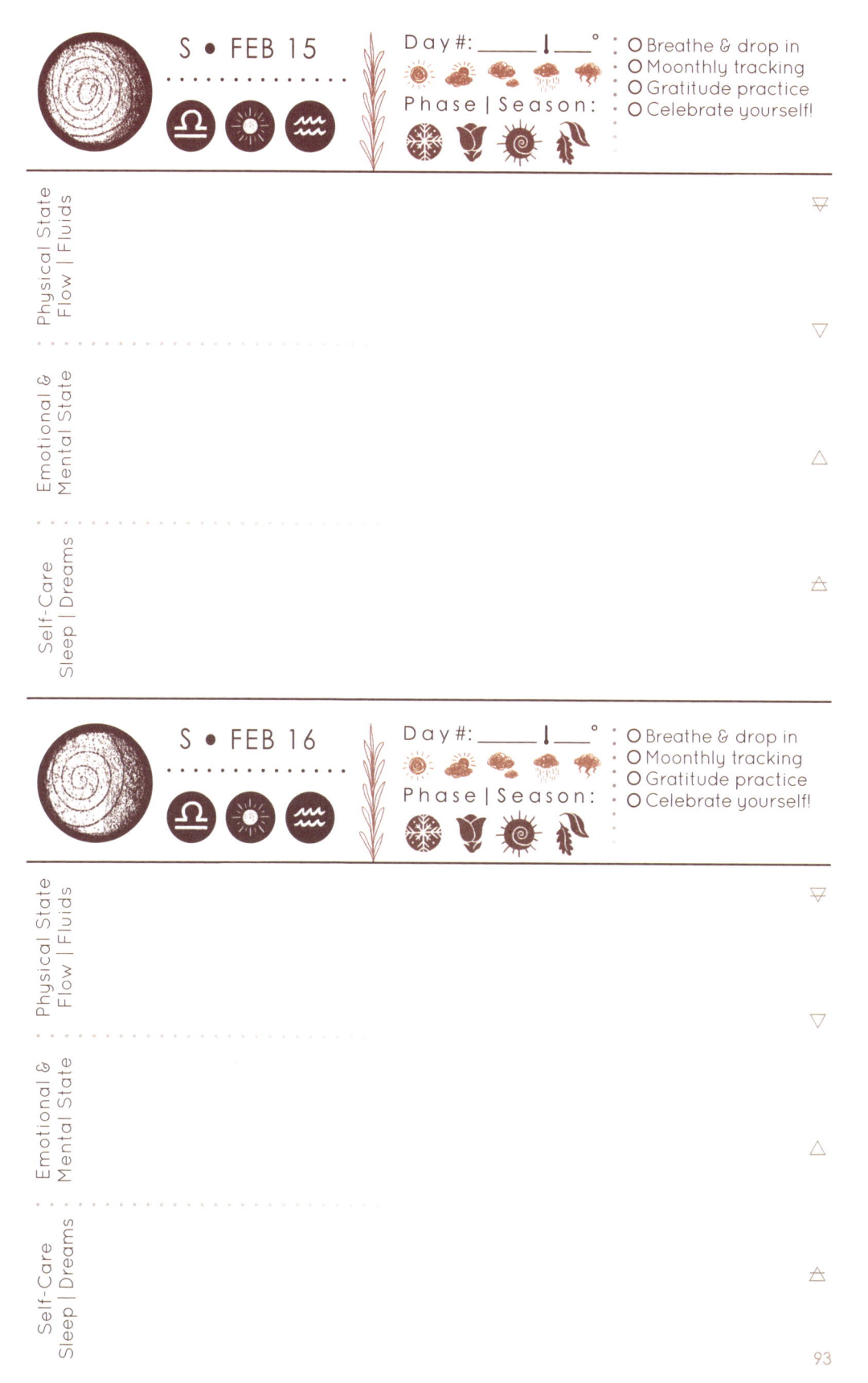

Day #: _____ | _____°

Phase | Season:

- ○ Breathe & drop in
- ○ Moonthly tracking
- ○ Gratitude practice
- ○ Celebrate yourself!

Physical State
Flow | Fluids

Emotional &
Mental State

Self-Care
Sleep | Dreams

S • FEB 16

Day #: _____ | _____°

Phase | Season:

- ○ Breathe & drop in
- ○ Moonthly tracking
- ○ Gratitude practice
- ○ Celebrate yourself!

Physical State
Flow | Fluids

Emotional &
Mental State

Self-Care
Sleep | Dreams

M • FEB 17

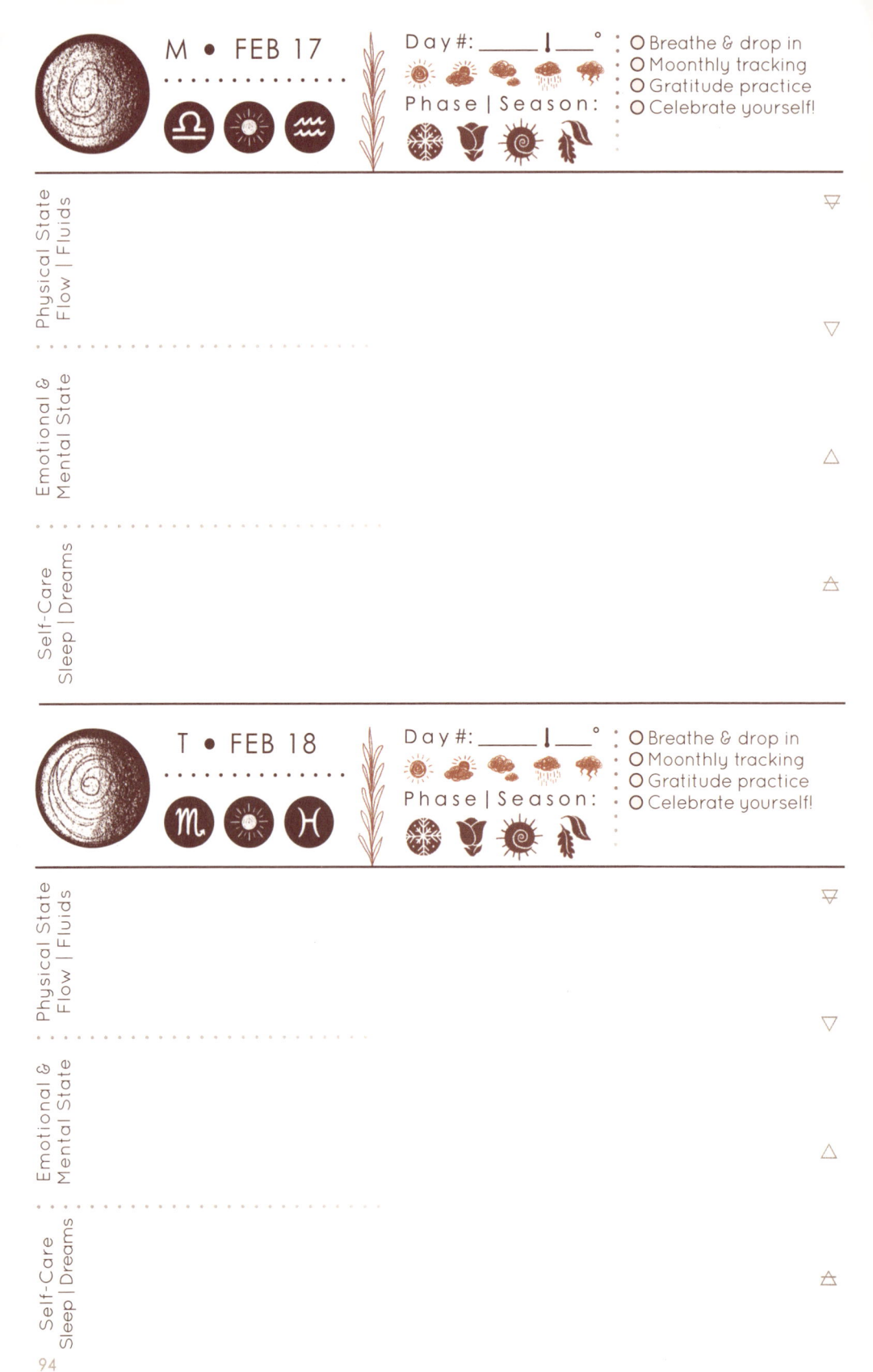

Day #: _____ | _____°

Phase | Season:

O Breathe & drop in
O Moonthly tracking
O Gratitude practice
O Celebrate yourself!

Physical State
Flow | Fluids

Emotional &
Mental State

Self-Care
Sleep | Dreams

T • FEB 18

Day #: _____ | _____°

Phase | Season:

O Breathe & drop in
O Moonthly tracking
O Gratitude practice
O Celebrate yourself!

Physical State
Flow | Fluids

Emotional &
Mental State

Self-Care
Sleep | Dreams

W • FEB 19

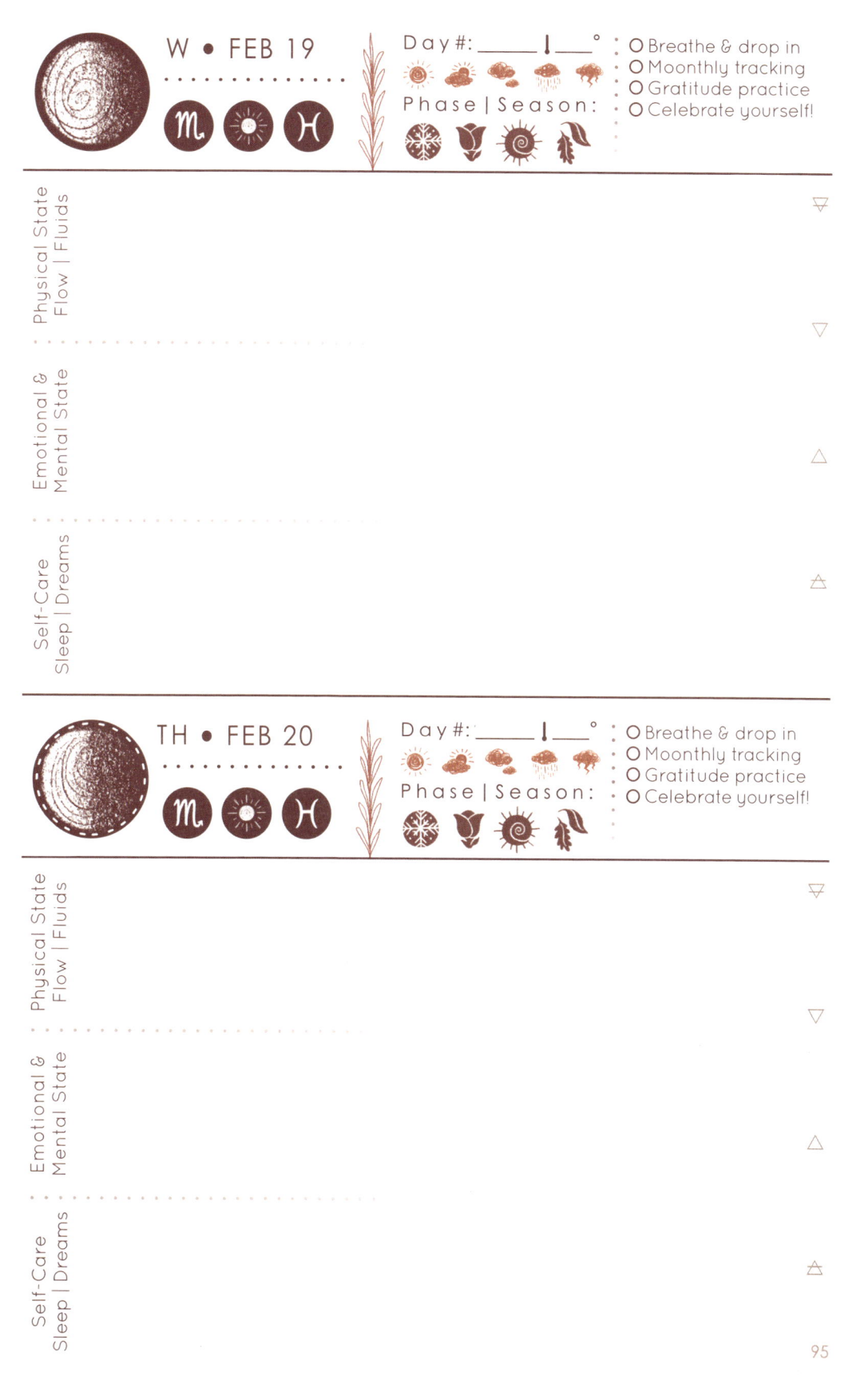

♏ ☉ ♓

Day #: _____ | _____°

Phase | Season:

- ◯ Breathe & drop in
- ◯ Moonthly tracking
- ◯ Gratitude practice
- ◯ Celebrate yourself!

Physical State / Flow | Fluids

Emotional & Mental State

Self-Care / Sleep | Dreams

TH • FEB 20

♏ ☉ ♓

Day #: _____ | _____°

Phase | Season:

- ◯ Breathe & drop in
- ◯ Moonthly tracking
- ◯ Gratitude practice
- ◯ Celebrate yourself!

Physical State / Flow | Fluids

Emotional & Mental State

Self-Care / Sleep | Dreams

95

LAST QUARTER IN SCORPIO

Instinctually clearing space to tune into subconscious desires

What am I leaving behind this lunar cycle?

Where can I make more space for reflection &/or integration?

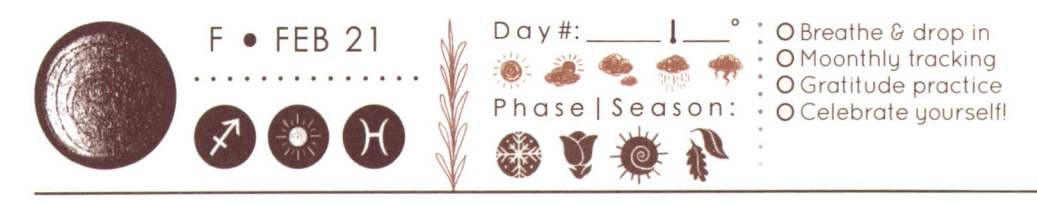

F • FEB 21

Day #: _____ | _____°

Phase | Season:

- ○ Breathe & drop in
- ○ Moonthly tracking
- ○ Gratitude practice
- ○ Celebrate yourself!

Physical State
Flow | Fluids

Emotional &
Mental State

Self-Care
Sleep | Dreams

96

S • FEB 22

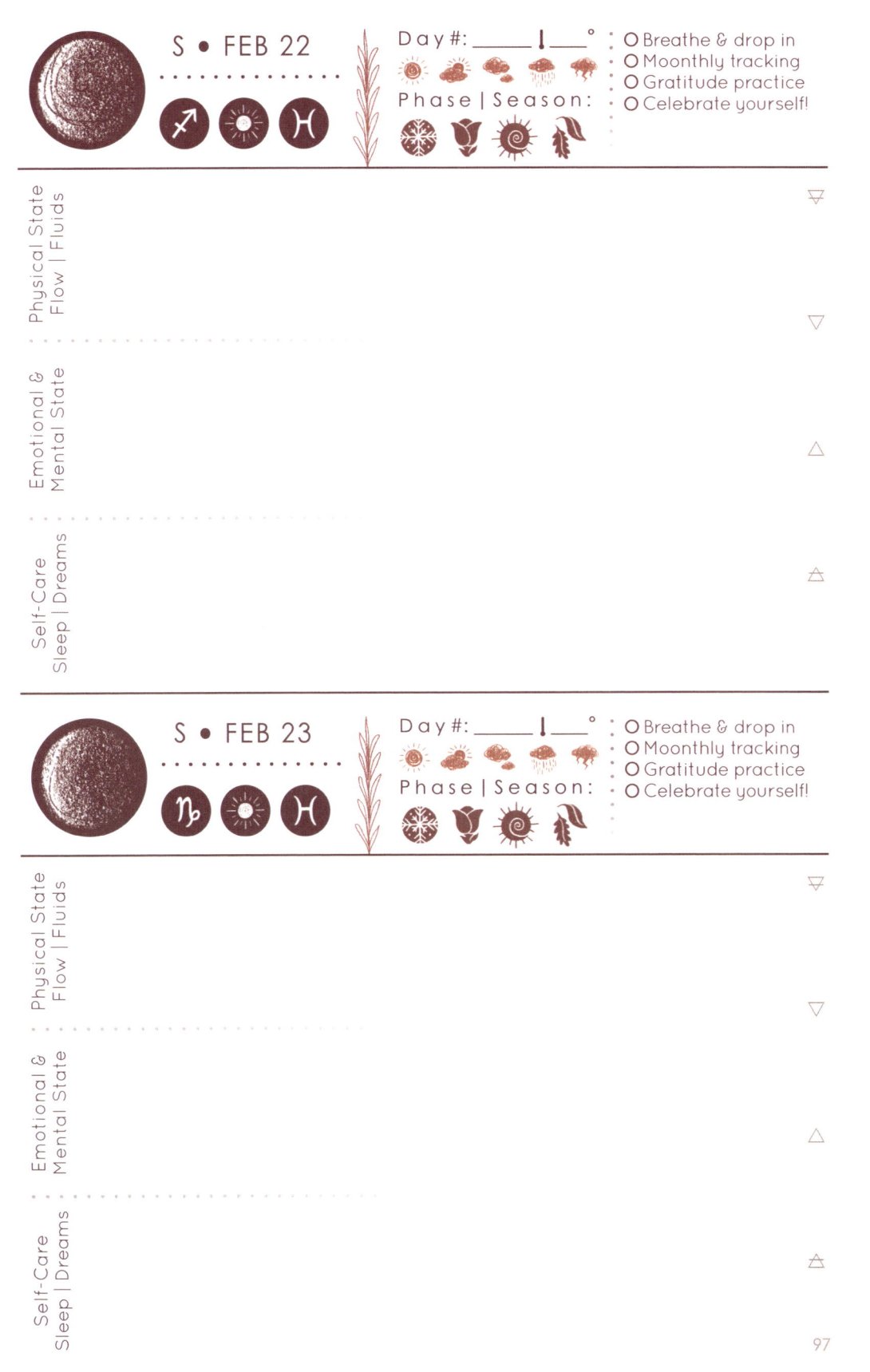

Day #: _____ | _____°

Phase | Season:

- ○ Breathe & drop in
- ○ Moonthly tracking
- ○ Gratitude practice
- ○ Celebrate yourself!

Physical State / Flow | Fluids

Emotional & Mental State

Self-Care / Sleep | Dreams

S • FEB 23

Day #: _____ | _____°

Phase | Season:

- ○ Breathe & drop in
- ○ Moonthly tracking
- ○ Gratitude practice
- ○ Celebrate yourself!

Physical State / Flow | Fluids

Emotional & Mental State

Self-Care / Sleep | Dreams

☾ 1st
01 | 29
02 | 26

CHECK IN & REFLECT

Last Cycle Day 1: _____

Last Cycle Length: _____

Use this space to reflect on your experiences & findings from this ending lunar cycle or your last menstrual cycle. Use cycle day #s if you bleed, or moon phases if you don't.

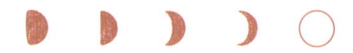

Circle the phase you bled near:

○ ☾ ☾ ☽ ☽ ● ● ☾ ☾ ☽ ☽ ○

Caution Days: (days I needed space)   **Bliss Days:** (days I felt great)

DAYS TO NOTE — Which cycle days stood out?

OBSERVATIONS — Notice any changes or patterns?

SELF-CARE — What was helpful & nourishing?

PLAN & PREPARE

Next Predicted Cycle:
🩸 ☾ _____

CHECKLIST

Add the following to any other planners or calendars for your next cycle, then check it off.

- ☐ Predicted "days to note" _____
- ☐ Days to slow down (pre-bleed) _____
- ☐ Rest day(s) (next bleed) _____
- ☐ Date with yourself _____
- ☐ _____

- ☐ Self chest/breast exam
- ☐ Meal plan with cycle
- ☐ _____
- ☐ _____
- ☐ _____

OPEN SPACE

Use this space how you wish, or print out one of our free templates to paste here for BBT charting, dream tracking, or something else:

Befriend Your Grief

by Marshall K Hammer (she/her) of Reiki for Today • Interspiritual Minister, Animal Reiki Practitioner • @reikifortoday • reikifortoday.com •

Grieving is a profound experience, yet modern society rushes us to "get over it" before we can fully process. Many employers don't allow time off for bereavement. We're expected to continue working as if nothing has changed.

Unexpected or sudden, traumatic loss is extra sticky. We struggle to relate with our loved ones who mean well but don't get it. We feel others' pressure to be over it, to be like we were before or to be, well, different than we are.

The truth is...loss changes us. And shouldn't it?

Grief has its own non-linear timeline. Grief needs space to breathe. Grief needs our presence, gentleness and care, just like other tender parts of us do.

Imagine you've invited your grief over for a cup of tea.

What questions would you ask?
Check what resonates and write your own.

- Why did this happen?

- What am I feeling guilty about?

- Will I ever feel like myself again?

- How can I grow from this loss?

- How can I best honor their memory?

Breathe, feel your feet on the ground, wiggle your toes.
Notice what feels alive in your body.

Ask yourself:
How can I thank myself for taking this time to sit with my grief?
How can I thank my grief for taking this time to sit with me?

By inviting grief in, asking questions, and allowing expression of those intense and uncomfortable emotions, we nurture our capacity to embody our process. We increase our inner resourcing and emotional fluency. Befriending grief is how we metabolize loss and begin to show up for our changed, enduring self.

Phasic Overview & In-Betweens

Use this space to focus on the phases of the moonth and the in-betweens of the peak lunations.

One way of using this space is to designate one column for your goal-planning, intention-setting or focus per phase/week. Use the other column for reflections, dream themes, nutrition tracking, cards pulls, etc!

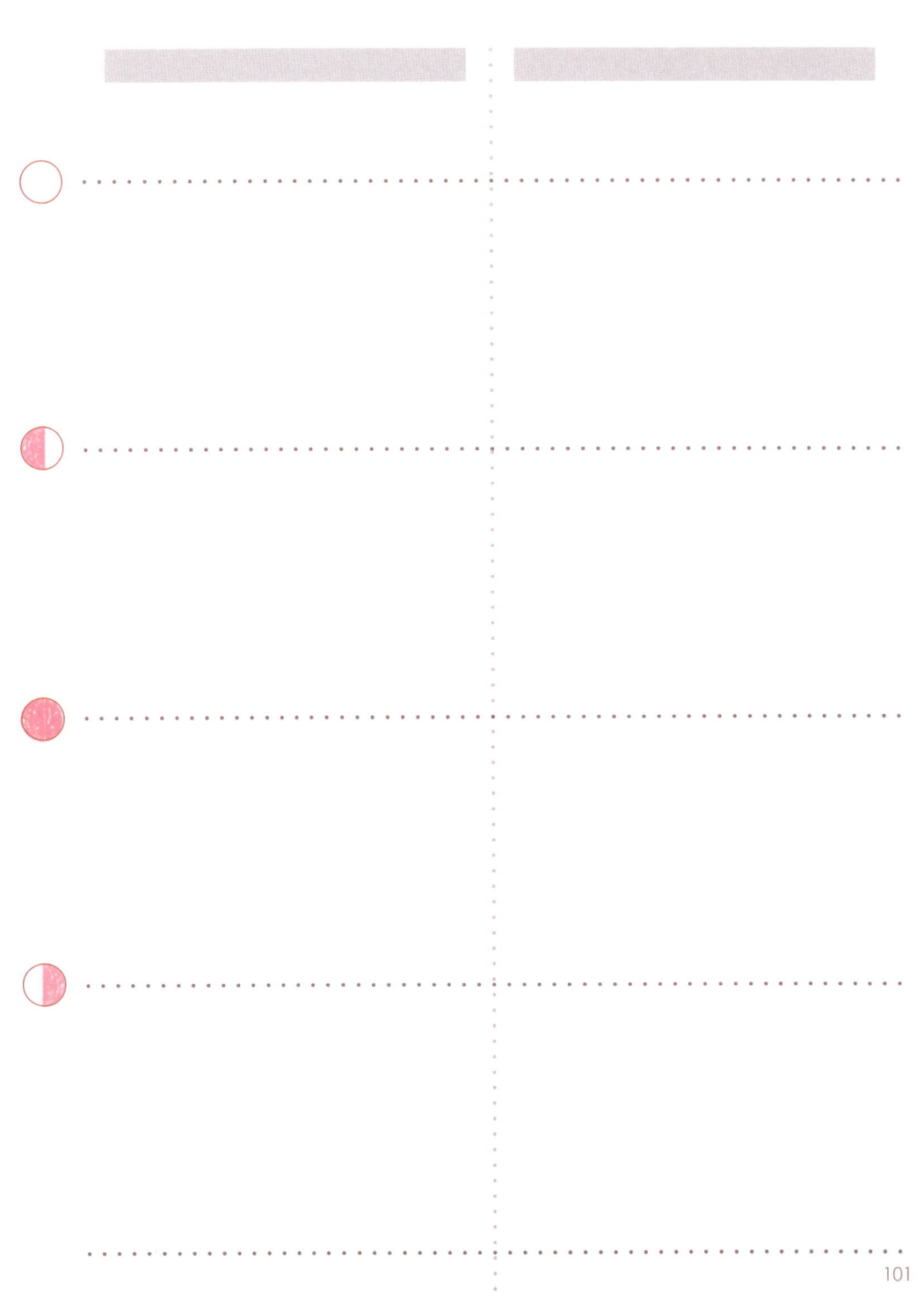

M • FEB 24

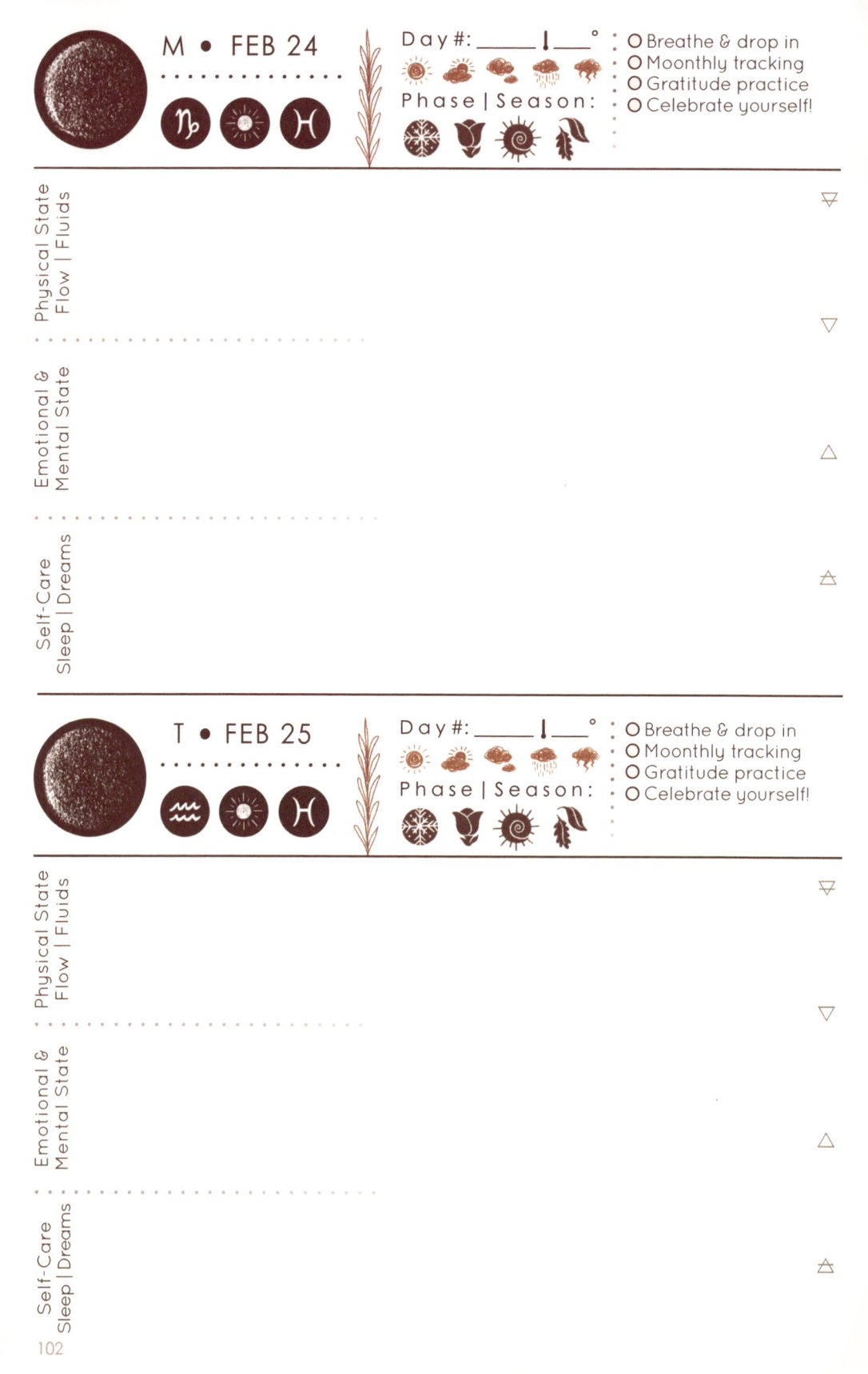

Day #: _____ | _____°
Phase | Season:

- Breathe & drop in
- Moonthly tracking
- Gratitude practice
- Celebrate yourself!

Physical State / Flow | Fluids

Emotional & Mental State

Self-Care / Sleep | Dreams

T • FEB 25

Day #: _____ | _____°
Phase | Season:

- Breathe & drop in
- Moonthly tracking
- Gratitude practice
- Celebrate yourself!

Physical State / Flow | Fluids

Emotional & Mental State

Self-Care / Sleep | Dreams

W • FEB 26

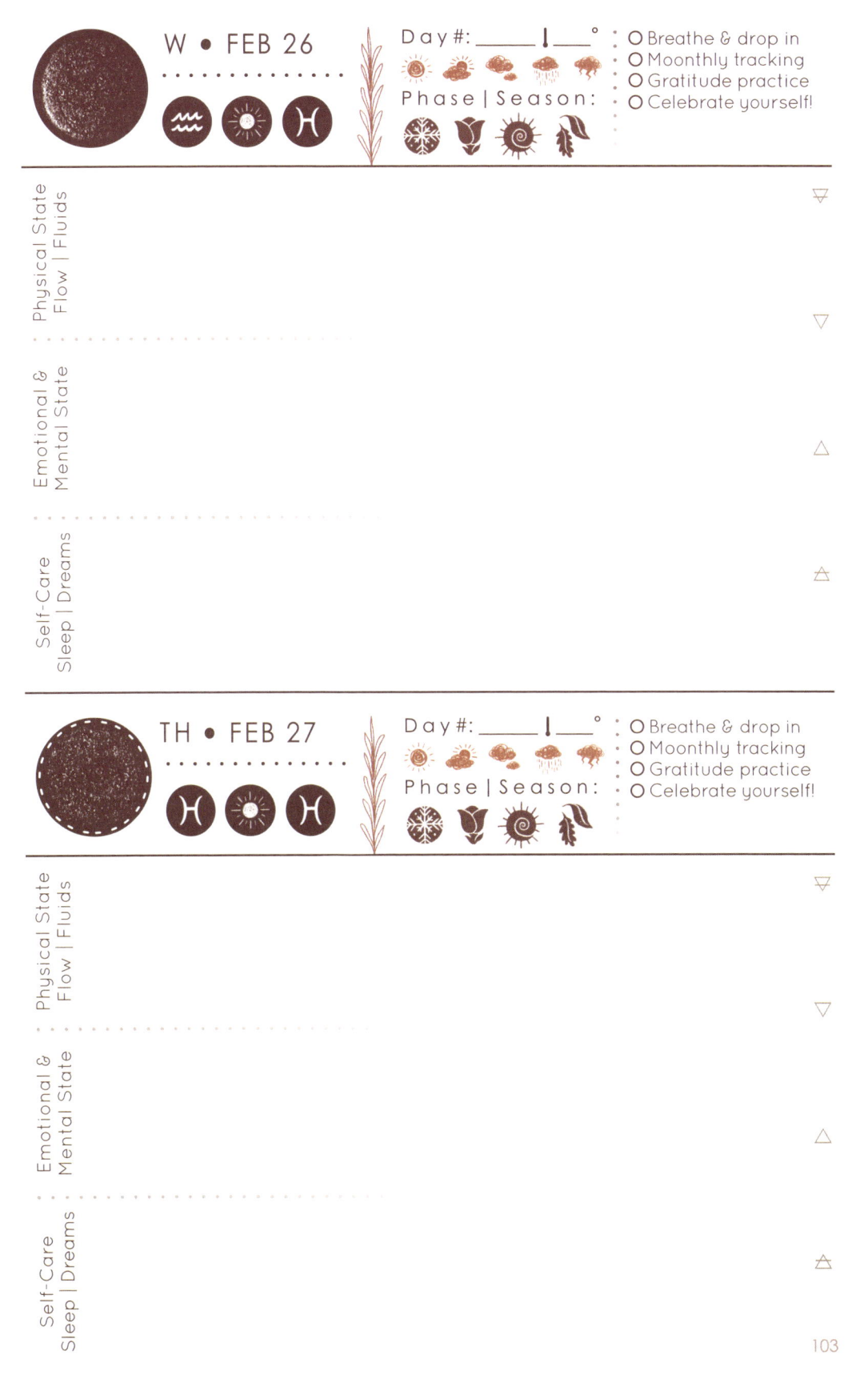

Day #: _____ | _____°

Phase | Season:

- ○ Breathe & drop in
- ○ Moonthly tracking
- ○ Gratitude practice
- ○ Celebrate yourself!

Physical State
Flow | Fluids

Emotional & Mental State

Self-Care
Sleep | Dreams

TH • FEB 27

Day #: _____ | _____°

Phase | Season:

- ○ Breathe & drop in
- ○ Moonthly tracking
- ○ Gratitude practice
- ○ Celebrate yourself!

Physical State
Flow | Fluids

Emotional & Mental State

Self-Care
Sleep | Dreams

NEW MOON IN PISCES

Opening up to new possibilities of inspiration & purpose

What do I want to grow & focus on during this lunar cycle?

How will I hold space for this?

F • FEB 28

Day #: _____ | _____°

Phase | Season:

- ○ Breathe & drop in
- ○ Moonthly tracking
- ○ Gratitude practice
- ○ Celebrate yourself!

Physical State / Flow | Fluids

Emotional & Mental State

Self-Care / Sleep | Dreams

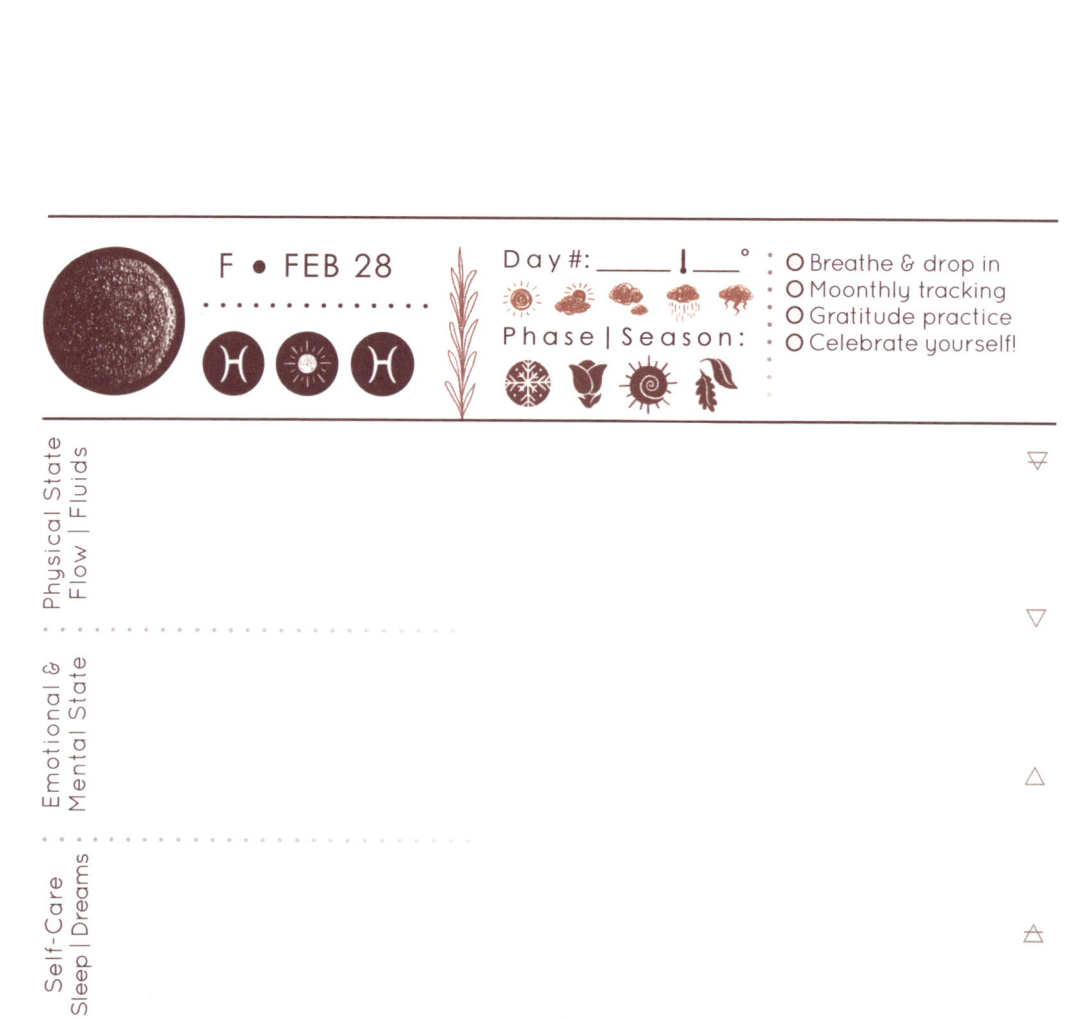

S • MAR 1

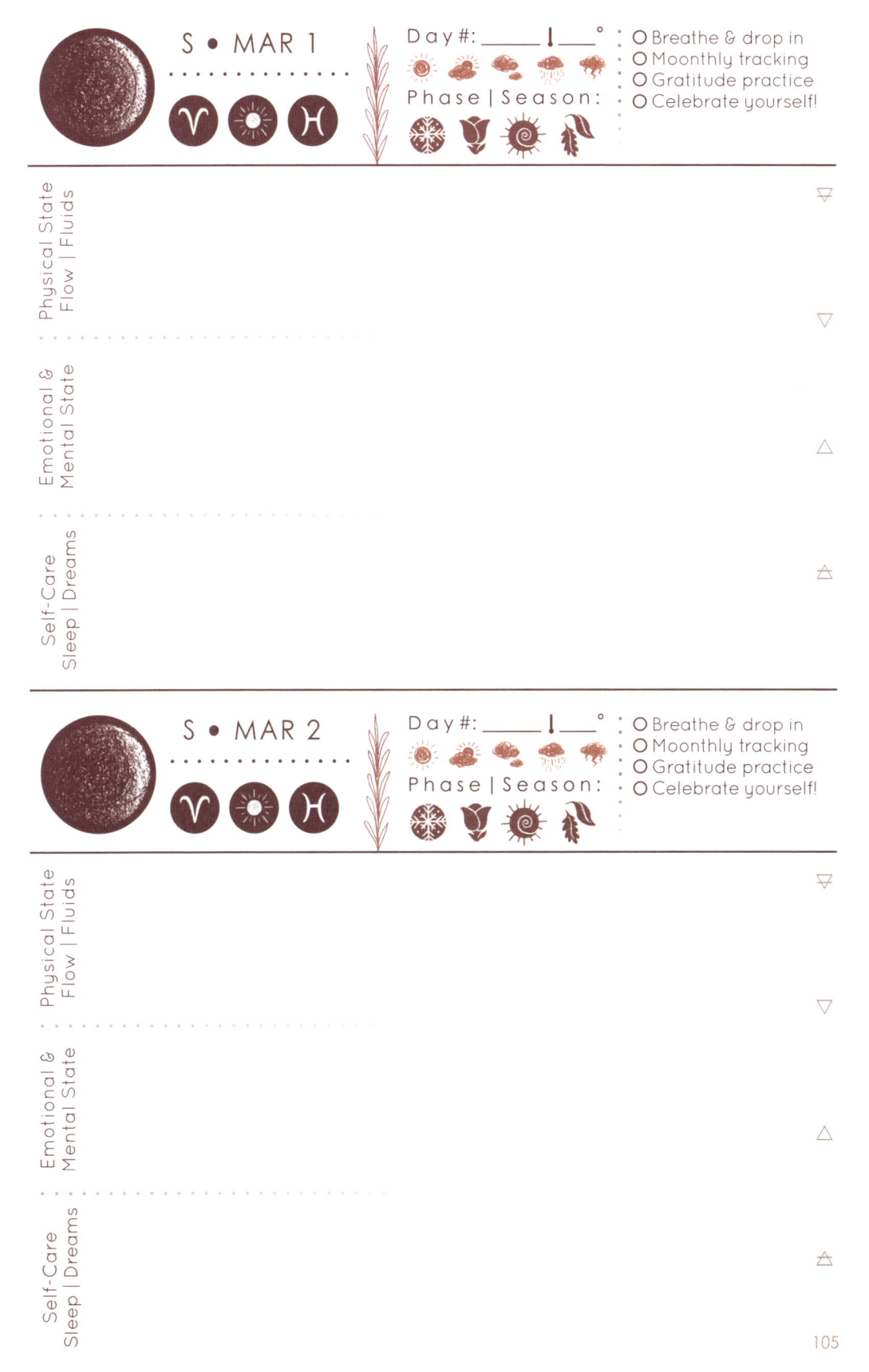

Day #: _____ | _____°
Phase | Season:

- ○ Breathe & drop in
- ○ Moonthly tracking
- ○ Gratitude practice
- ○ Celebrate yourself!

Physical State
Flow | Fluids

Emotional &
Mental State

Self-Care
Sleep | Dreams

S • MAR 2

Day #: _____ | _____°
Phase | Season:

- ○ Breathe & drop in
- ○ Moonthly tracking
- ○ Gratitude practice
- ○ Celebrate yourself!

Physical State
Flow | Fluids

Emotional &
Mental State

Self-Care
Sleep | Dreams

M • MAR 3

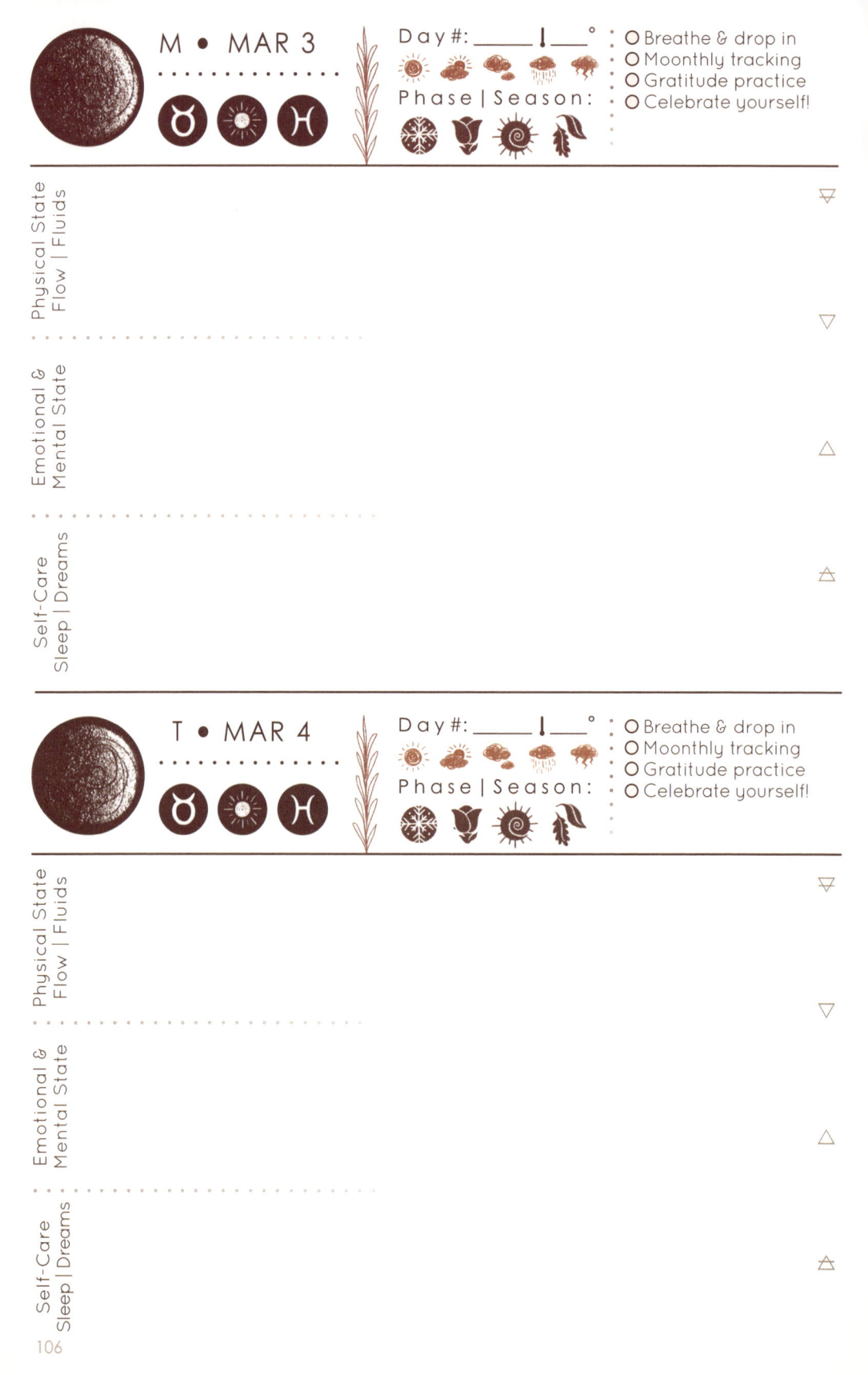

Day #: _____ | _____°

Phase | Season:

- Breathe & drop in
- Moonthly tracking
- Gratitude practice
- Celebrate yourself!

Physical State
Flow | Fluids

Emotional & Mental State

Self-Care
Sleep | Dreams

T • MAR 4

Day #: _____ | _____°

Phase | Season:

- Breathe & drop in
- Moonthly tracking
- Gratitude practice
- Celebrate yourself!

Physical State
Flow | Fluids

Emotional & Mental State

Self-Care
Sleep | Dreams

W • MAR 5

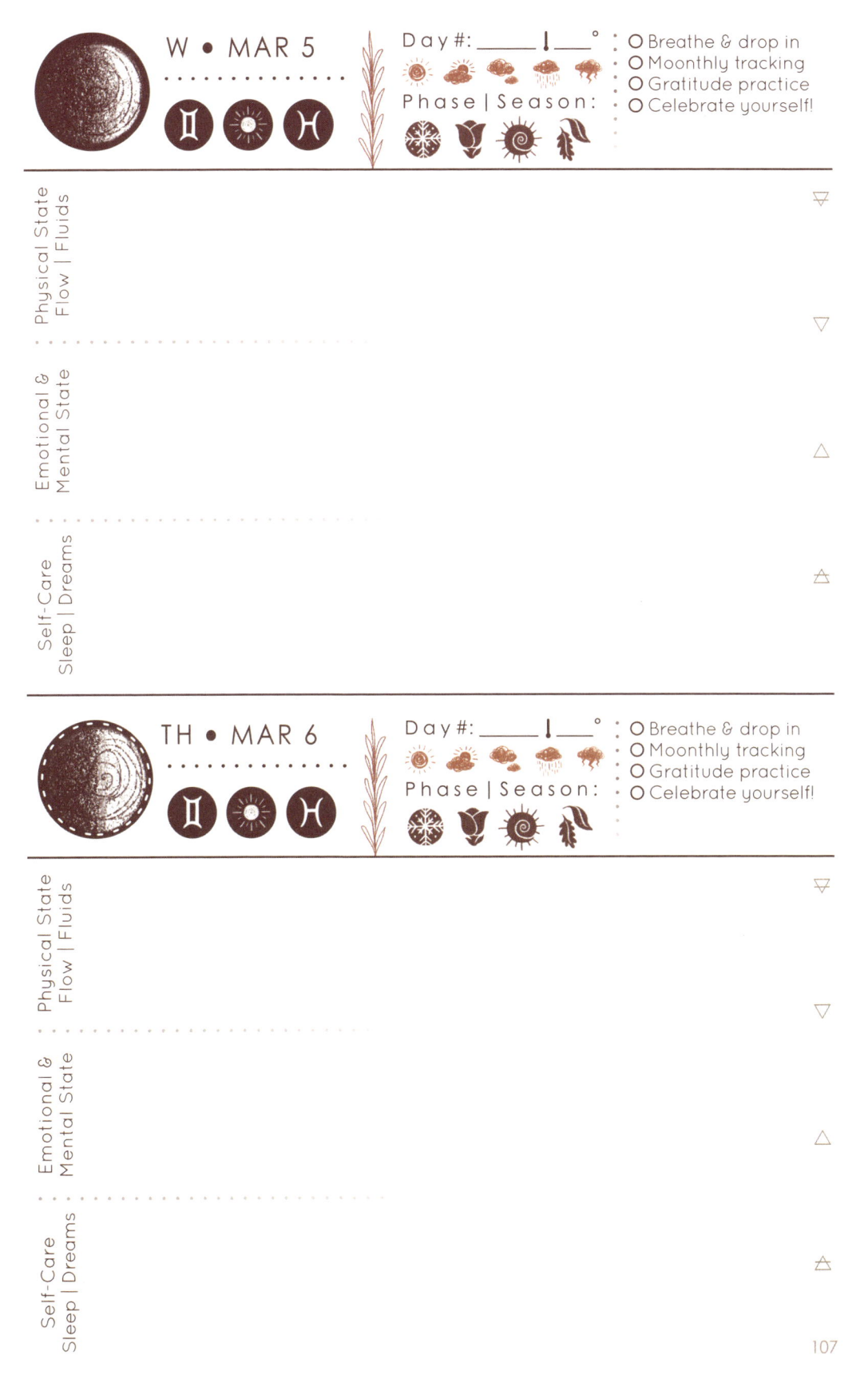

Day #: _____ | _____°

Phase | Season:

- ○ Breathe & drop in
- ○ Moonthly tracking
- ○ Gratitude practice
- ○ Celebrate yourself!

Physical State / Flow | Fluids

Emotional & Mental State

Self-Care / Sleep | Dreams

TH • MAR 6

Day #: _____ | _____°

Phase | Season:

- ○ Breathe & drop in
- ○ Moonthly tracking
- ○ Gratitude practice
- ○ Celebrate yourself!

Physical State / Flow | Fluids

Emotional & Mental State

Self-Care / Sleep | Dreams

FIRST QUARTER IN GEMINI

A growing awareness of intentional ideation

What is sprouting & coming into awareness?

What can I release to make space for further growth & grounding?

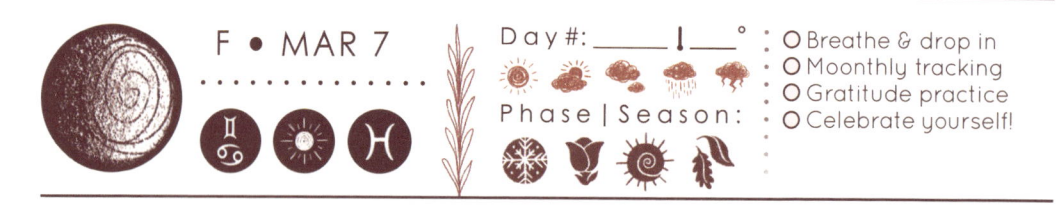

F • MAR 7

Day #: _____ | _____°

Phase | Season:

○ Breathe & drop in
○ Moonthly tracking
○ Gratitude practice
○ Celebrate yourself!

Physical State
Flow | Fluids

Emotional &
Mental State

Self-Care
Sleep | Dreams

108

S • MAR 8

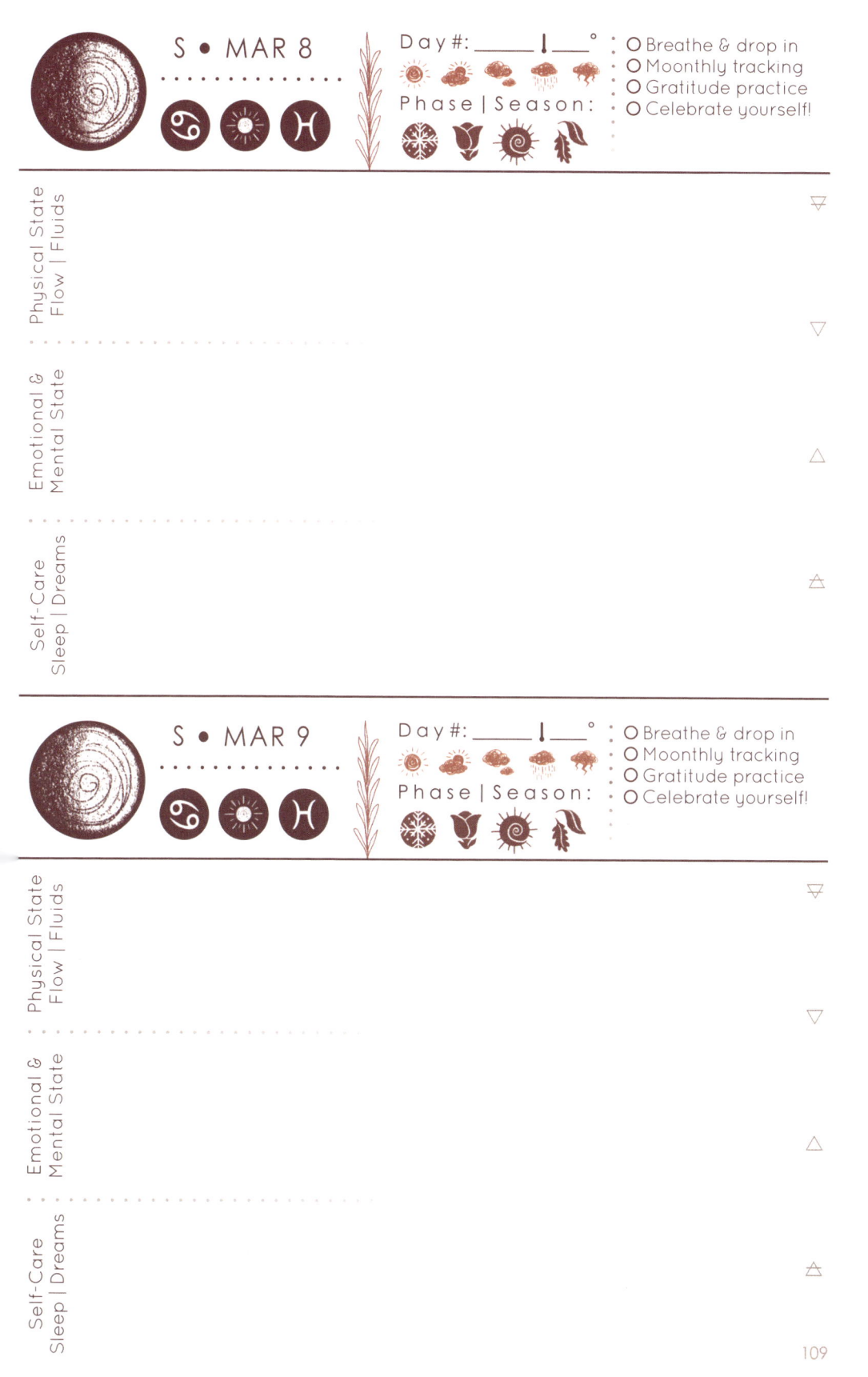

Day #: _____ | _____°

Phase | Season:

- ○ Breathe & drop in
- ○ Moonthly tracking
- ○ Gratitude practice
- ○ Celebrate yourself!

Physical State / Flow | Fluids

Emotional & Mental State

Self-Care / Sleep | Dreams

S • MAR 9

Day #: _____ | _____°

Phase | Season:

- ○ Breathe & drop in
- ○ Moonthly tracking
- ○ Gratitude practice
- ○ Celebrate yourself!

Physical State / Flow | Fluids

Emotional & Mental State

Self-Care / Sleep | Dreams

M • MAR 10

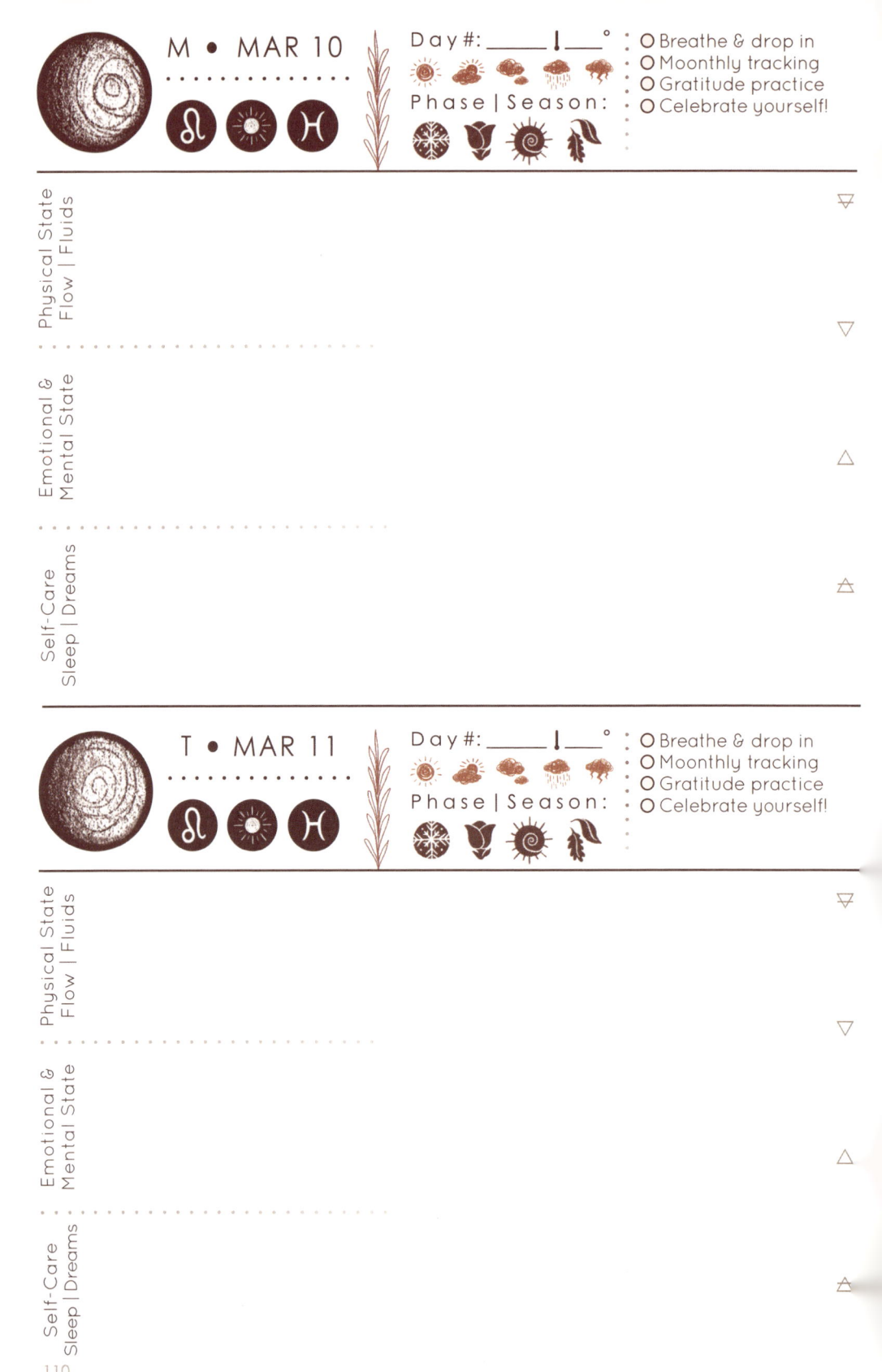

♌ ☉ ♓

Day #: _____ | _____°

Phase | Season:

- ○ Breathe & drop in
- ○ Moonthly tracking
- ○ Gratitude practice
- ○ Celebrate yourself!

Physical State / Flow | Fluids

Emotional & Mental State

Self-Care / Sleep | Dreams

T • MAR 11

♌ ☉ ♓

Day #: _____ | _____°

Phase | Season:

- ○ Breathe & drop in
- ○ Moonthly tracking
- ○ Gratitude practice
- ○ Celebrate yourself!

Physical State / Flow | Fluids

Emotional & Mental State

Self-Care / Sleep | Dreams

W • MAR 12

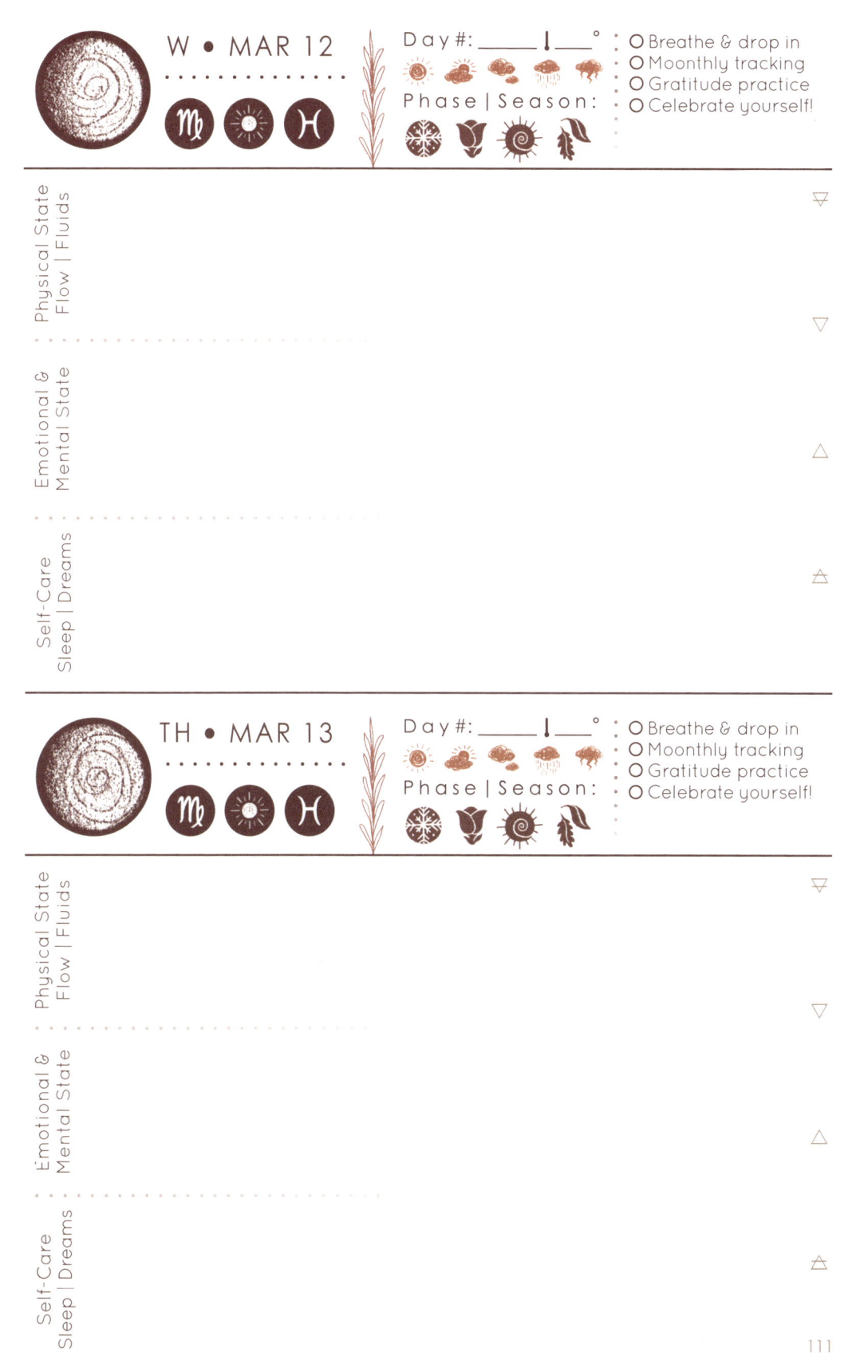

♍ ☉ ♓

Day #: _____ | _____°

Phase | Season:

- ○ Breathe & drop in
- ○ Moonthly tracking
- ○ Gratitude practice
- ○ Celebrate yourself!

Physical State
Flow | Fluids

Emotional &
Mental State

Self-Care
Sleep | Dreams

TH • MAR 13

♍ ☉ ♓

Day #: _____ | _____°

Phase | Season:

- ○ Breathe & drop in
- ○ Moonthly tracking
- ○ Gratitude practice
- ○ Celebrate yourself!

Physical State
Flow | Fluids

Emotional &
Mental State

Self-Care
Sleep | Dreams

F • MAR 14

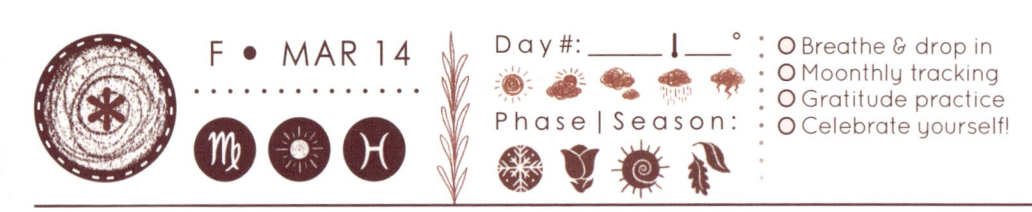

Day #: _____ | _____°

Phase | Season:

- Breathe & drop in
- Moonthly tracking
- Gratitude practice
- Celebrate yourself!

Physical State / Flow | Fluids

Emotional & Mental State

Self-Care / Sleep | Dreams

FULL MOON LUNAR ECLIPSE IN VIRGO

A call towards more reflection in the realm of inner consciousness

What is being illuminated?

I give gratitude for what is & what is becoming:

W • MAR 12

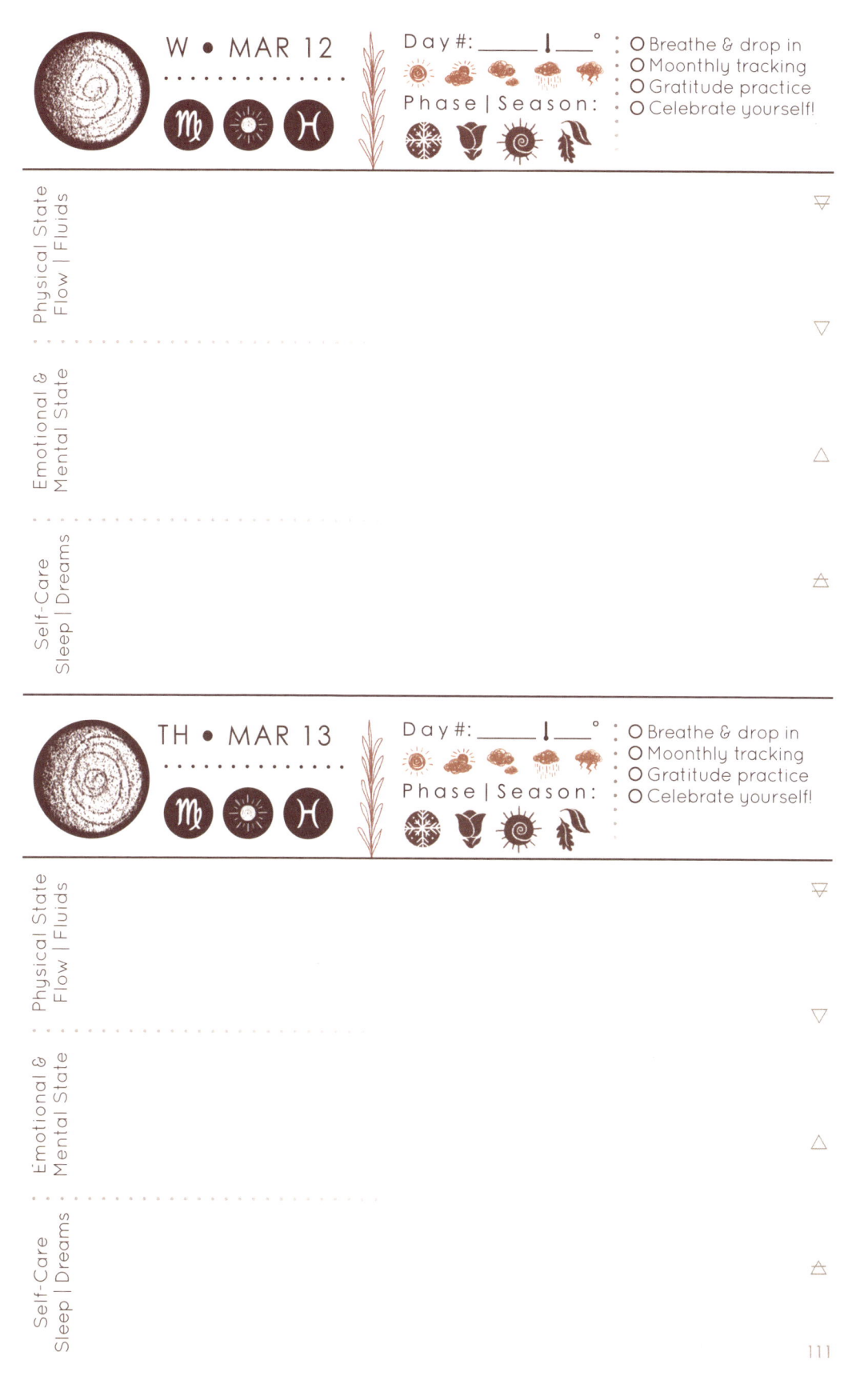

♍ ☀ ♓

Day #: _____ | _____°

Phase | Season:

- Breathe & drop in
- Moonthly tracking
- Gratitude practice
- Celebrate yourself!

Physical State
Flow | Fluids

Emotional & Mental State

Self-Care
Sleep | Dreams

TH • MAR 13

♍ ☀ ♓

Day #: _____ | _____°

Phase | Season:

- Breathe & drop in
- Moonthly tracking
- Gratitude practice
- Celebrate yourself!

Physical State
Flow | Fluids

Emotional & Mental State

Self-Care
Sleep | Dreams

F • MAR 14

Day #: _____ | _____°

Phase | Season:

- ○ Breathe & drop in
- ○ Moonthly tracking
- ○ Gratitude practice
- ○ Celebrate yourself!

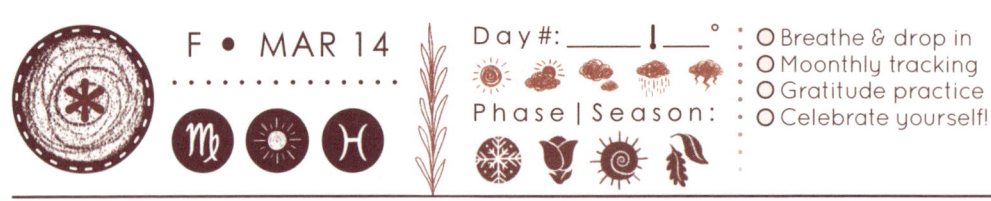

Physical State
Flow | Fluids

Emotional & Mental State

Self-Care
Sleep | Dreams

FULL MOON LUNAR ECLIPSE IN VIRGO

A call towards more reflection in the realm of inner consciousness

---

What is being illuminated?

I give gratitude for what is & what is becoming:

S • MAR 15

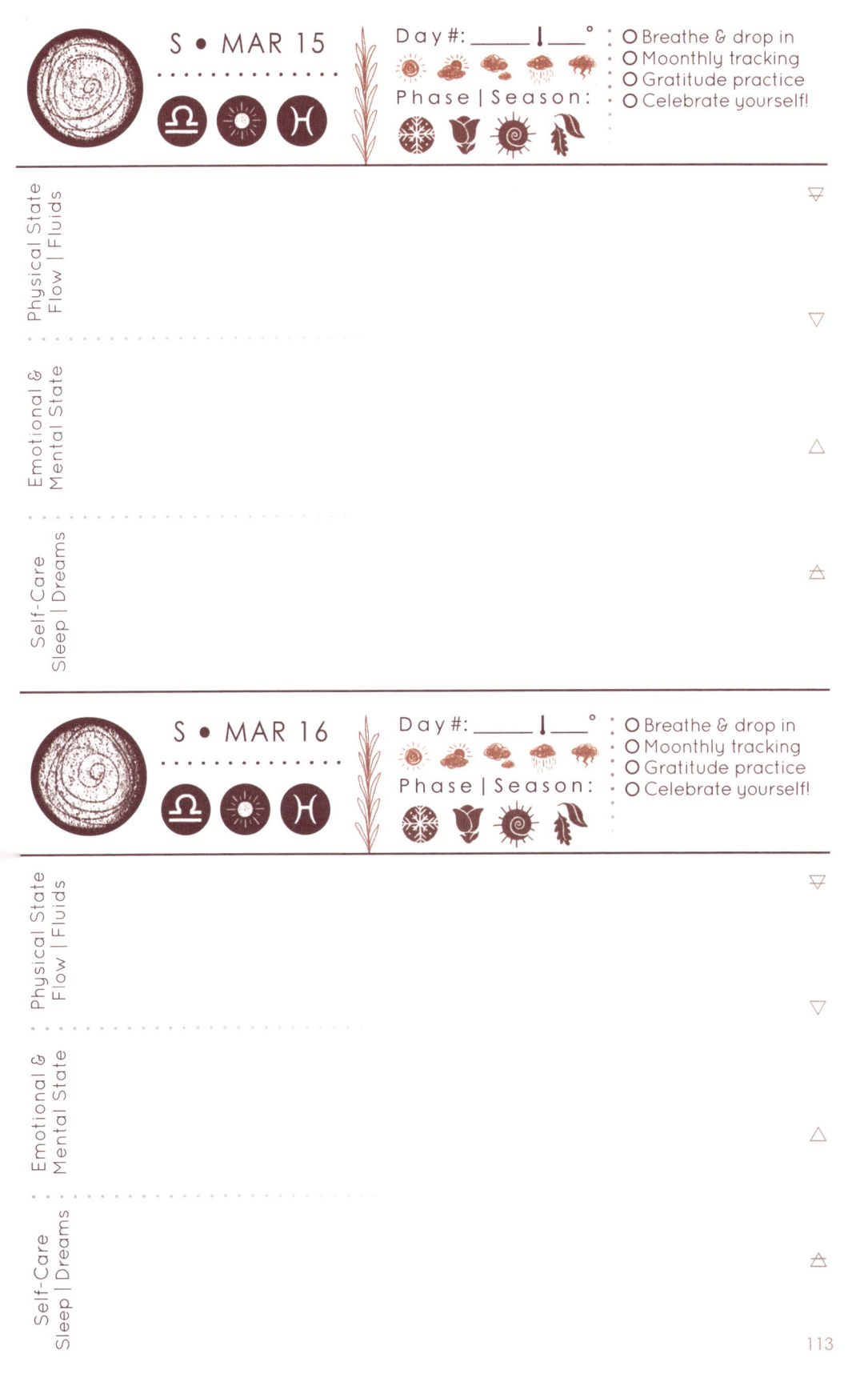

Day #: _____ | _____°

Phase | Season:

- ○ Breathe & drop in
- ○ Moonthly tracking
- ○ Gratitude practice
- ○ Celebrate yourself!

Physical State / Flow | Fluids

Emotional & Mental State

Self-Care / Sleep | Dreams

S • MAR 16

Day #: _____ | _____°

Phase | Season:

- ○ Breathe & drop in
- ○ Moonthly tracking
- ○ Gratitude practice
- ○ Celebrate yourself!

Physical State / Flow | Fluids

Emotional & Mental State

Self-Care / Sleep | Dreams

M • MAR 17

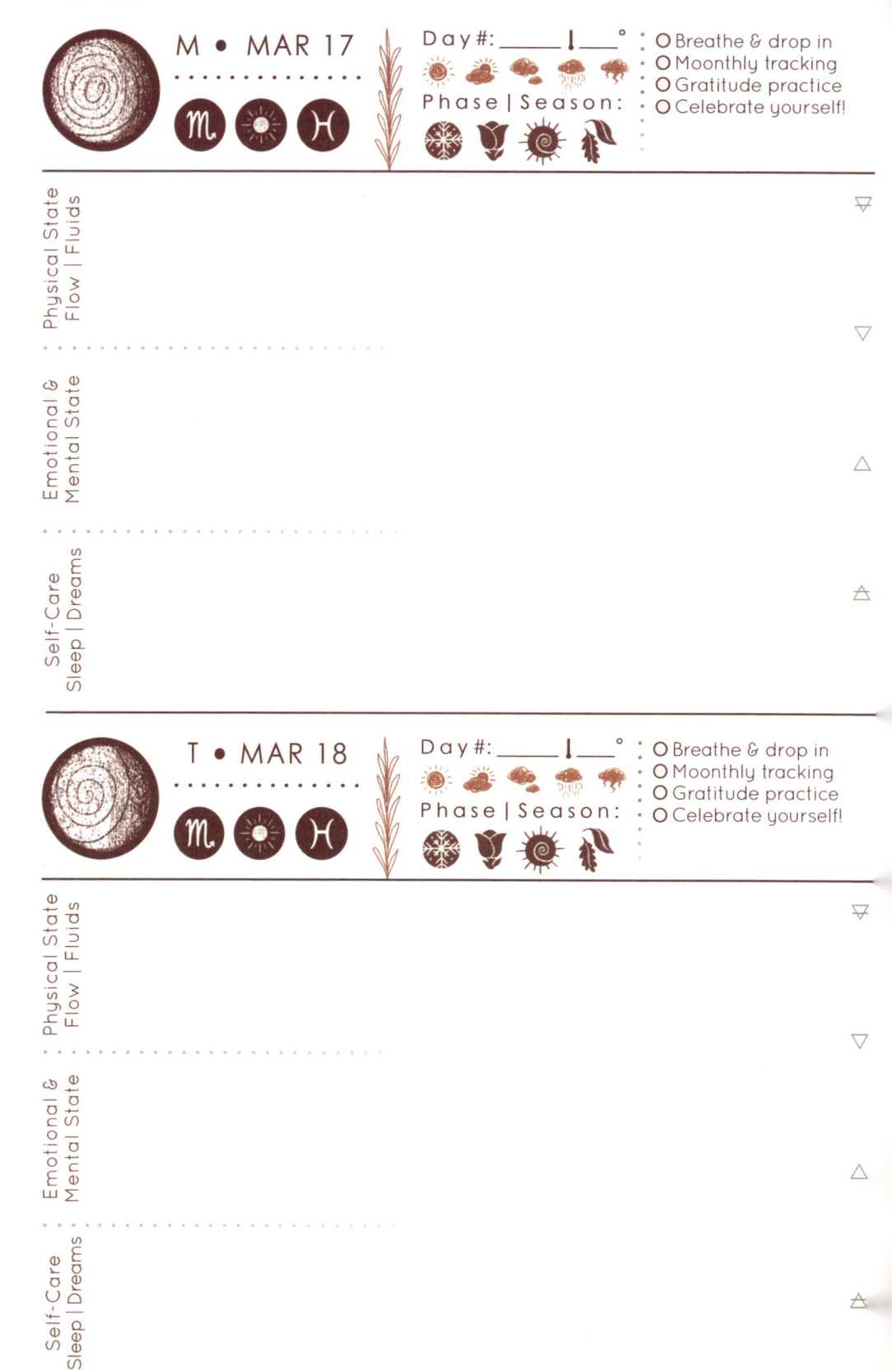

Day #: _____ | _____°

Phase | Season:

- ○ Breathe & drop in
- ○ Moonthly tracking
- ○ Gratitude practice
- ○ Celebrate yourself!

Physical State
Flow | Fluids

Emotional &
Mental State

Self-Care
Sleep | Dreams

T • MAR 18

Day #: _____ | _____°

Phase | Season:

- ○ Breathe & drop in
- ○ Moonthly tracking
- ○ Gratitude practice
- ○ Celebrate yourself!

Physical State
Flow | Fluids

Emotional &
Mental State

Self-Care
Sleep | Dreams

W • MAR 19

Day #: _____ | ____°

Phase | Season:

- O Breathe & drop in
- O Moonthly tracking
- O Gratitude practice
- O Celebrate yourself!

Physical State / Flow | Fluids

Emotional & Mental State

Self-Care / Sleep | Dreams

TH • MAR 20 •• EQUINOX ••

Day #: _____ | ____°

Phase | Season:

- O Breathe & drop in
- O Moonthly tracking
- O Gratitude practice
- O Celebrate yourself!

Physical State / Flow | Fluids

Emotional & Mental State

Self-Care / Sleep | Dreams

F • MAR 21

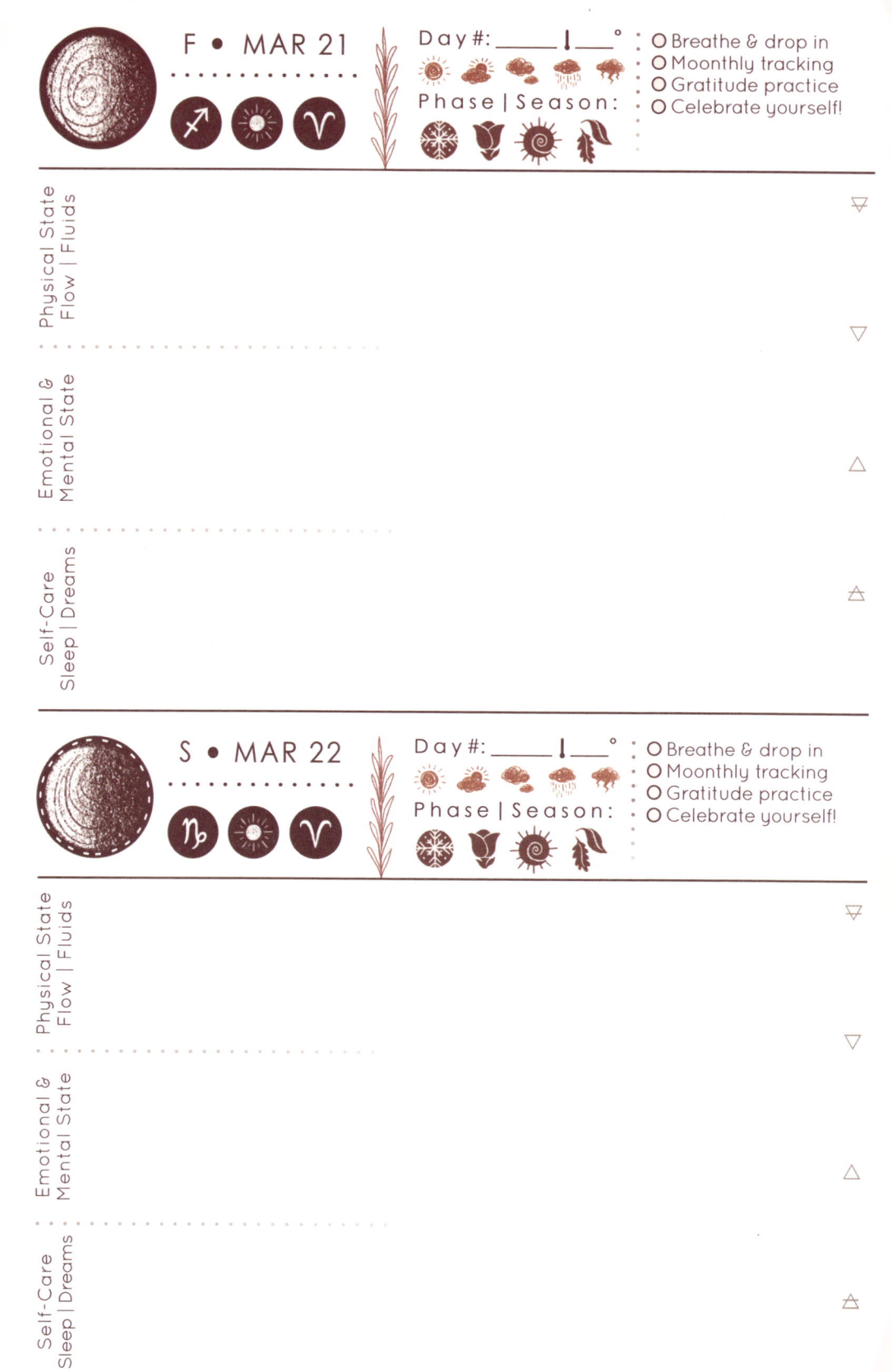

Day #: _____ | _____°

Phase | Season:

- ○ Breathe & drop in
- ○ Moonthly tracking
- ○ Gratitude practice
- ○ Celebrate yourself!

Physical State / Flow | Fluids

Emotional & Mental State

Self-Care / Sleep | Dreams

S • MAR 22

Day #: _____ | _____°

Phase | Season:

- ○ Breathe & drop in
- ○ Moonthly tracking
- ○ Gratitude practice
- ○ Celebrate yourself!

Physical State / Flow | Fluids

Emotional & Mental State

Self-Care / Sleep | Dreams

LAST QUARTER IN CAPRICORN

A deep surrender to dismantling unsupportive structures

What am I leaving behind this lunar cycle?

Where can I make more space for reflection &/or integration?

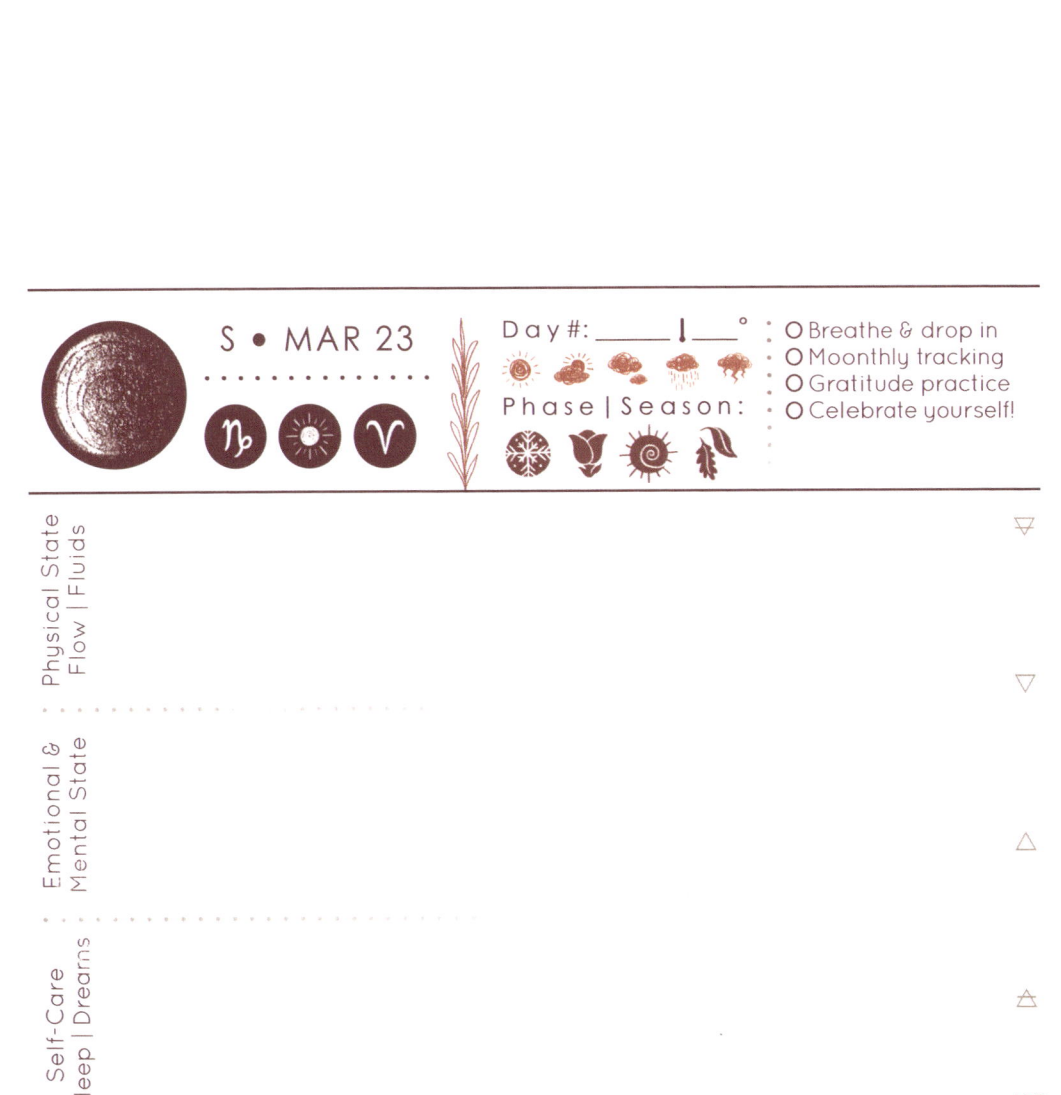

S • MAR 23

Day #: _____ | _____°

Phase | Season:

- ○ Breathe & drop in
- ○ Moonthly tracking
- ○ Gratitude practice
- ○ Celebrate yourself!

Physical State
Flow | Fluids

Emotional &
Mental State

Self-Care
Sleep | Dreams

M • MAR 24

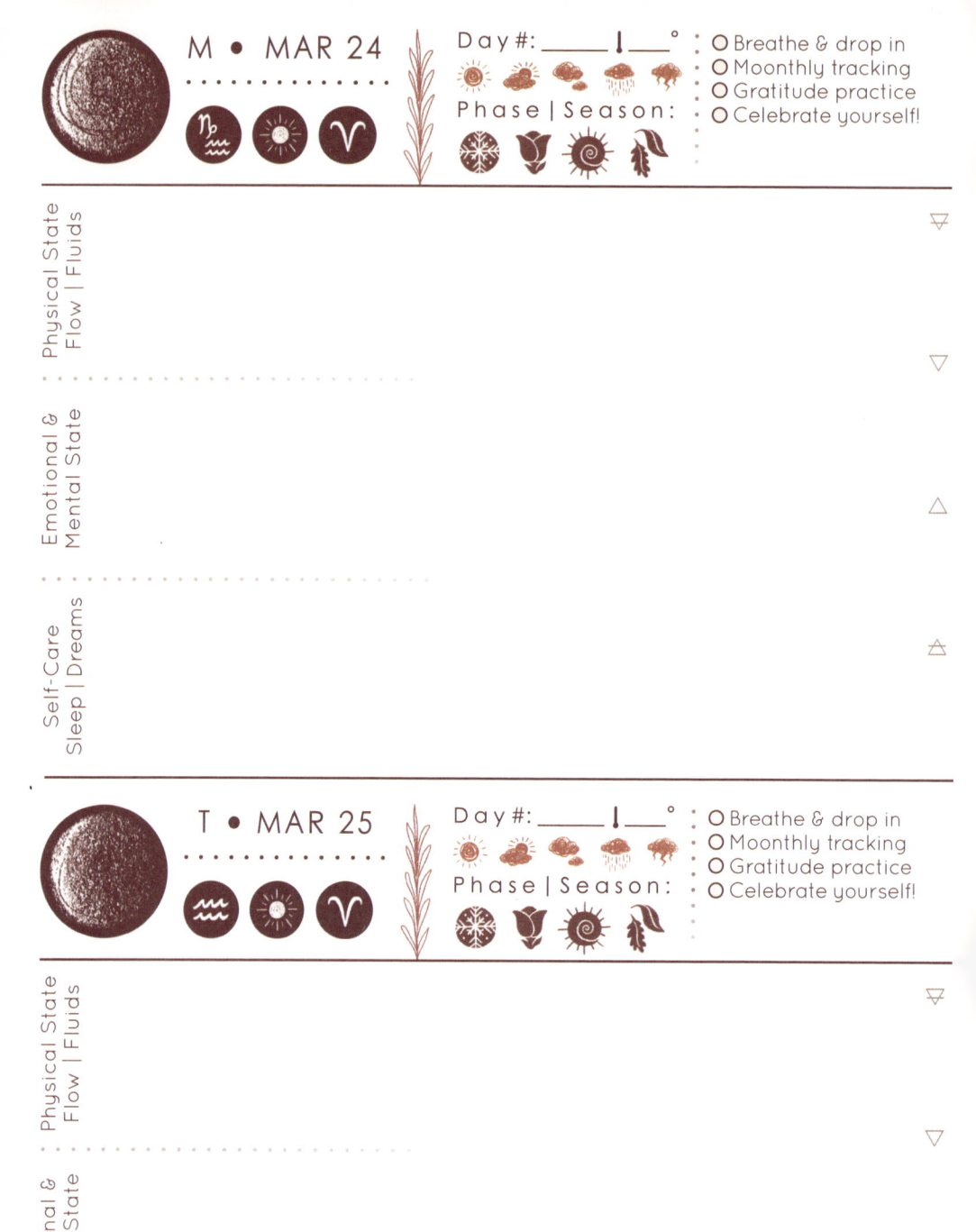

♑ ☀ ♈

Day #: _____ | _____°

Phase | Season:

- ○ Breathe & drop in
- ○ Moonthly tracking
- ○ Gratitude practice
- ○ Celebrate yourself!

Physical State
Flow | Fluids

Emotional & Mental State

Self-Care
Sleep | Dreams

T • MAR 25

♒ ☀ ♈

Day #: _____ | _____°

Phase | Season:

- ○ Breathe & drop in
- ○ Moonthly tracking
- ○ Gratitude practice
- ○ Celebrate yourself!

Physical State
Flow | Fluids

Emotional & Mental State

Self-Care
Sleep | Dreams

W • MAR 26

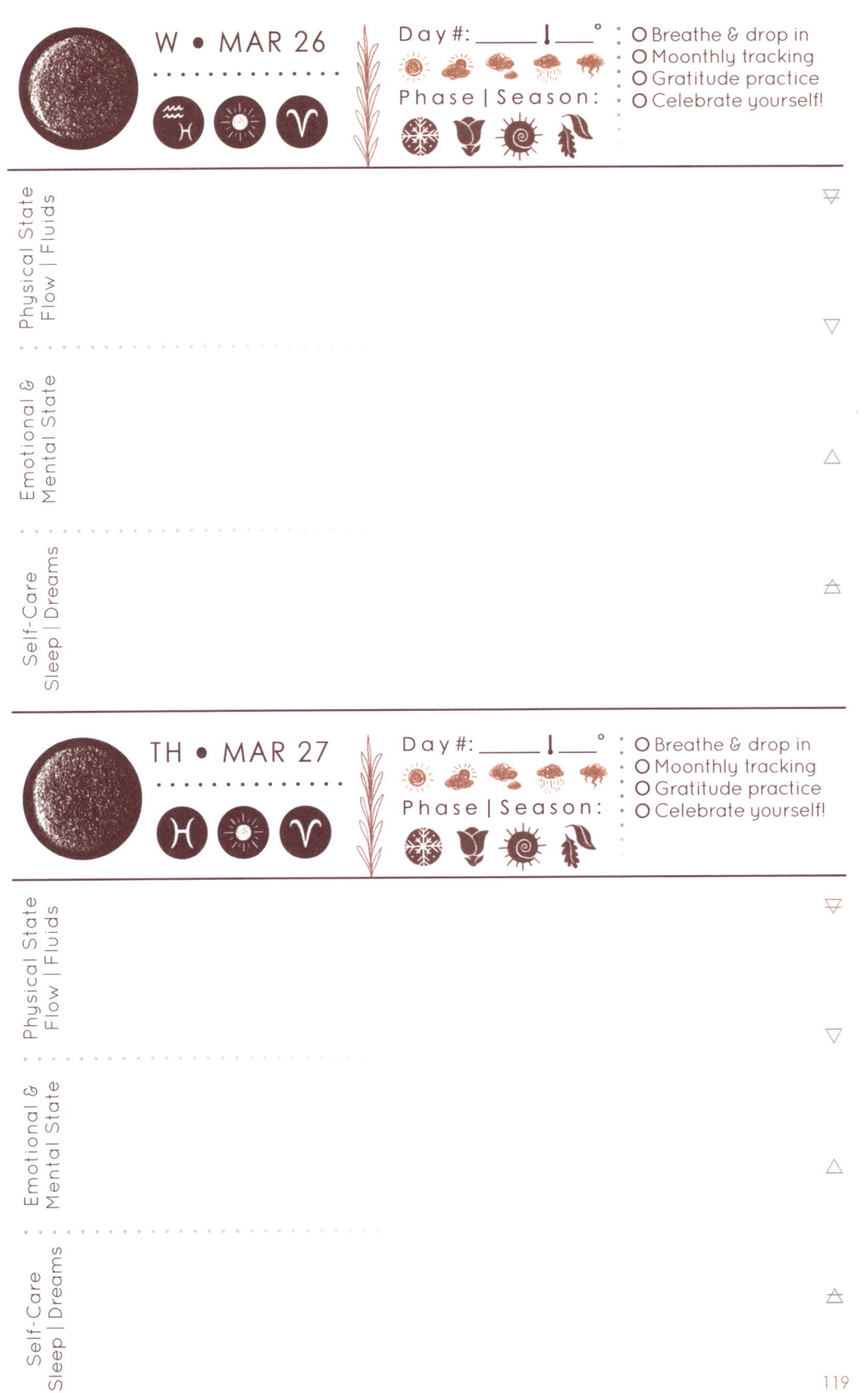

Day #: _____ | ____°

Phase | Season:

- ○ Breathe & drop in
- ○ Moonthly tracking
- ○ Gratitude practice
- ○ Celebrate yourself!

Physical State
Flow | Fluids

Emotional & Mental State

Self-Care
Sleep | Dreams

TH • MAR 27

Day #: _____ | ____°

Phase | Season:

- ○ Breathe & drop in
- ○ Moonthly tracking
- ○ Gratitude practice
- ○ Celebrate yourself!

Physical State
Flow | Fluids

Emotional & Mental State

Self-Care
Sleep | Dreams

CHECK IN & REFLECT

Use this space to reflect on your experiences & findings from this ending lunar cycle or your last menstrual cycle. Use cycle day #s if you bleed, or moon phases if you don't.

Last Cycle Day 1: _____

Last Cycle Length: _____

Circle the phase you bled near:

○ ☾ ☾ ☾ ☾ ● ● ● ☽ ☽ ☽ ○

Caution Days: (days I needed space)

Bliss Days: (days I felt great)

DAYS TO NOTE — Which cycle days stood out?

OBSERVATIONS — Notice any changes or patterns?

SELF-CARE — What was helpful & nourishing?

PLAN & PREPARE

Next Predicted Cycle:
🩸 ☾ _____

CHECKLIST

Add the following to any other planners or calendars for your next cycle, then check it off.

- ☐ Predicted "days to note" _____
- ☐ Days to slow down (pre-bleed) _____
- ☐ Rest day(s) (next bleed) _____
- ☐ Date with yourself _____
- ☐ _____

- ☐ Self chest/breast exam
- ☐ Meal plan with cycle
- ☐ _____
- ☐ _____
- ☐ _____

OPEN SPACE

Use this space how you wish, or print out one of our free templates to paste here for BBT charting, dream tracking, or something else:

Embodied Activism: Radically Rooted Collective Change

by Tamsin Fagan (she/they) of Zami Healing • Embodiment Educator and Womb Practitioner • @zamihealing • zamihealing.com •

Create a sacred space to explore this work, head out into nature or sit by your altar and call in the elements. Start to feel into the prompts below and get creative at each stage; meditate, journal, move, sing, create art or pull cards.

Do this practice all in one or you can sync each prompt with the correlating phase of your menstrual or moon cycle. We start here with luteal as this phase is the most stigmatized, but is the most needed during these times.

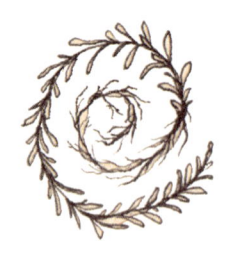

1. **CONNECTION** - Take deep breaths. Inhale to draw up grounding, supportive energy from the earth into your body. Exhale to send gratitude back. Repeat for as long as needed.

2. **RADICAL HONESTY** - Luteal/Waning Moon - What am I currently embodying that is keeping me in collusion with oppressive systems?

(after exploring, inhale COMPASSION into your body from the earth, to meet these parts of yourself with love and exhale gratitude back)

3. **RENEWAL** - Menstrual/New Moon - Which of these colluding parts am I ready to release? AND As I allow these parts to die and decompose, what wisdom emerges from this death?

(after exploring, inhale NOURISHMENT from the earth to feed you after this release and exhale gratitude back)

4. **CREATION** - Follicular/Waxing Moon - Using this deep wisdom, what seeds can I start to sow into this fertile soil I have created, in order to support collective change?

(after exploring, inhale EMPOWERMENT from the earth so that you can bravely take radical responsibility for what you are to grow, and exhale gratitude back)

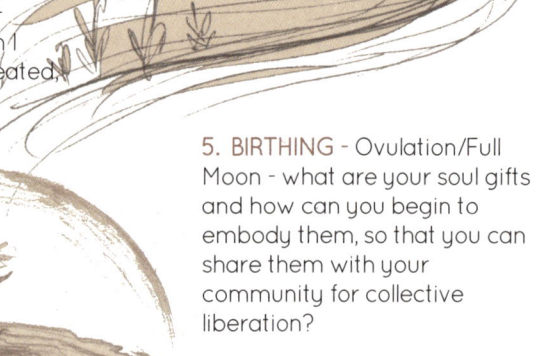

5. **BIRTHING** - Ovulation/Full Moon - what are your soul gifts and how can you begin to embody them, so that you can share them with your community for collective liberation?

(After exploration, inhale these soul gifts from your core and exhale to birth them down into the earth coming into a space of RECIPROCITY)

Phasic Overview & In-Betweens

Use this space to focus on the phases of the moonth and the in-betweens of the peak lunations.

One way of using this space is to designate one column for your goal-planning, intention-setting or focus per phase/week. Use the other column for reflections, dream themes, nutrition tracking, cards pulls, etc!

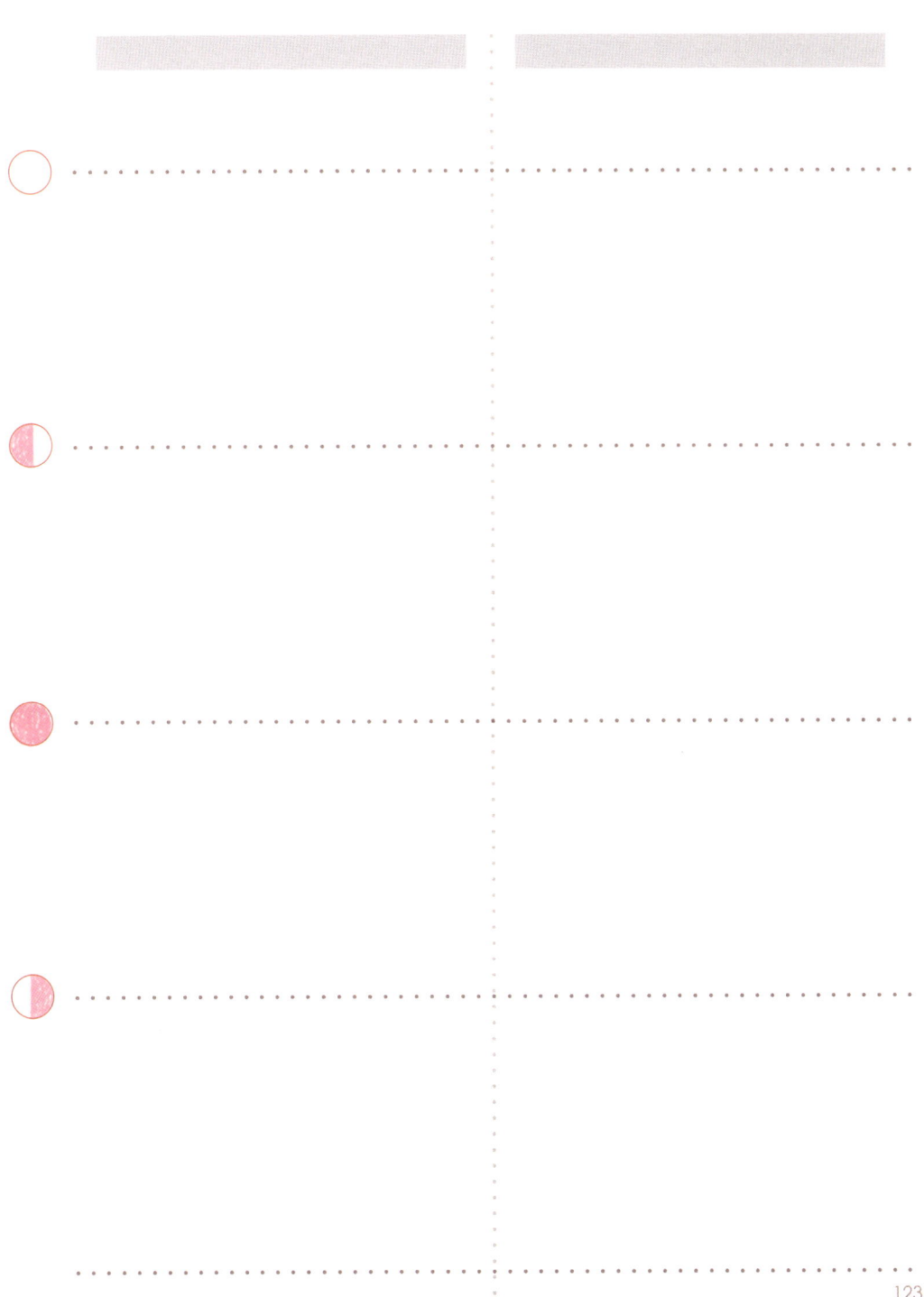

F • MAR 28

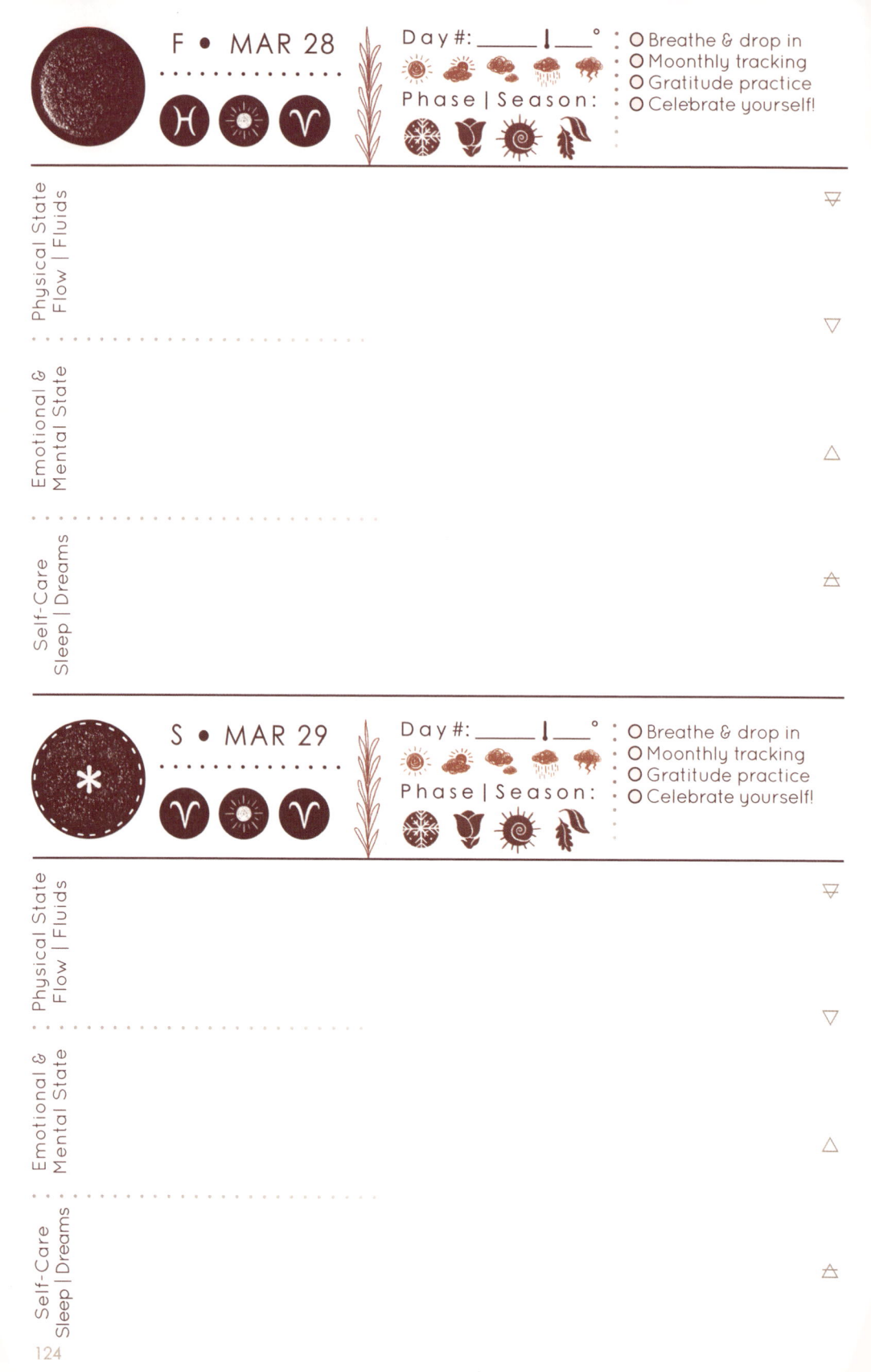

Day #: _____ | _____°
Phase | Season:

- Breathe & drop in
- Moonthly tracking
- Gratitude practice
- Celebrate yourself!

Physical State
Flow | Fluids

Emotional & Mental State

Self-Care
Sleep | Dreams

S • MAR 29

Day #: _____ | _____°
Phase | Season:

- Breathe & drop in
- Moonthly tracking
- Gratitude practice
- Celebrate yourself!

Physical State
Flow | Fluids

Emotional & Mental State

Self-Care
Sleep | Dreams

NEW MOON SOLAR ECLIPSE IN ARIES

Clarifying your unique avenue of action and awe

What do I want to grow & focus on during this lunar cycle?

How will I hold space for this?

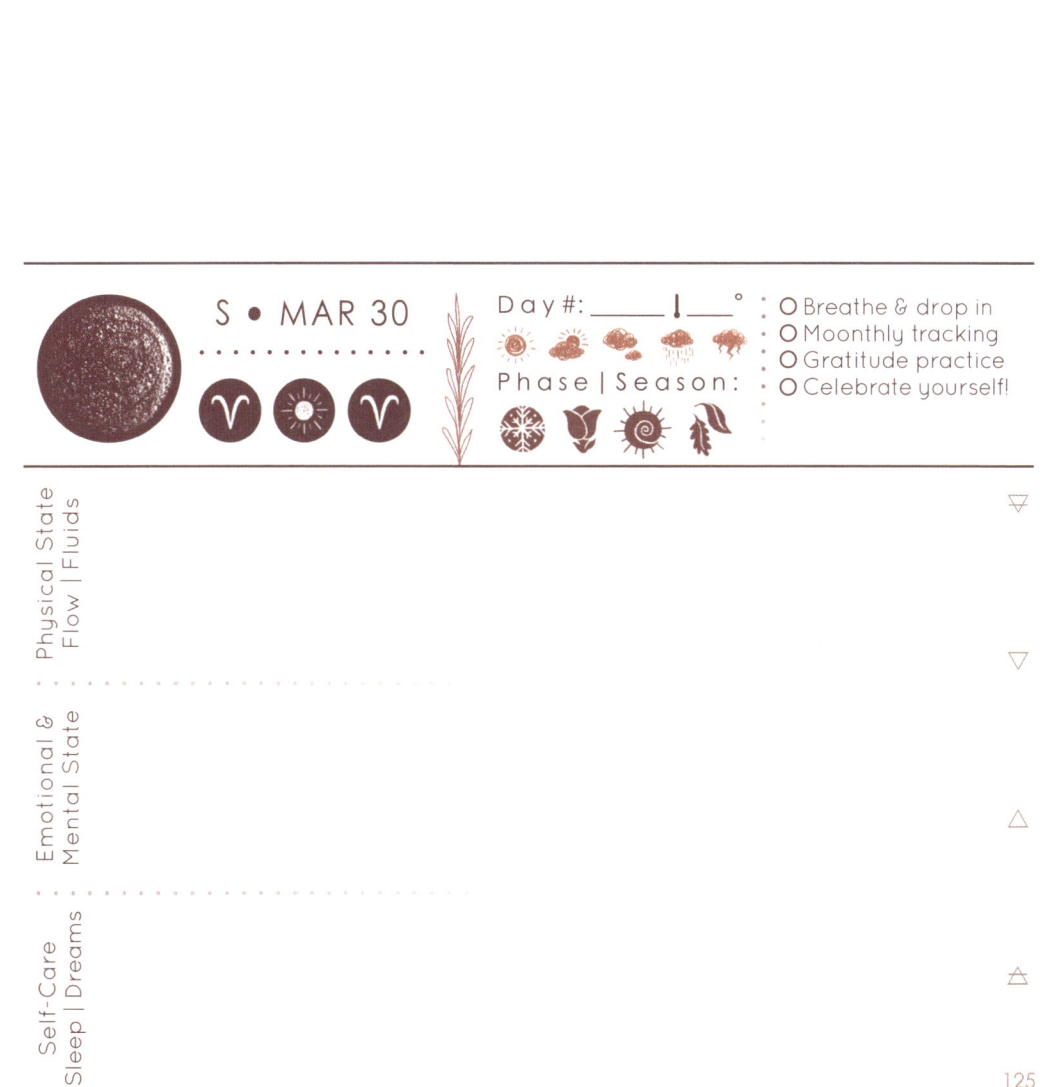

S • MAR 30

Day #: _____ | ___°

Phase | Season:

- ○ Breathe & drop in
- ○ Moonthly tracking
- ○ Gratitude practice
- ○ Celebrate yourself!

Physical State
Flow | Fluids

Emotional &
Mental State

Self-Care
Sleep | Dreams

M • MAR 31

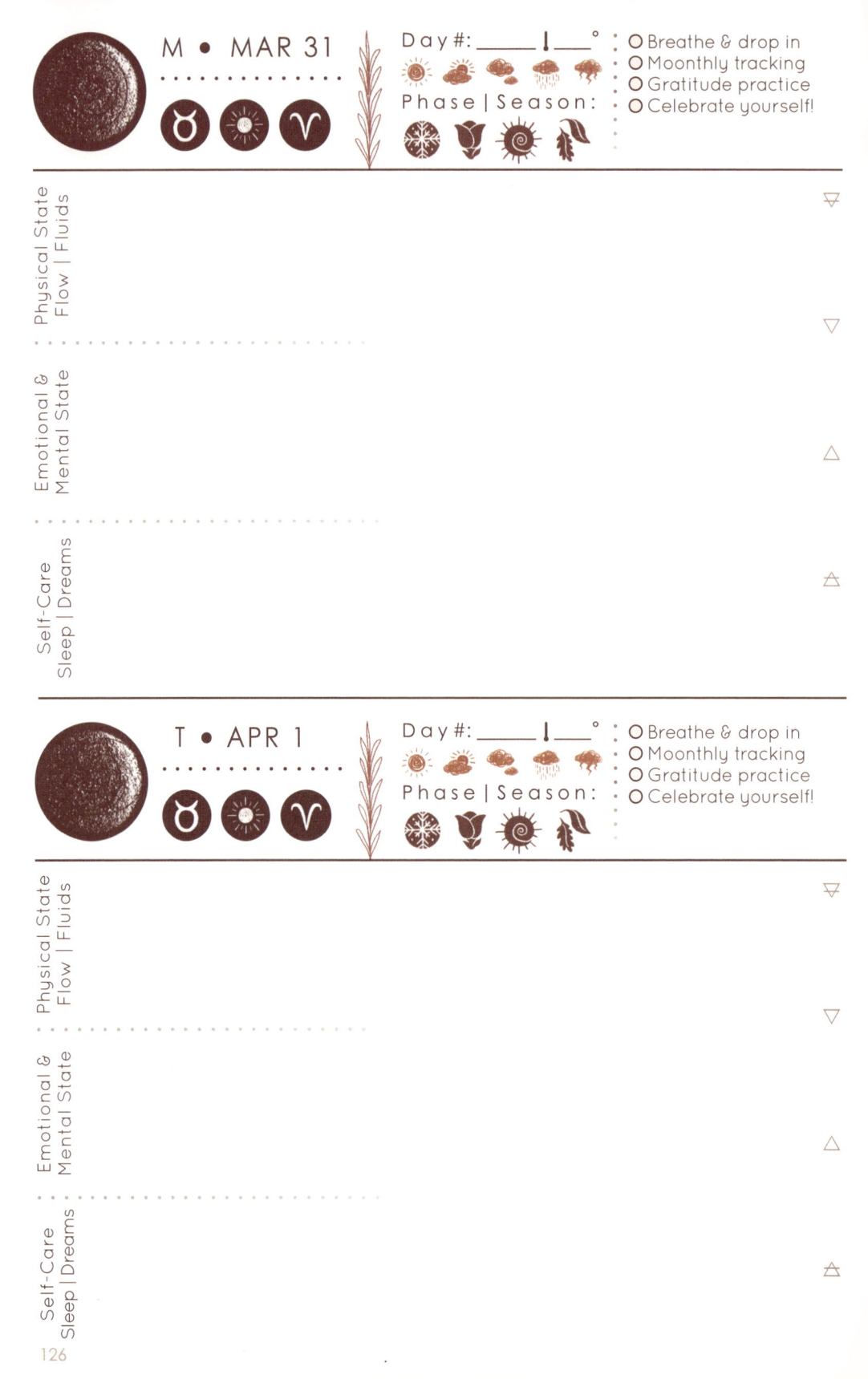

Day #: _____ | _____°

Phase | Season:

- ○ Breathe & drop in
- ○ Moonthly tracking
- ○ Gratitude practice
- ○ Celebrate yourself!

Physical State
Flow | Fluids

Emotional &
Mental State

Self-Care
Sleep | Dreams

T • APR 1

Day #: _____ | _____°

Phase | Season:

- ○ Breathe & drop in
- ○ Moonthly tracking
- ○ Gratitude practice
- ○ Celebrate yourself!

Physical State
Flow | Fluids

Emotional &
Mental State

Self-Care
Sleep | Dreams

W • APR 2

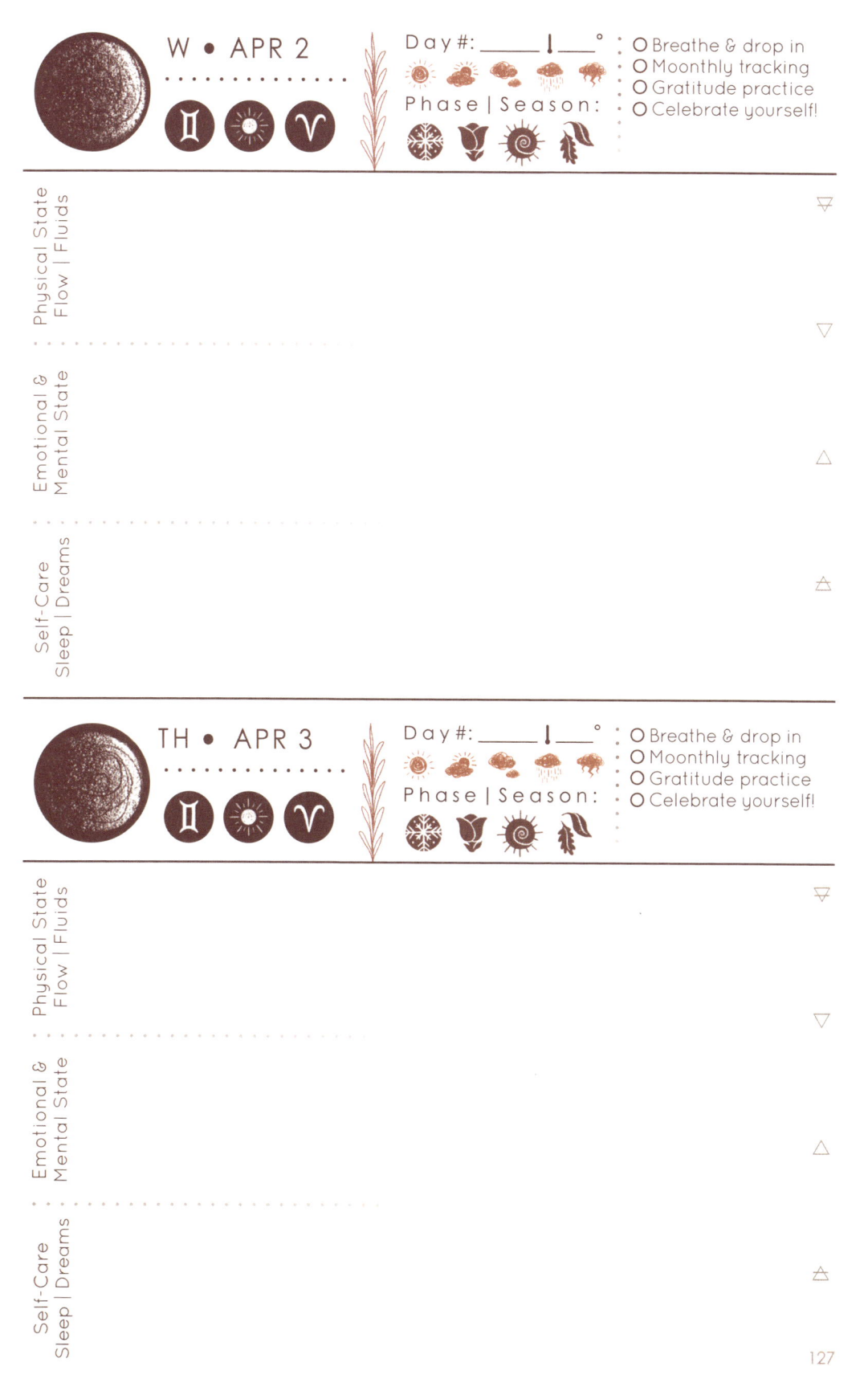

Day #: _____ | _____°

Phase | Season:

- ○ Breathe & drop in
- ○ Moonthly tracking
- ○ Gratitude practice
- ○ Celebrate yourself!

Physical State
Flow | Fluids

Emotional & Mental State

Self-Care
Sleep | Dreams

TH • APR 3

Day #: _____ | _____°

Phase | Season:

- ○ Breathe & drop in
- ○ Moonthly tracking
- ○ Gratitude practice
- ○ Celebrate yourself!

Physical State
Flow | Fluids

Emotional & Mental State

Self-Care
Sleep | Dreams

F • APR 4

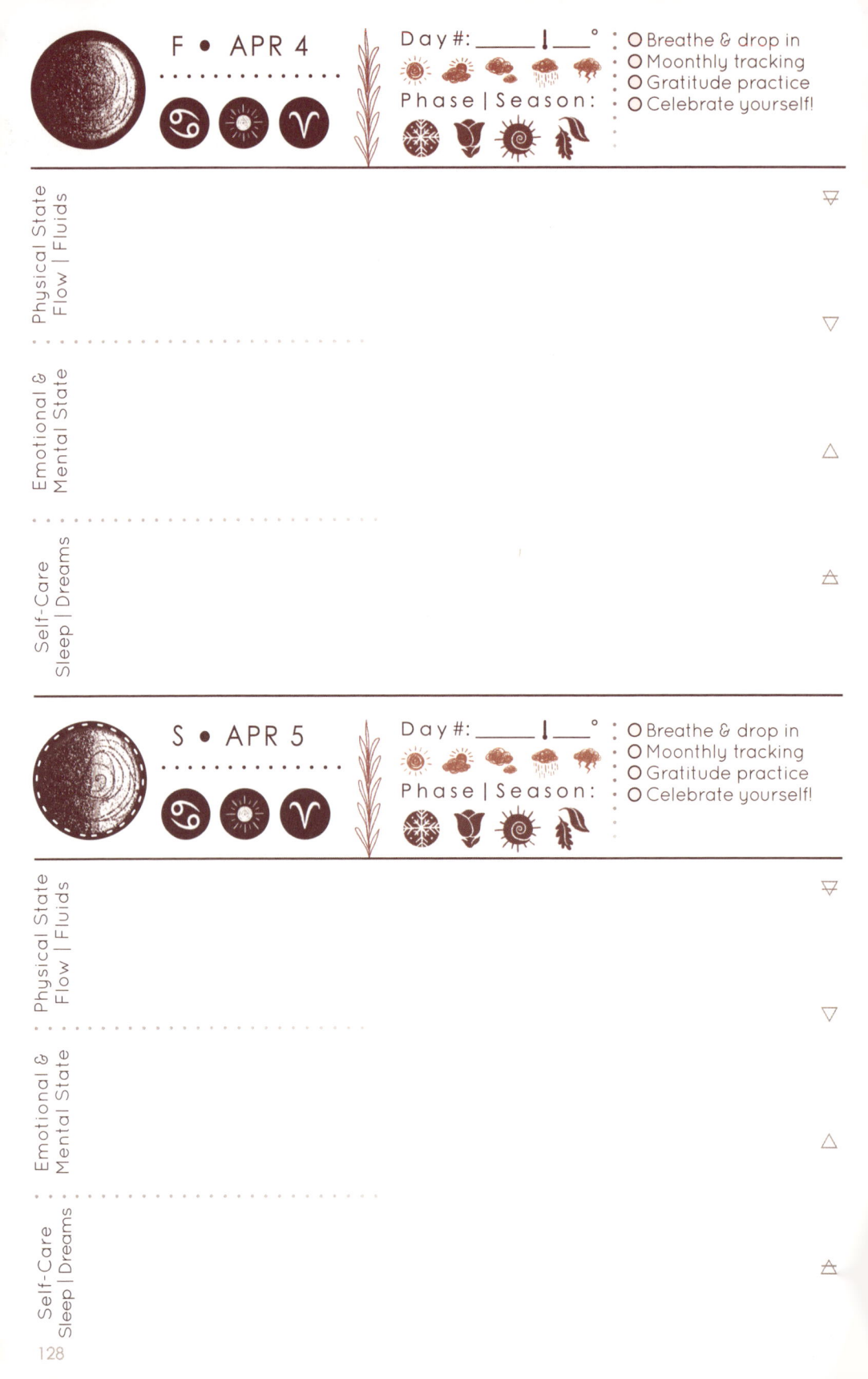

Day #: _____ | _____°

Phase | Season:

- ○ Breathe & drop in
- ○ Moonthly tracking
- ○ Gratitude practice
- ○ Celebrate yourself!

Physical State / Flow | Fluids

Emotional & Mental State

Self-Care / Sleep | Dreams

S • APR 5

Day #: _____ | _____°

Phase | Season:

- ○ Breathe & drop in
- ○ Moonthly tracking
- ○ Gratitude practice
- ○ Celebrate yourself!

Physical State / Flow | Fluids

Emotional & Mental State

Self-Care / Sleep | Dreams

FIRST QUARTER IN CANCER

Recognizing the potential for self-inquiry in each expanding moment

What is sprouting & coming into awareness?

What can I release to make space for further growth & grounding?

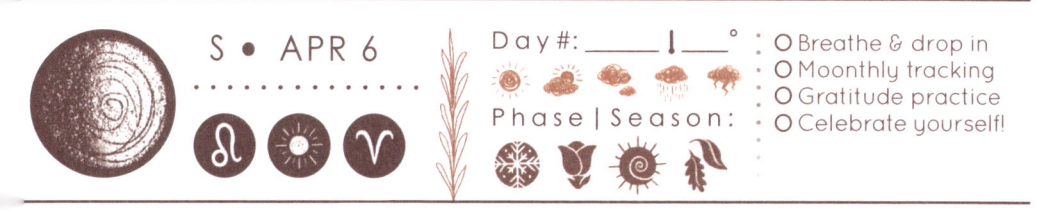

S • APR 6

Day #: _____ | _____°

Phase | Season:

- ○ Breathe & drop in
- ○ Moonthly tracking
- ○ Gratitude practice
- ○ Celebrate yourself!

Physical State
Flow | Fluids

Emotional &
Mental State

Self-Care
Sleep | Dreams

M • APR 7

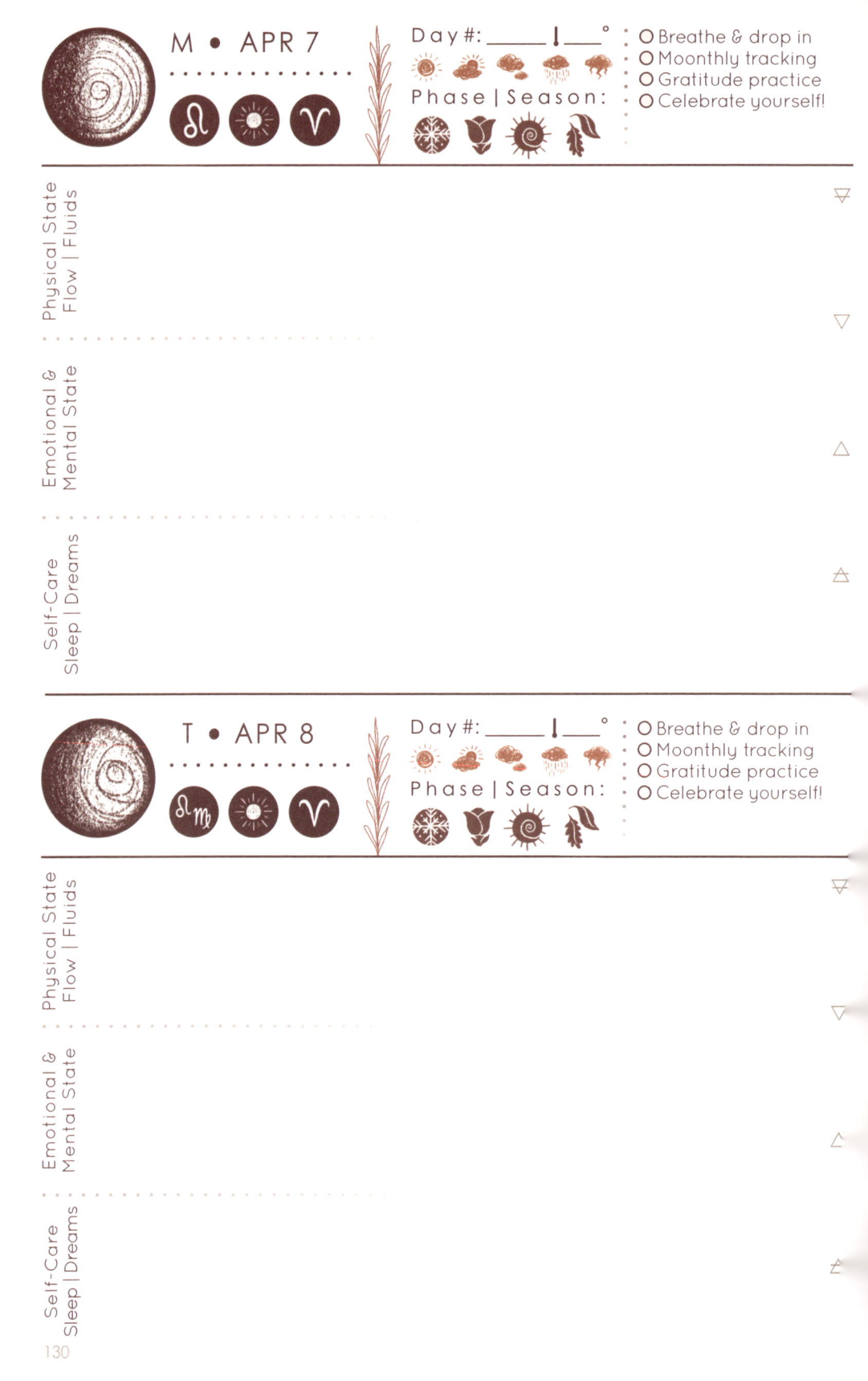

♌ ☉ ♈

Day #: _____ | _____°

Phase | Season:

- ○ Breathe & drop in
- ○ Moonthly tracking
- ○ Gratitude practice
- ○ Celebrate yourself!

Physical State
Flow | Fluids

Emotional & Mental State

Self-Care
Sleep | Dreams

T • APR 8

♍ ☉ ♈

Day #: _____ | _____°

Phase | Season:

- ○ Breathe & drop in
- ○ Moonthly tracking
- ○ Gratitude practice
- ○ Celebrate yourself!

Physical State
Flow | Fluids

Emotional & Mental State

Self-Care
Sleep | Dreams

W • APR 9

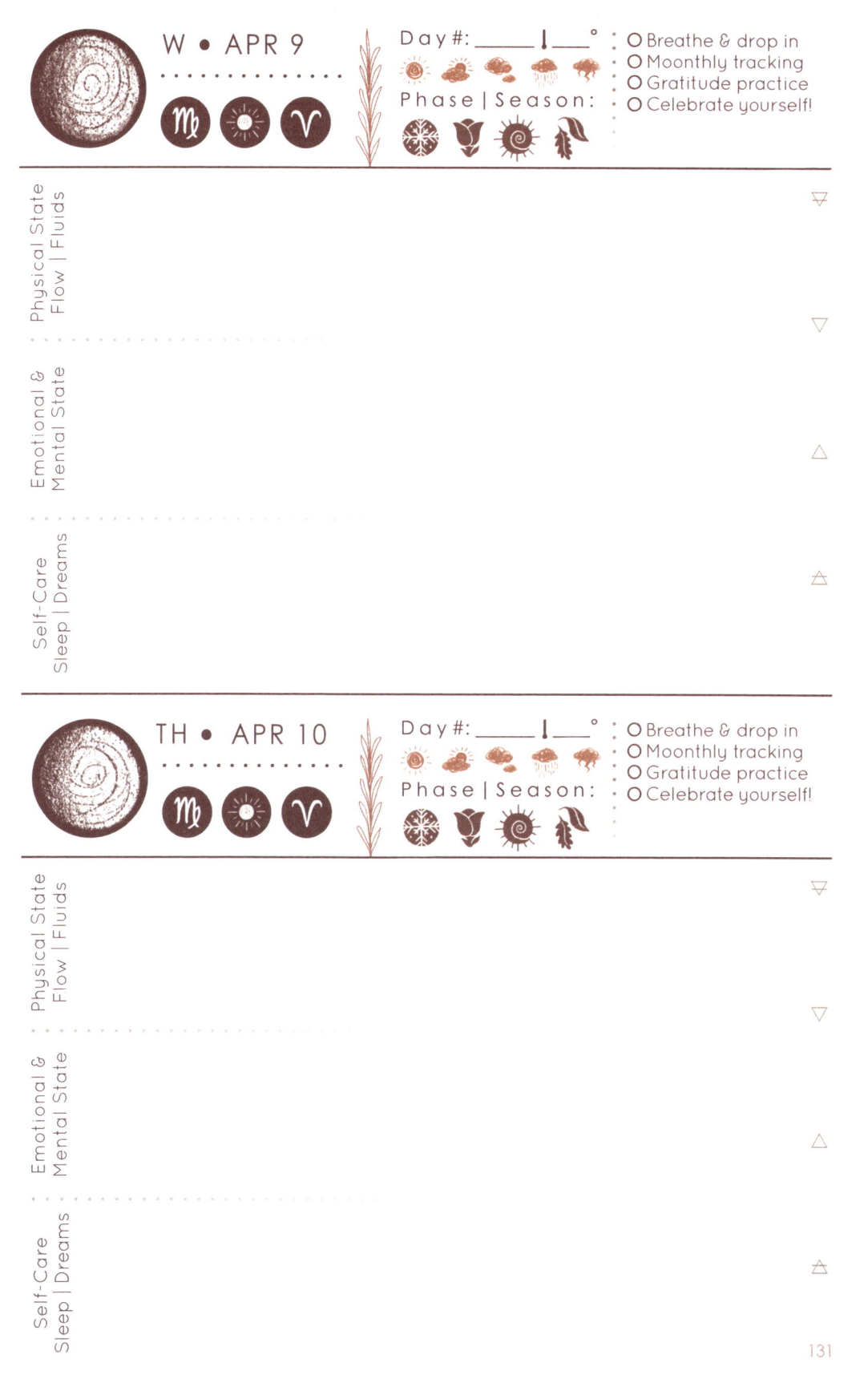

Day #: _____ | _____°

Phase | Season:

- ○ Breathe & drop in
- ○ Moonthly tracking
- ○ Gratitude practice
- ○ Celebrate yourself!

Physical State / Flow | Fluids

Emotional & Mental State

Self-Care / Sleep | Dreams

TH • APR 10

Day #: _____ | _____°

Phase | Season:

- ○ Breathe & drop in
- ○ Moonthly tracking
- ○ Gratitude practice
- ○ Celebrate yourself!

Physical State / Flow | Fluids

Emotional & Mental State

Self-Care / Sleep | Dreams

F • APR 11

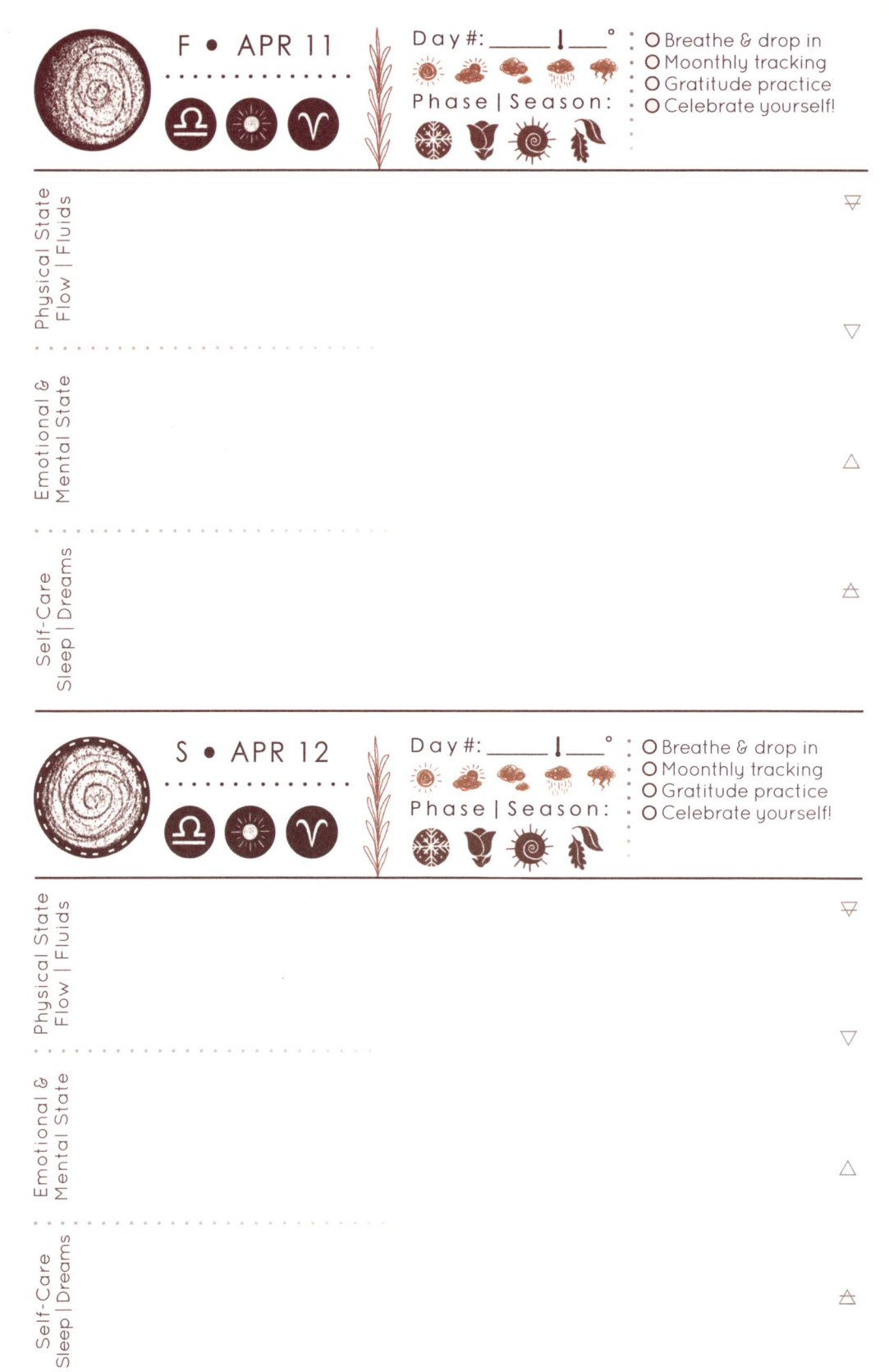

Day #: _____ | ____°

Phase | Season:

- ○ Breathe & drop in
- ○ Moonthly tracking
- ○ Gratitude practice
- ○ Celebrate yourself!

Physical State
Flow | Fluids

Emotional & Mental State

Self-Care
Sleep | Dreams

S • APR 12

Day #: _____ | ____°

Phase | Season:

- ○ Breathe & drop in
- ○ Moonthly tracking
- ○ Gratitude practice
- ○ Celebrate yourself!

Physical State
Flow | Fluids

Emotional & Mental State

Self-Care
Sleep | Dreams

FULL MOON IN LIBRA

Embracing the inherent stability in the ever-changing nature of it all

What is being illuminated?

I give gratitude for what is & what is becoming:

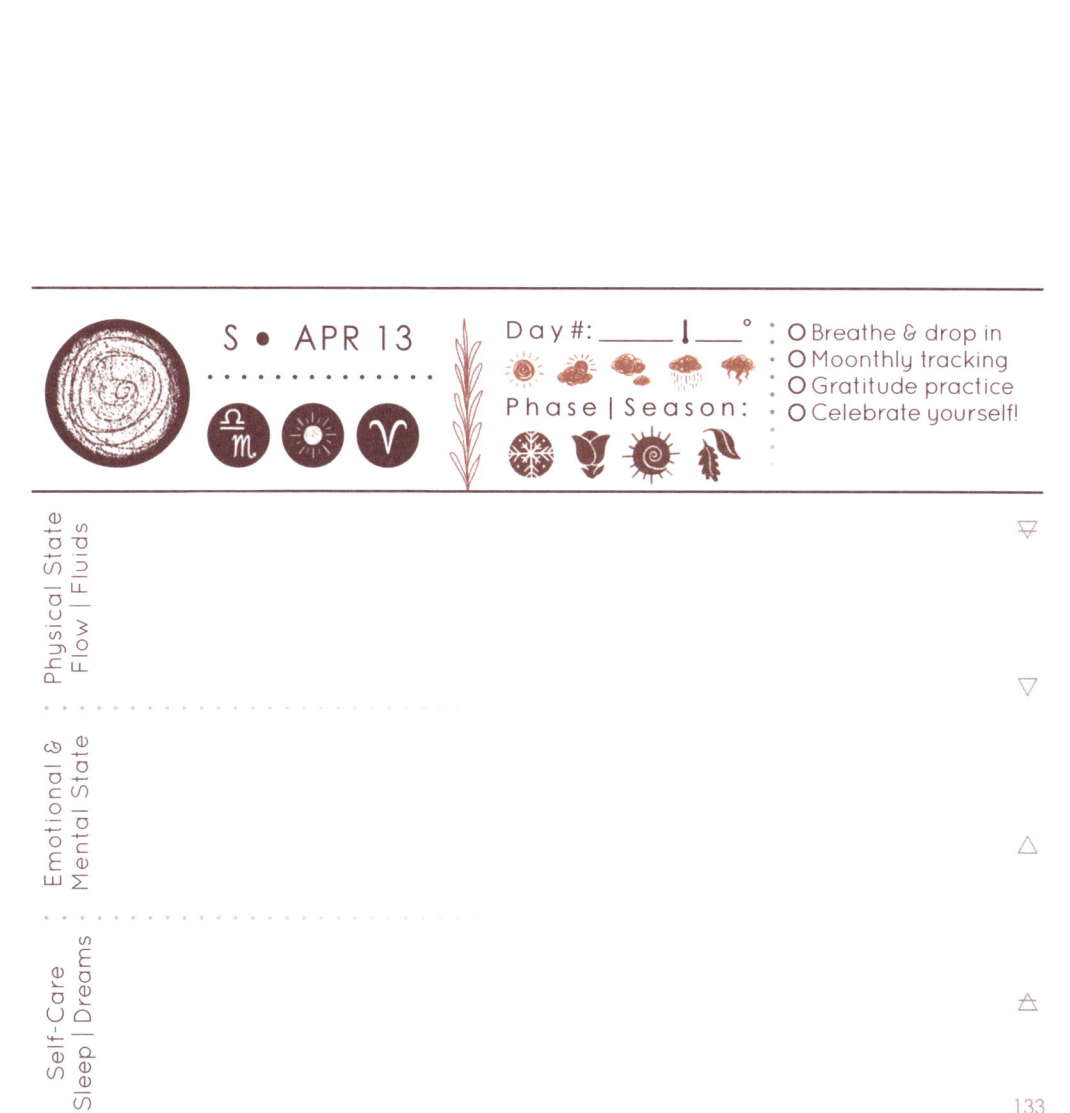

S • APR 13

Day #: _____ | _____°

Phase | Season:

- ○ Breathe & drop in
- ○ Moonthly tracking
- ○ Gratitude practice
- ○ Celebrate yourself!

Physical State / Flow | Fluids

Emotional & Mental State

Self-Care / Sleep | Dreams

M • APR 14

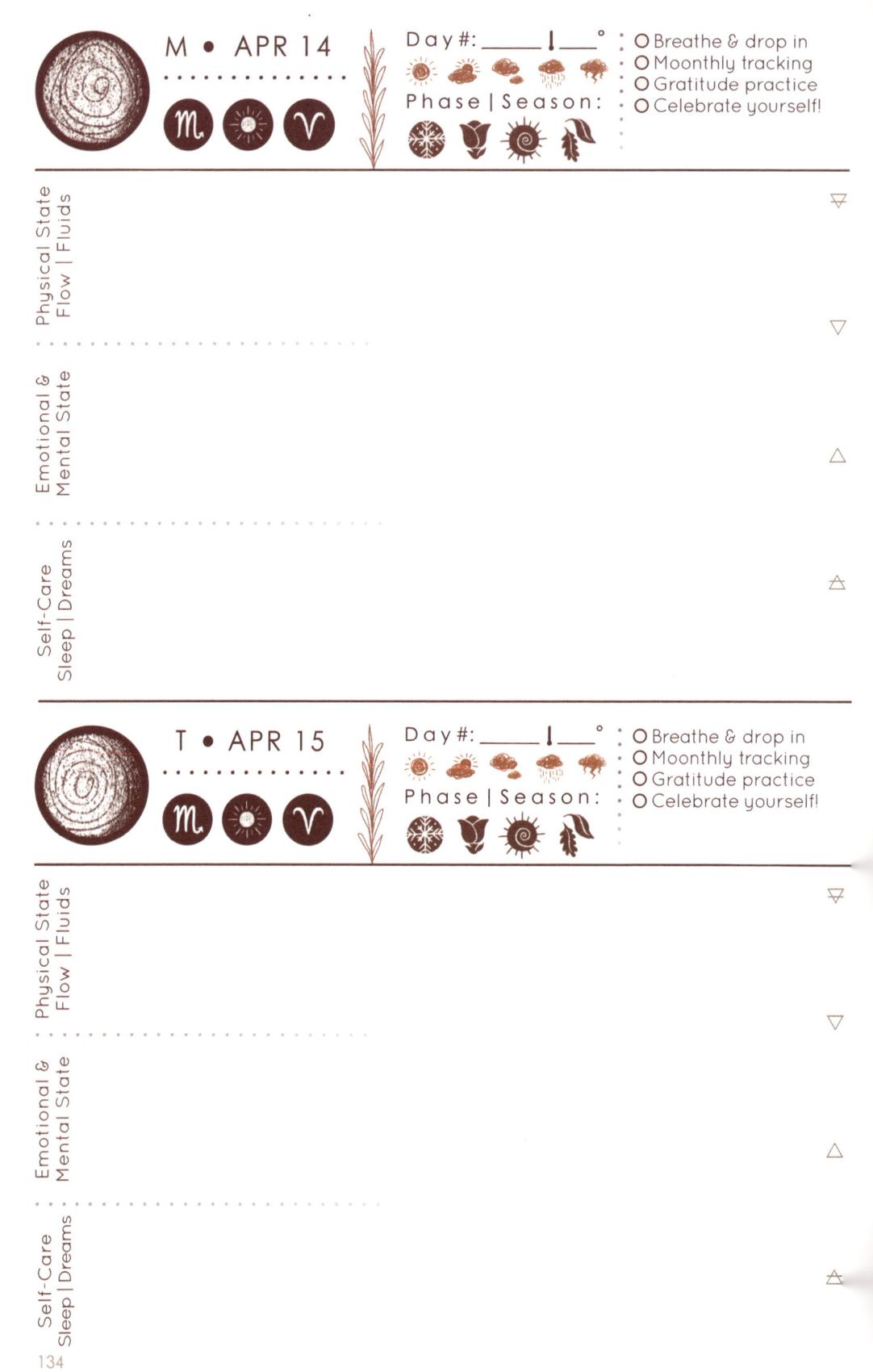

♏ ☉ ♈

Day #: _____ | _____°

Phase | Season:

- ○ Breathe & drop in
- ○ Moonthly tracking
- ○ Gratitude practice
- ○ Celebrate yourself!

Physical State
Flow | Fluids

Emotional & Mental State

Self-Care
Sleep | Dreams

T • APR 15

♏ ☉ ♈

Day #: _____ | _____°

Phase | Season:

- ○ Breathe & drop in
- ○ Moonthly tracking
- ○ Gratitude practice
- ○ Celebrate yourself!

Physical State
Flow | Fluids

Emotional & Mental State

Self-Care
Sleep | Dreams

W • APR 16

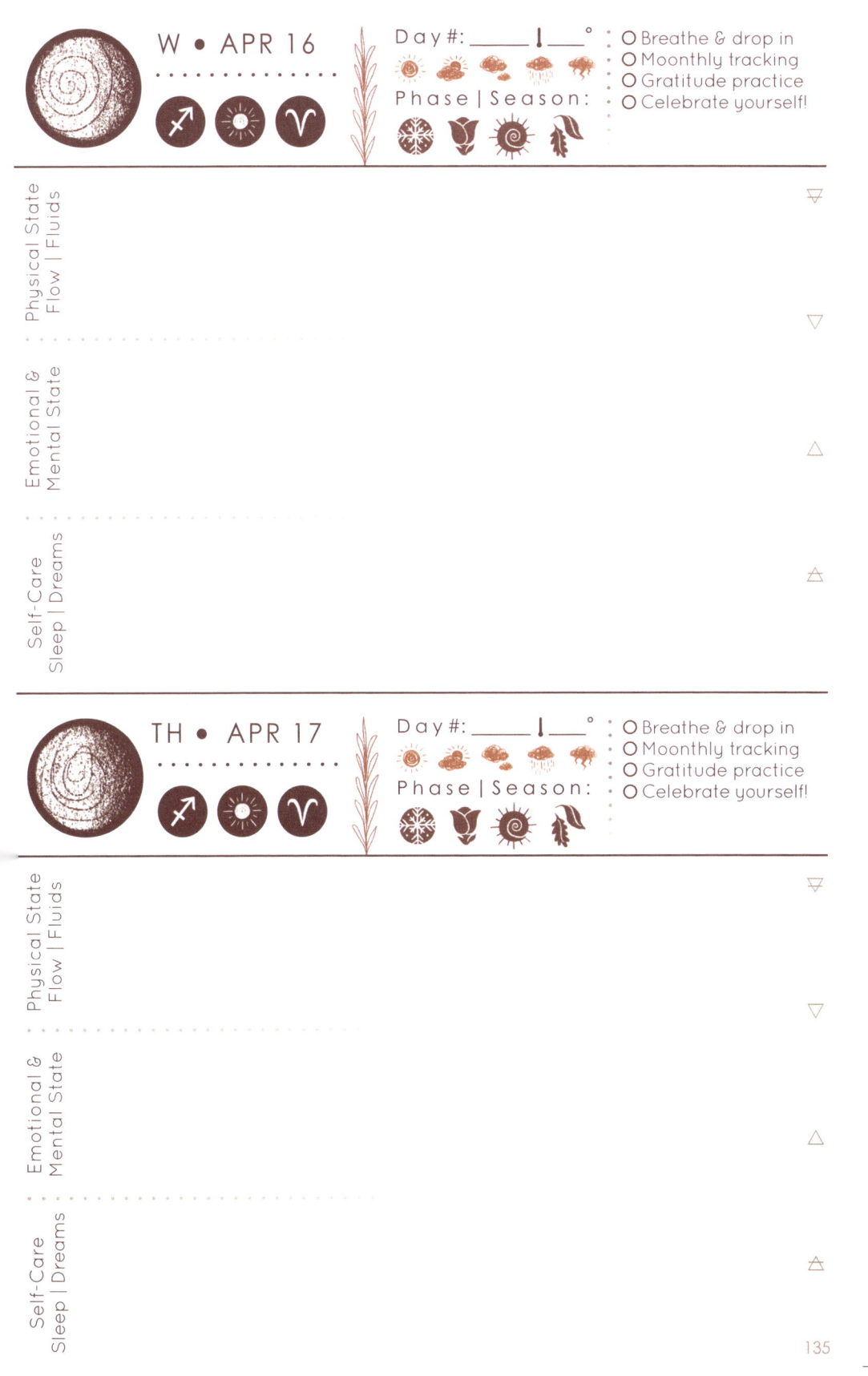

Day #: _____ | _____°

Phase | Season:

- ○ Breathe & drop in
- ○ Moonthly tracking
- ○ Gratitude practice
- ○ Celebrate yourself!

Physical State
Flow | Fluids

Emotional &
Mental State

Self-Care
Sleep | Dreams

TH • APR 17

Day #: _____ | _____°

Phase | Season:

- ○ Breathe & drop in
- ○ Moonthly tracking
- ○ Gratitude practice
- ○ Celebrate yourself!

Physical State
Flow | Fluids

Emotional &
Mental State

Self-Care
Sleep | Dreams

F • APR 18

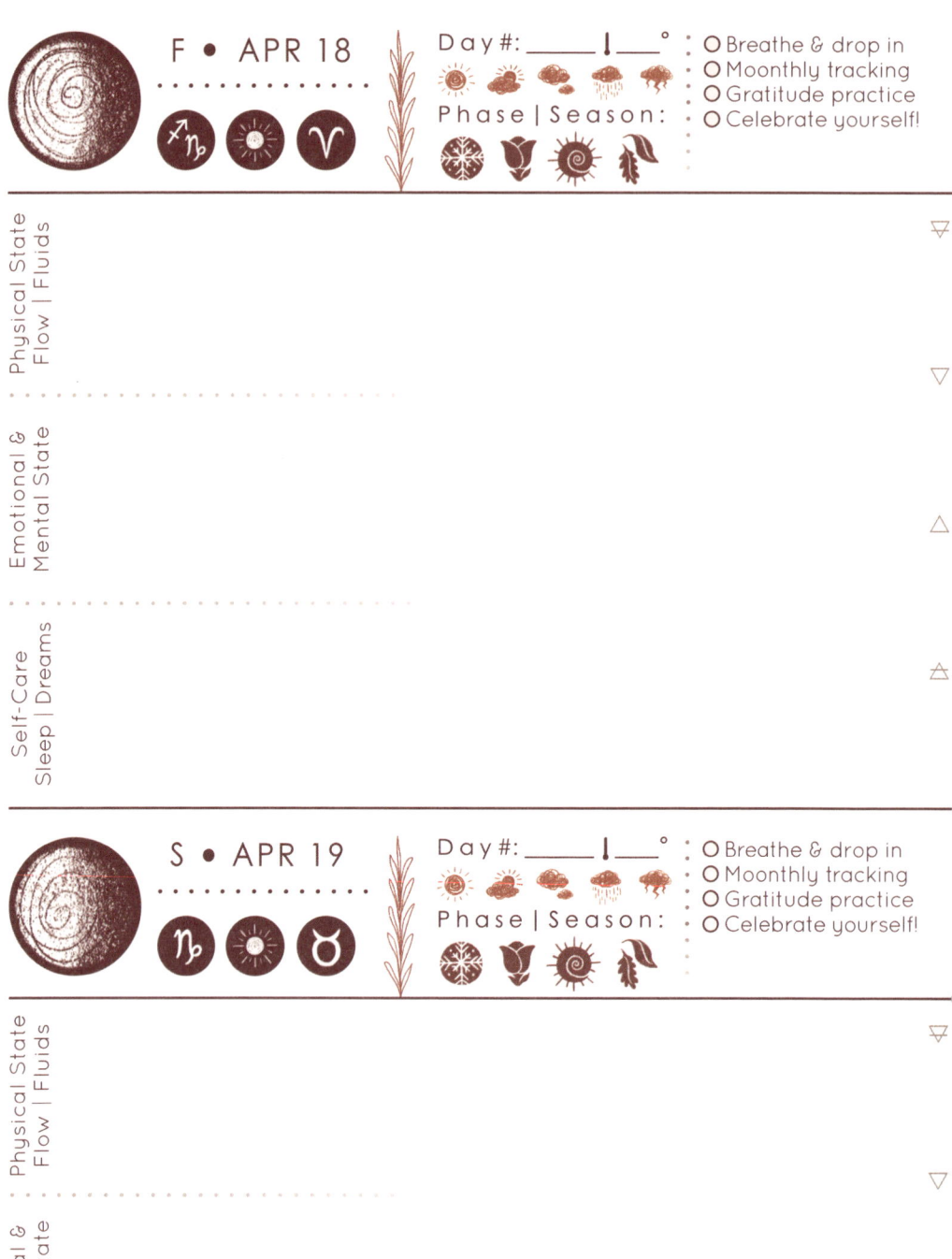

Day #: _____ | _____°

Phase | Season:

- ○ Breathe & drop in
- ○ Moonthly tracking
- ○ Gratitude practice
- ○ Celebrate yourself!

Physical State / Flow | Fluids

Emotional & Mental State

Self-Care / Sleep | Dreams

S • APR 19

Day #: _____ | _____°

Phase | Season:

- ○ Breathe & drop in
- ○ Moonthly tracking
- ○ Gratitude practice
- ○ Celebrate yourself!

Physical State / Flow | Fluids

Emotional & Mental State

Self-Care / Sleep | Dreams

S • APR 20

Day #: ____ | ____°

Phase | Season:

- ○ Breathe & drop in
- ○ Moonthly tracking
- ○ Gratitude practice
- ○ Celebrate yourself!

Physical State / Flow | Fluids

Emotional & Mental State

Self-Care / Sleep | Dreams

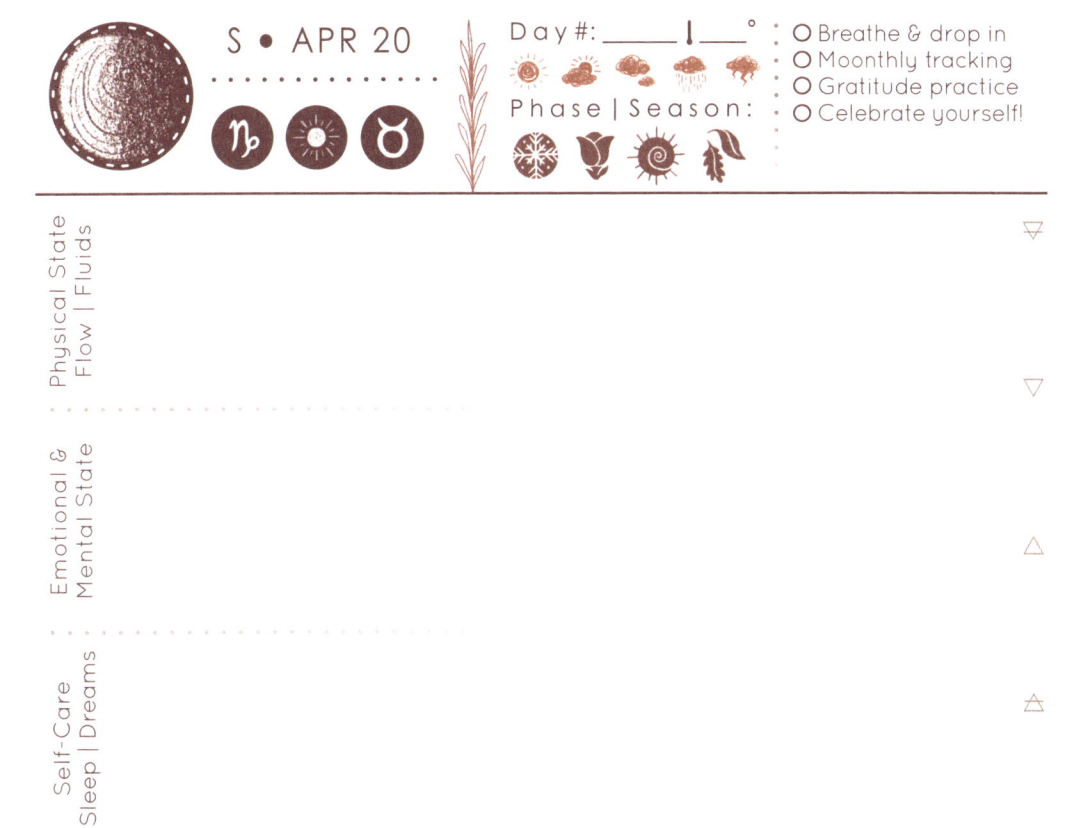

LAST QUARTER IN CAPRICORN

Dissolving pre-established notions that bypass reality

What am I leaving behind this lunar cycle?

Where can I make more space for reflection &/or integration?

M • APR 21

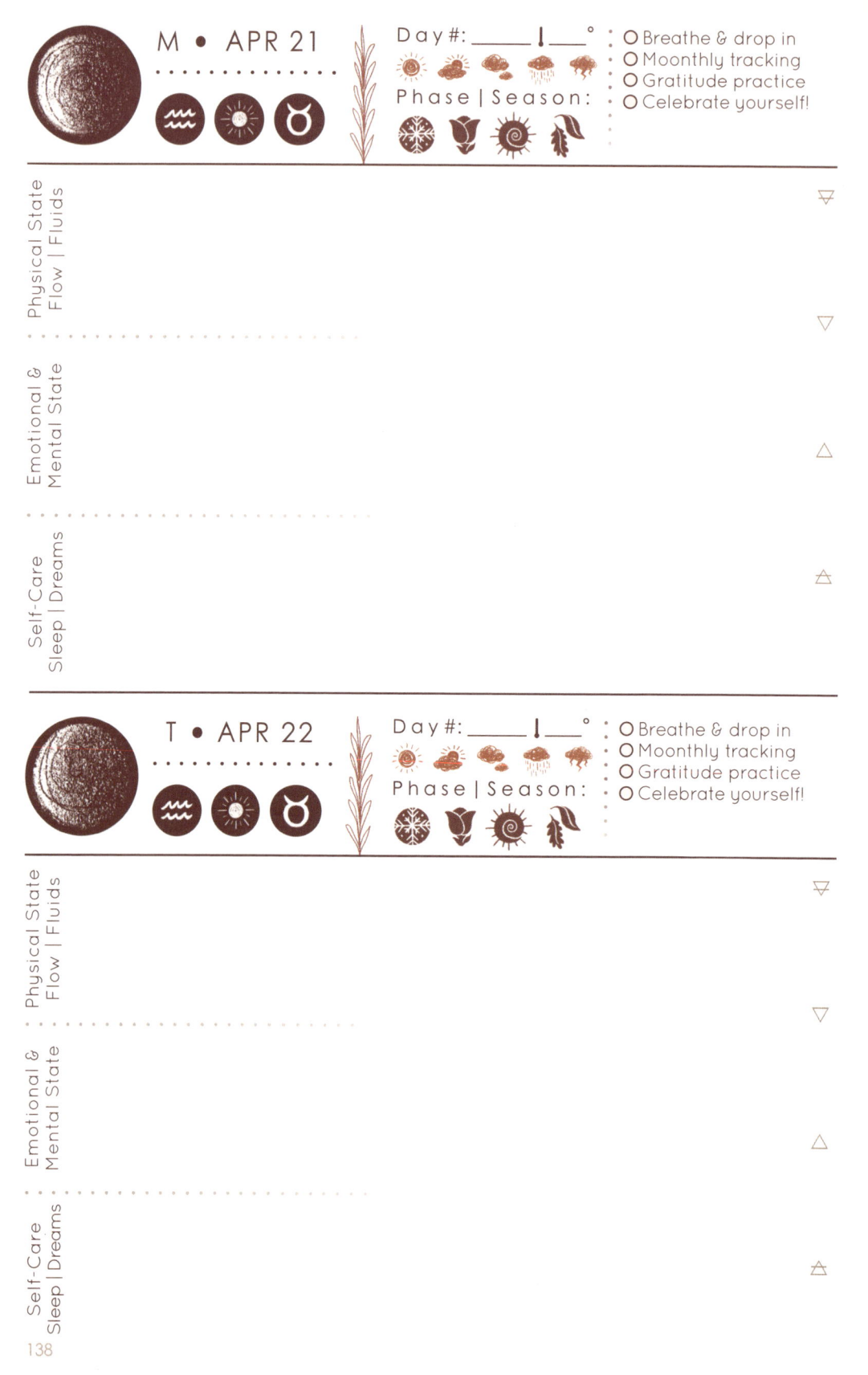

Day #: _____ | ____°

Phase | Season:

- ○ Breathe & drop in
- ○ Moonthly tracking
- ○ Gratitude practice
- ○ Celebrate yourself!

Physical State
Flow | Fluids

Emotional & Mental State

Self-Care
Sleep | Dreams

T • APR 22

Day #: _____ | ____°

Phase | Season:

- ○ Breathe & drop in
- ○ Moonthly tracking
- ○ Gratitude practice
- ○ Celebrate yourself!

Physical State
Flow | Fluids

Emotional & Mental State

Self-Care
Sleep | Dreams

W • APR 23

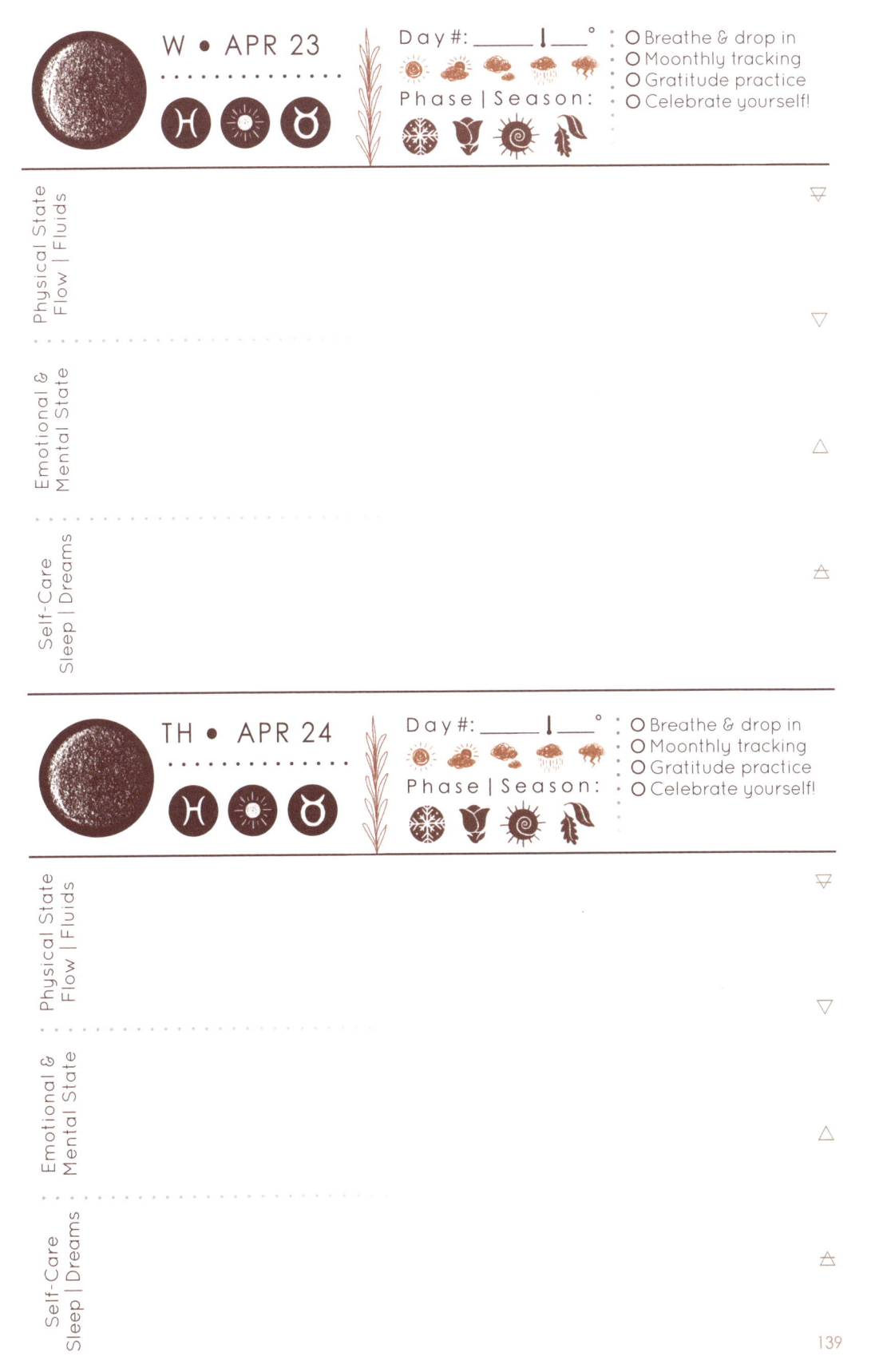

Day #: _____ | _____°

Phase | Season:

- ○ Breathe & drop in
- ○ Moonthly tracking
- ○ Gratitude practice
- ○ Celebrate yourself!

Physical State
Flow | Fluids

Emotional &
Mental State

Self-Care
Sleep | Dreams

TH • APR 24

Day #: _____ | _____°

Phase | Season:

- ○ Breathe & drop in
- ○ Moonthly tracking
- ○ Gratitude practice
- ○ Celebrate yourself!

Physical State
Flow | Fluids

Emotional &
Mental State

Self-Care
Sleep | Dreams

☾ 3rd
03 | 29
04 | 26

CHECK IN & REFLECT

Use this space to reflect on your experiences & findings from this ending lunar cycle or your last menstrual cycle. Use cycle day #s if you bleed, or moon phases if you don't.

Last Cycle Day 1: _____

Last Cycle Length: _____

Circle the phase you bled near:

○ ☽ ☽ ☽ ☽ ☽ ● ☾ ☾ ☾ ☾ ○

Caution Days: (days I needed space)

Bliss Days: (days I felt great)

DAYS TO NOTE — Which cycle days stood out?

OBSERVATIONS — Notice any changes or patterns?

SELF-CARE — What was helpful & nourishing?

PLAN & PREPARE

Next Predicted Cycle:
🩸 ☾ _____

CHECKLIST

Add the following to any other planners or calendars for your next cycle, then check it off.

- ☐ Predicted "days to note" _____
- ☐ Days to slow down (pre-bleed) _____
- ☐ Rest day(s) (next bleed) _____
- ☐ Date with yourself _____
- ☐ _____

- ☐ Self chest/breast exam
- ☐ Meal plan with cycle
- ☐ _____
- ☐ _____
- ☐ _____

OPEN SPACE

Use this space how you wish, or print out one of our free templates to paste here for BBT charting, dream tracking, or something else:

The Roots of PMDD

by Mandy Rother (she/her) • Functional Dietitian + Functional Medicine Nutrition Specialist • @mandyrother.RD • revealfunctionalnutrition.com

---

Premenstrual Dysphoric Disorder (PMDD) is a hormone-based mood disorder with psychological and physical symptoms occurring during the luteal phase of the menstrual cycle. It is caused by a negative reaction in the brain to the normal rise and fall of hormones throughout the cycle. PMDD is NOT PMS. It is different in both the severity and the cause.

It's biology, not a behavior choice.

PMDD is suspected to be a hormone sensitivity in the brain. Each person with PMDD has a unique set of factors that contribute to or trigger symptoms. Genetics, structural brain differences, inflammation, and stress response may all play a role. PMDD is real with a biological basis. It's not your fault or "all in your head."

Same diagnosis. Unique root cause.

First-line conventional treatments often include oral contraceptives and antidepressants. While they work for some, at least 40% of people with PMDD do not respond favorably to those treatments. Why? Because we are not all the same. What works for someone else, even with similar symptoms, may not be what YOU need. There may be unique causal factors that impact why some respond to treatments and others do not.

Root-cause Approach

Single remedies, whether medications or natural supplements, often fall short because they merely mask symptoms without addressing YOUR unique set of underlying factors to bring those systems back into balance. Each person has different interwoven factors such as genetics, brain chemistry, co-existing hormonal imbalances, nutrient insufficiencies, stress, trauma, and more. If that list feels daunting, know that you don't need to go it alone. Cut out the guesswork and partner with a functional medicine practitioner familiar with the intricacies of PMDD.

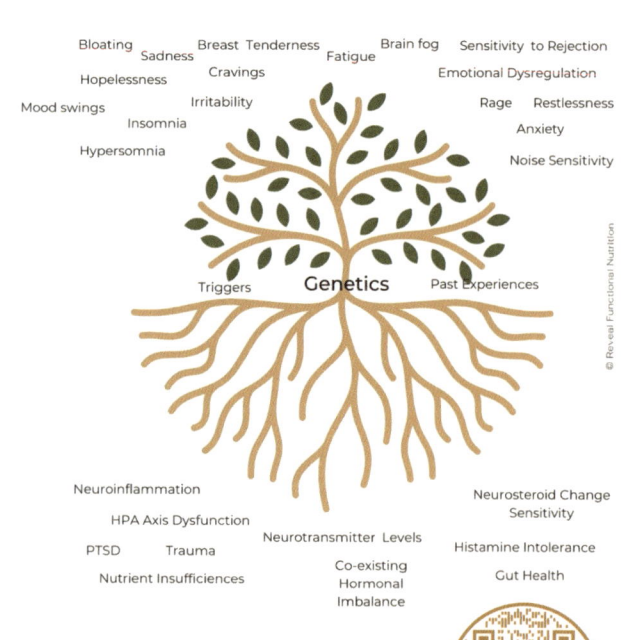

Tree leaves (symptoms): Bloating, Sadness, Breast Tenderness, Fatigue, Brain fog, Sensitivity to Rejection, Hopelessness, Cravings, Emotional Dysregulation, Mood swings, Irritability, Rage, Restlessness, Insomnia, Anxiety, Hypersomnia, Noise Sensitivity

Tree trunk: Triggers, Genetics, Past Experiences

Tree roots (root causes): Neuroinflammation, HPA Axis Dysfunction, PTSD, Trauma, Nutrient Insufficiencies, Neurotransmitter Levels, Co-existing Hormonal Imbalance, Neurosteroid Change Sensitivity, Histamine Intolerance, Gut Health

© Reveal Functional Nutrition

Ready to ditch band-aid solutions and explore a whole-person, root-cause approach? Scan the QR code.

Phasic Overview & In-Betweens

Use this space to focus on the phases of the moonth and the in-betweens of the peak lunations.

One way of using this space is to designate one column for your goal-planning, intention-setting or focus per phase/week. Use the other column for reflections, dream themes, nutrition tracking, cards pulls, etc!

F • APR 25

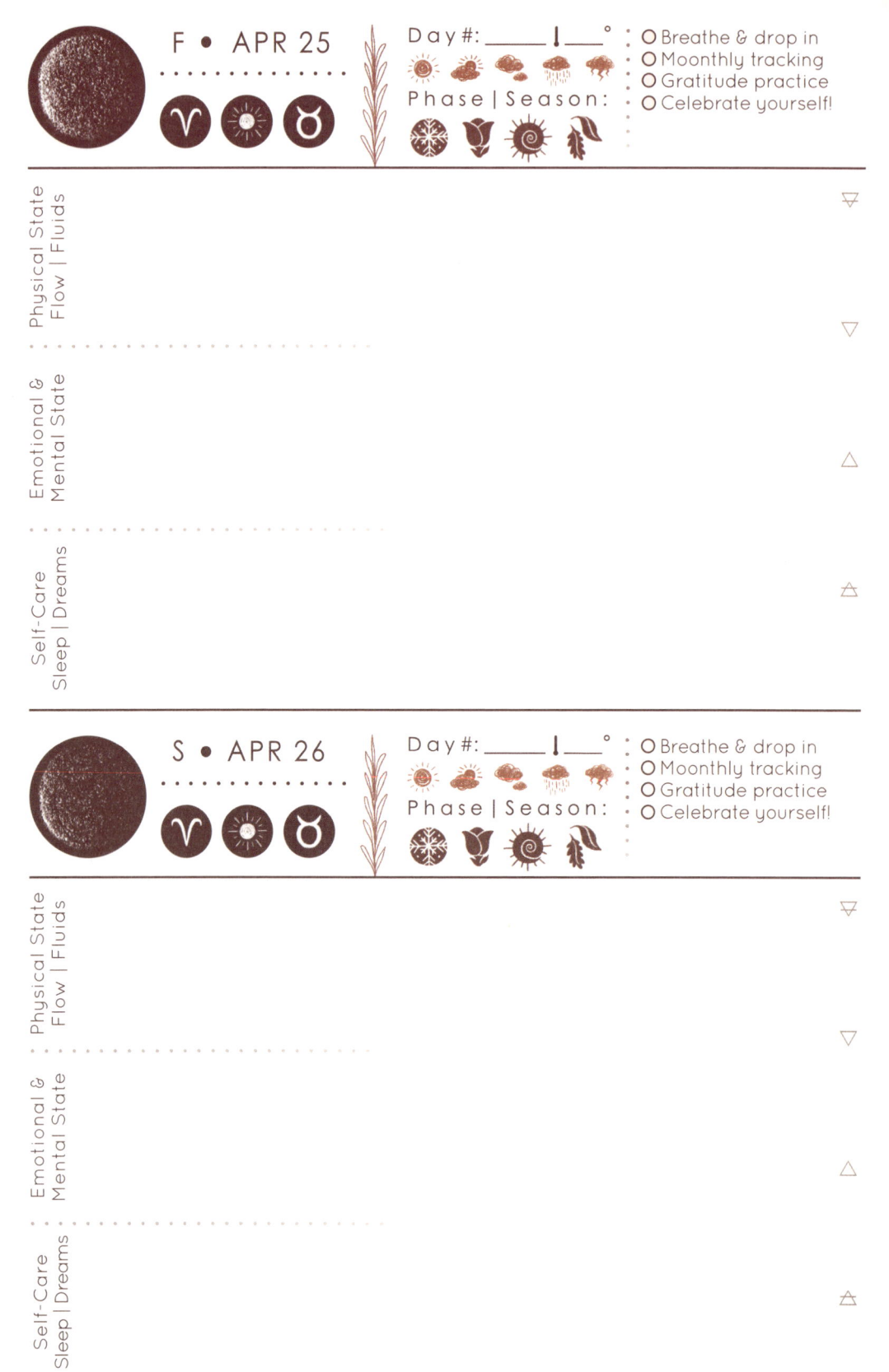

Day #: _____ | _____°
Phase | Season:

○ Breathe & drop in
○ Moonthly tracking
○ Gratitude practice
○ Celebrate yourself!

Physical State
Flow | Fluids

Emotional &
Mental State

Self-Care
Sleep | Dreams

S • APR 26

Day #: _____ | _____°
Phase | Season:

○ Breathe & drop in
○ Moonthly tracking
○ Gratitude practice
○ Celebrate yourself!

Physical State
Flow | Fluids

Emotional &
Mental State

Self-Care
Sleep | Dreams

S • APR 27

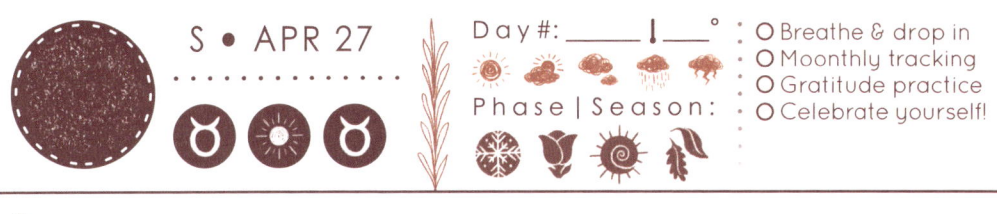

Day #: _____ | ___°

Phase | Season:

- ○ Breathe & drop in
- ○ Moonthly tracking
- ○ Gratitude practice
- ○ Celebrate yourself!

Physical State
Flow | Fluids

Emotional &
Mental State

Self-Care
Sleep | Dreams

NEW MOON IN TAURUS

Planting seeds in spaces of comfort & nourishment

What do I want to grow & focus on during this lunar cycle?

How will I hold space for this?

M • APR 28

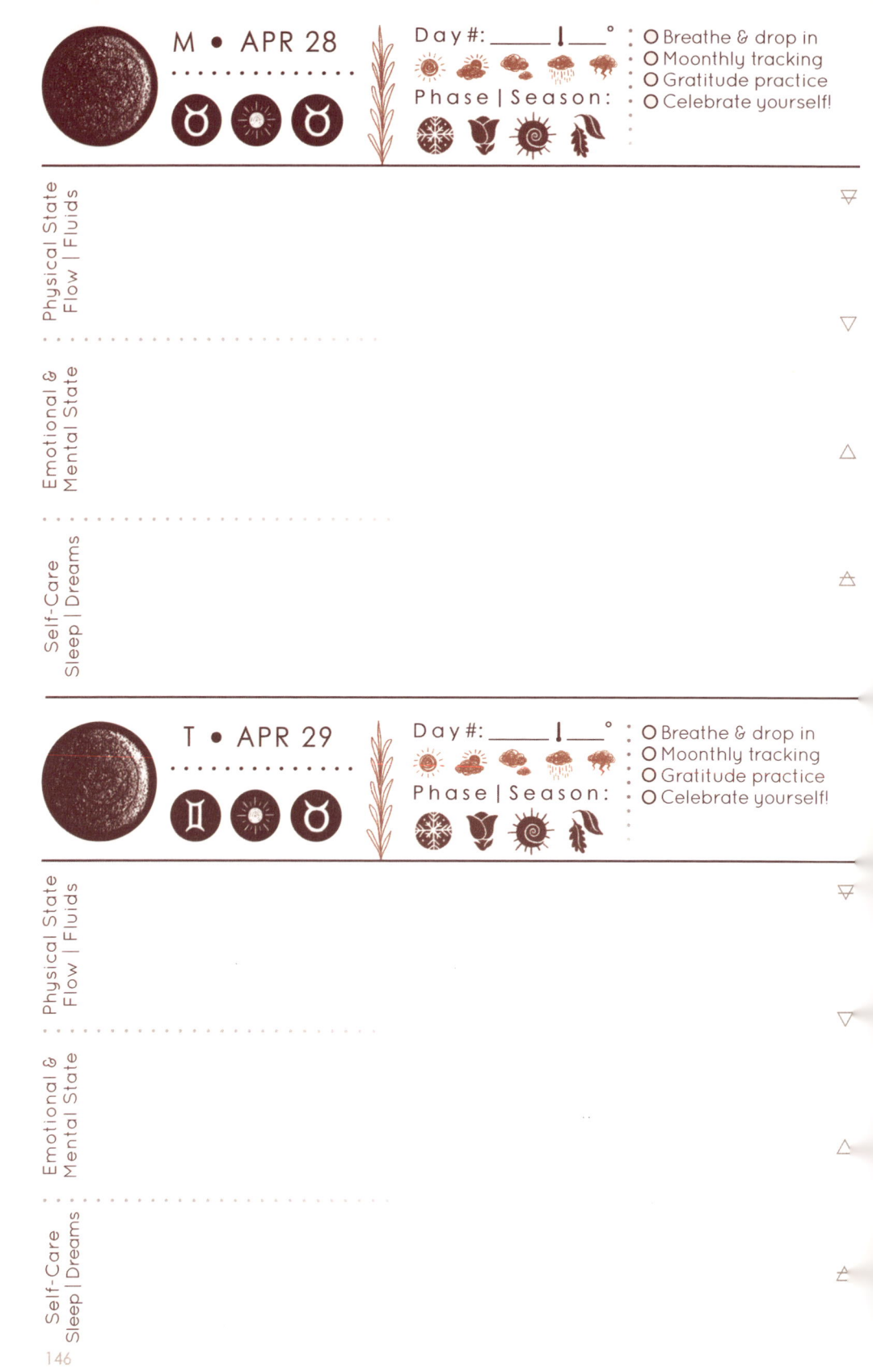

Day #: _____ | _____°

Phase | Season:

- Breathe & drop in
- Moonthly tracking
- Gratitude practice
- Celebrate yourself!

Physical State / Flow | Fluids

Emotional & Mental State

Self-Care / Sleep | Dreams

T • APR 29

Day #: _____ | _____°

Phase | Season:

- Breathe & drop in
- Moonthly tracking
- Gratitude practice
- Celebrate yourself!

Physical State / Flow | Fluids

Emotional & Mental State

Self-Care / Sleep | Dreams

W • APR 30

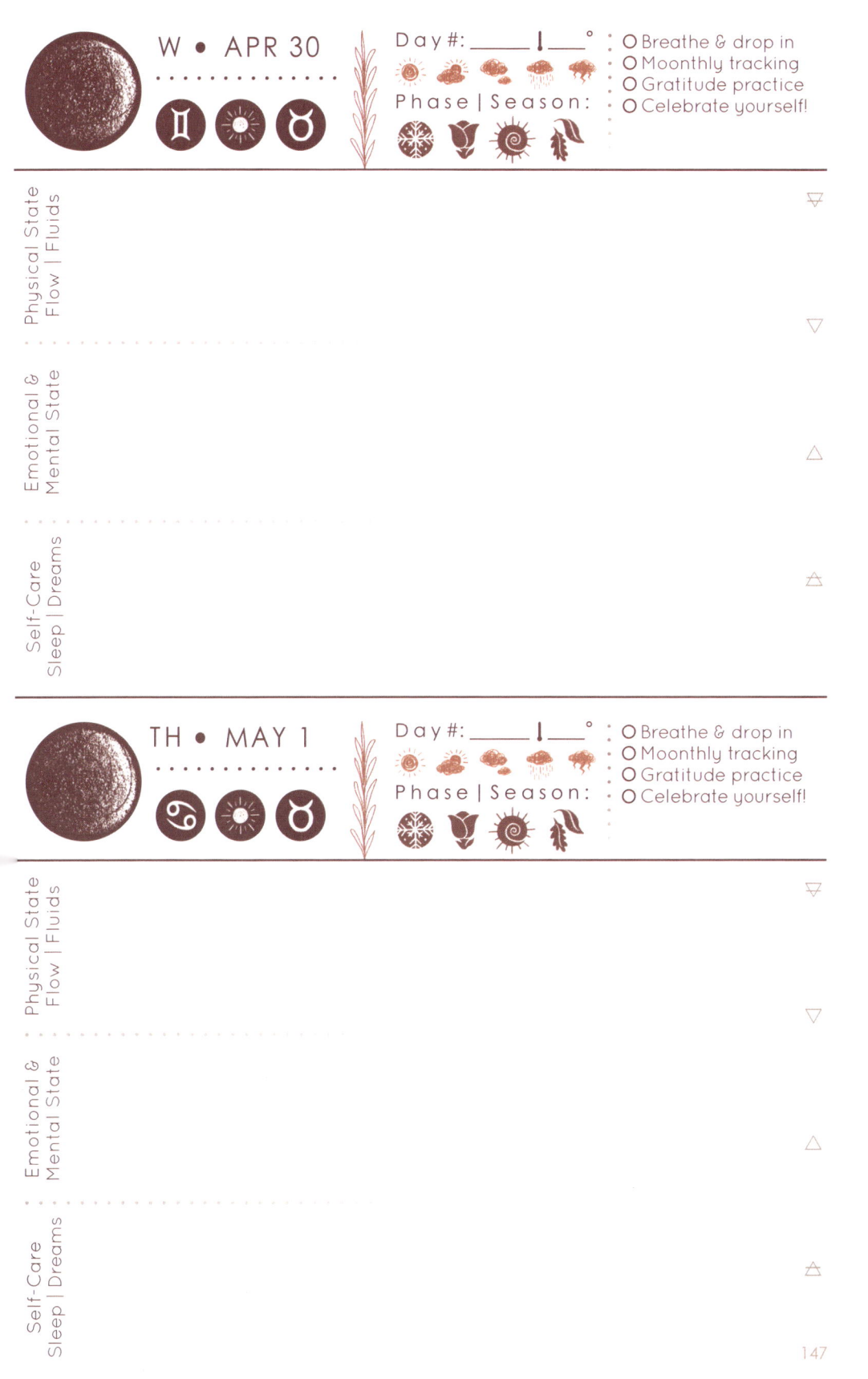

Day #: _____ | ___°

Phase | Season:

- ○ Breathe & drop in
- ○ Moonthly tracking
- ○ Gratitude practice
- ○ Celebrate yourself!

Physical State — Flow | Fluids

Emotional & Mental State

Self-Care — Sleep | Dreams

TH • MAY 1

Day #: _____ | ___°

Phase | Season:

- ○ Breathe & drop in
- ○ Moonthly tracking
- ○ Gratitude practice
- ○ Celebrate yourself!

Physical State — Flow | Fluids

Emotional & Mental State

Self-Care — Sleep | Dreams

F • MAY 2

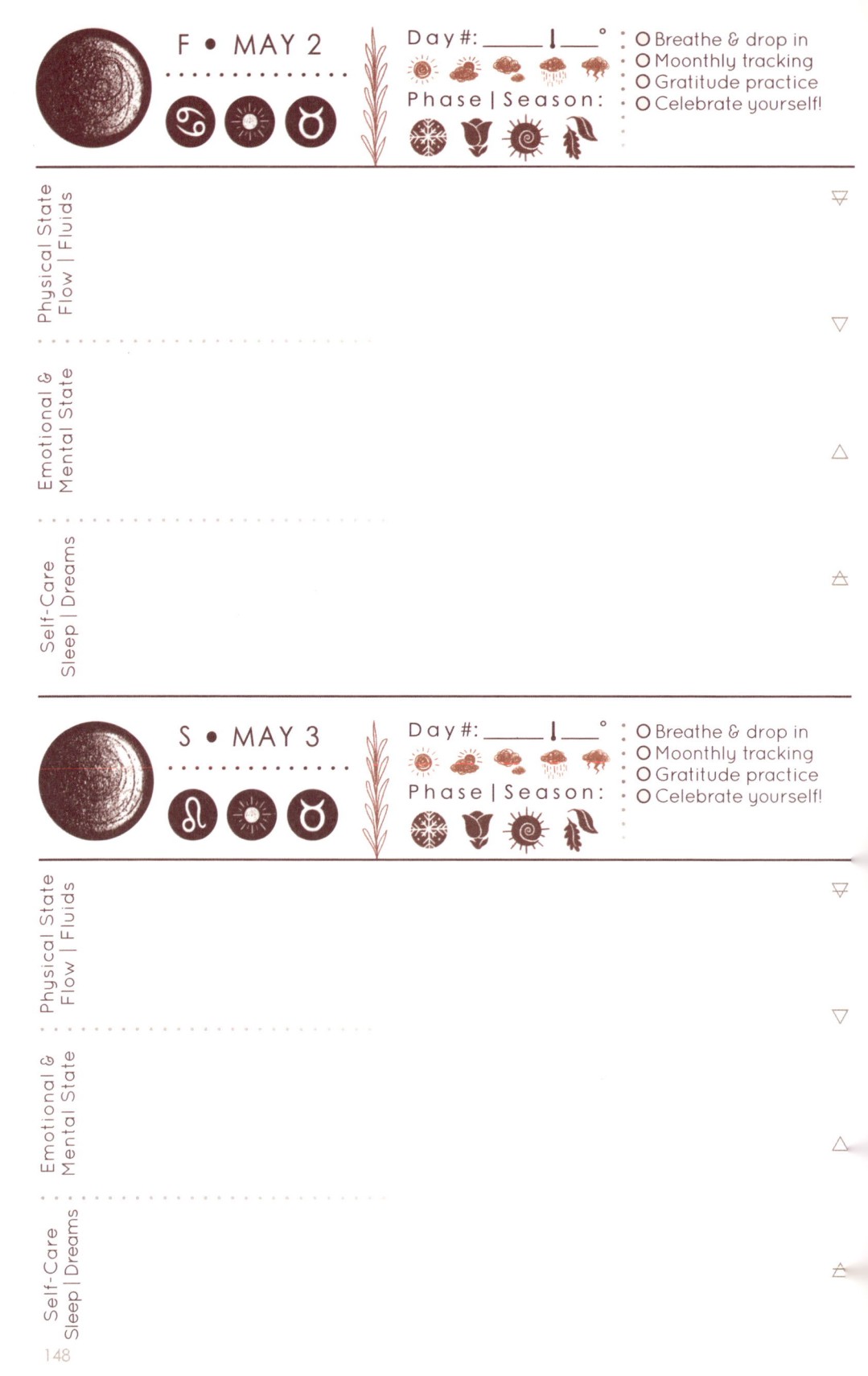

Day #: _____ | ___°

Phase | Season:

- ○ Breathe & drop in
- ○ Moonthly tracking
- ○ Gratitude practice
- ○ Celebrate yourself!

Physical State
Flow | Fluids

Emotional &
Mental State

Self-Care
Sleep | Dreams

S • MAY 3

Day #: _____ | ___°

Phase | Season:

- ○ Breathe & drop in
- ○ Moonthly tracking
- ○ Gratitude practice
- ○ Celebrate yourself!

Physical State
Flow | Fluids

Emotional &
Mental State

Self-Care
Sleep | Dreams

S • MAY 4

Day #: _____ | ___°
Phase | Season:

- ○ Breathe & drop in
- ○ Moonthly tracking
- ○ Gratitude practice
- ○ Celebrate yourself!

Physical State
Flow | Fluids

Emotional & Mental State

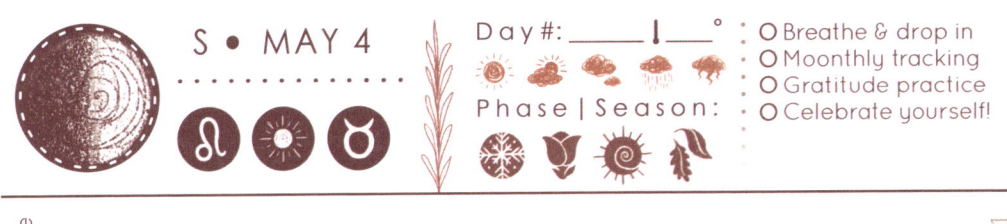

Self-Care
Sleep | Dreams

FIRST QUARTER IN LEO

Growing towards open expression & fulfillment

What is sprouting & coming into awareness?

What can I release to make space for further growth & grounding?

M • MAY 5

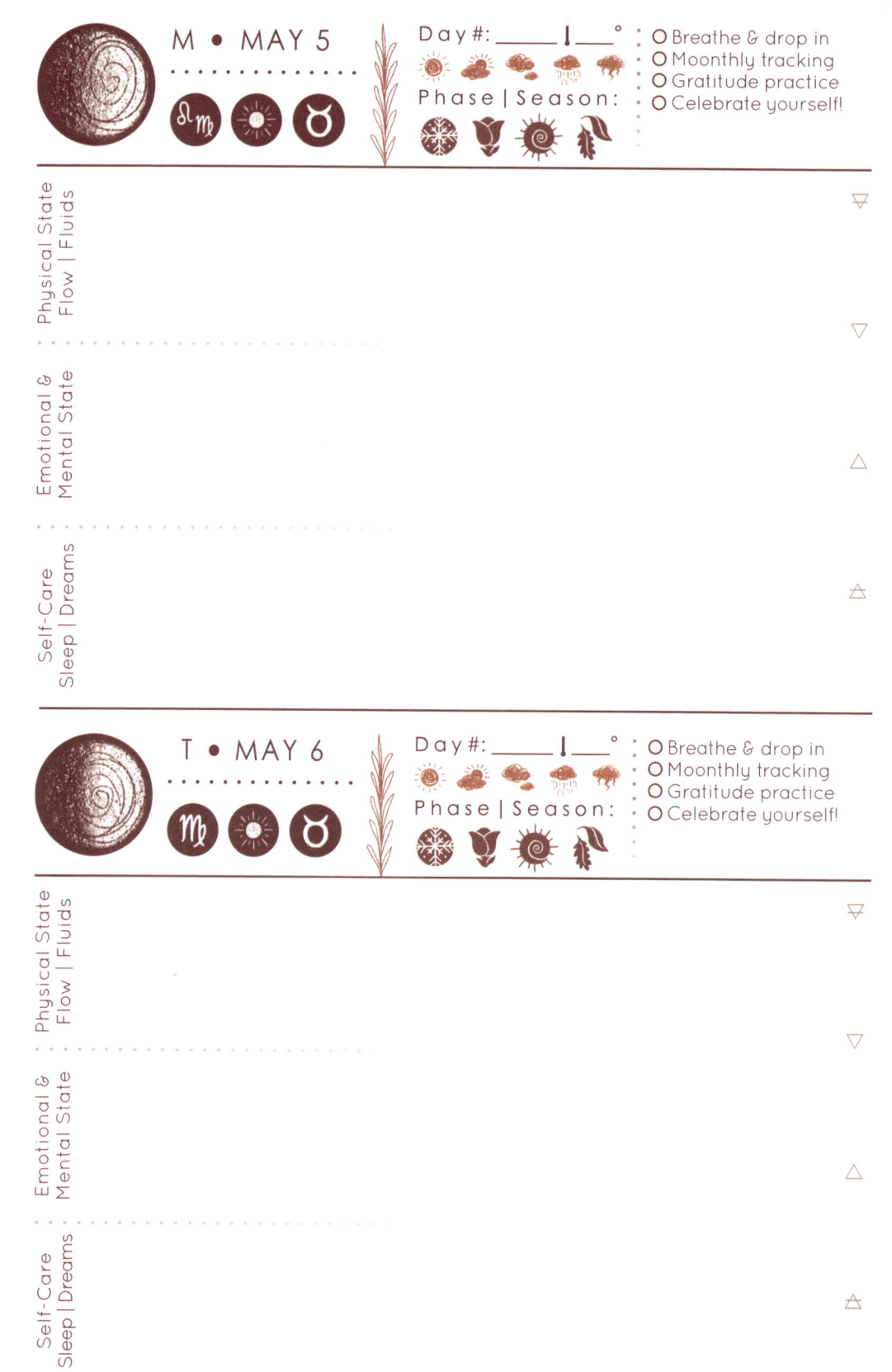

Day #: _____ | _____°

Phase | Season:

- ○ Breathe & drop in
- ○ Moonthly tracking
- ○ Gratitude practice
- ○ Celebrate yourself!

Physical State — Flow | Fluids

Emotional & Mental State

Self-Care — Sleep | Dreams

T • MAY 6

Day #: _____ | _____°

Phase | Season:

- ○ Breathe & drop in
- ○ Moonthly tracking
- ○ Gratitude practice
- ○ Celebrate yourself!

Physical State — Flow | Fluids

Emotional & Mental State

Self-Care — Sleep | Dreams

W • MAY 7

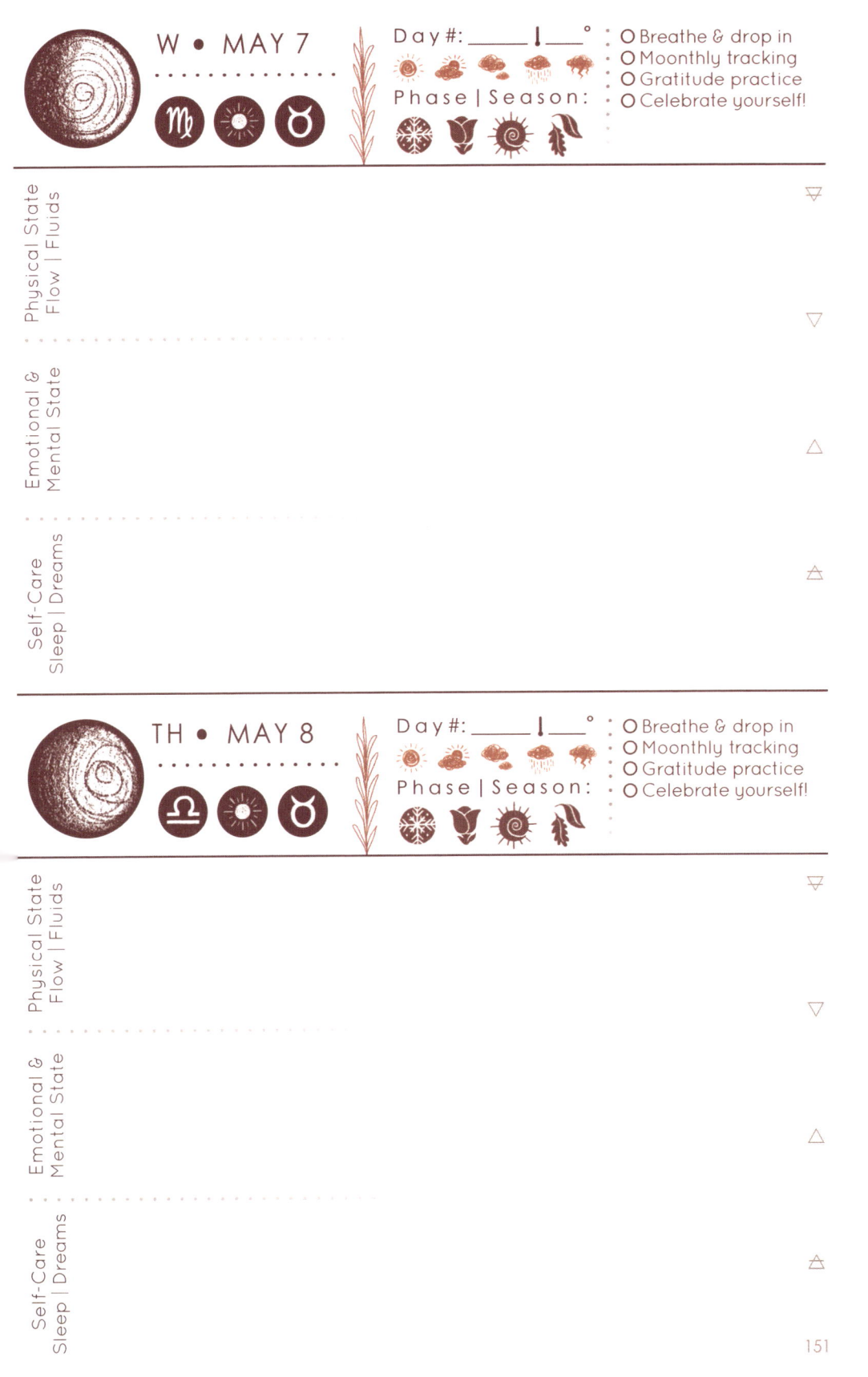

Day #: _____ | ___°

Phase | Season:

- Breathe & drop in
- Moonthly tracking
- Gratitude practice
- Celebrate yourself!

Physical State
Flow | Fluids

Emotional &
Mental State

Self-Care
Sleep | Dreams

TH • MAY 8

Day #: _____ | ___°

Phase | Season:

- Breathe & drop in
- Moonthly tracking
- Gratitude practice
- Celebrate yourself!

Physical State
Flow | Fluids

Emotional &
Mental State

Self-Care
Sleep | Dreams

F • MAY 9

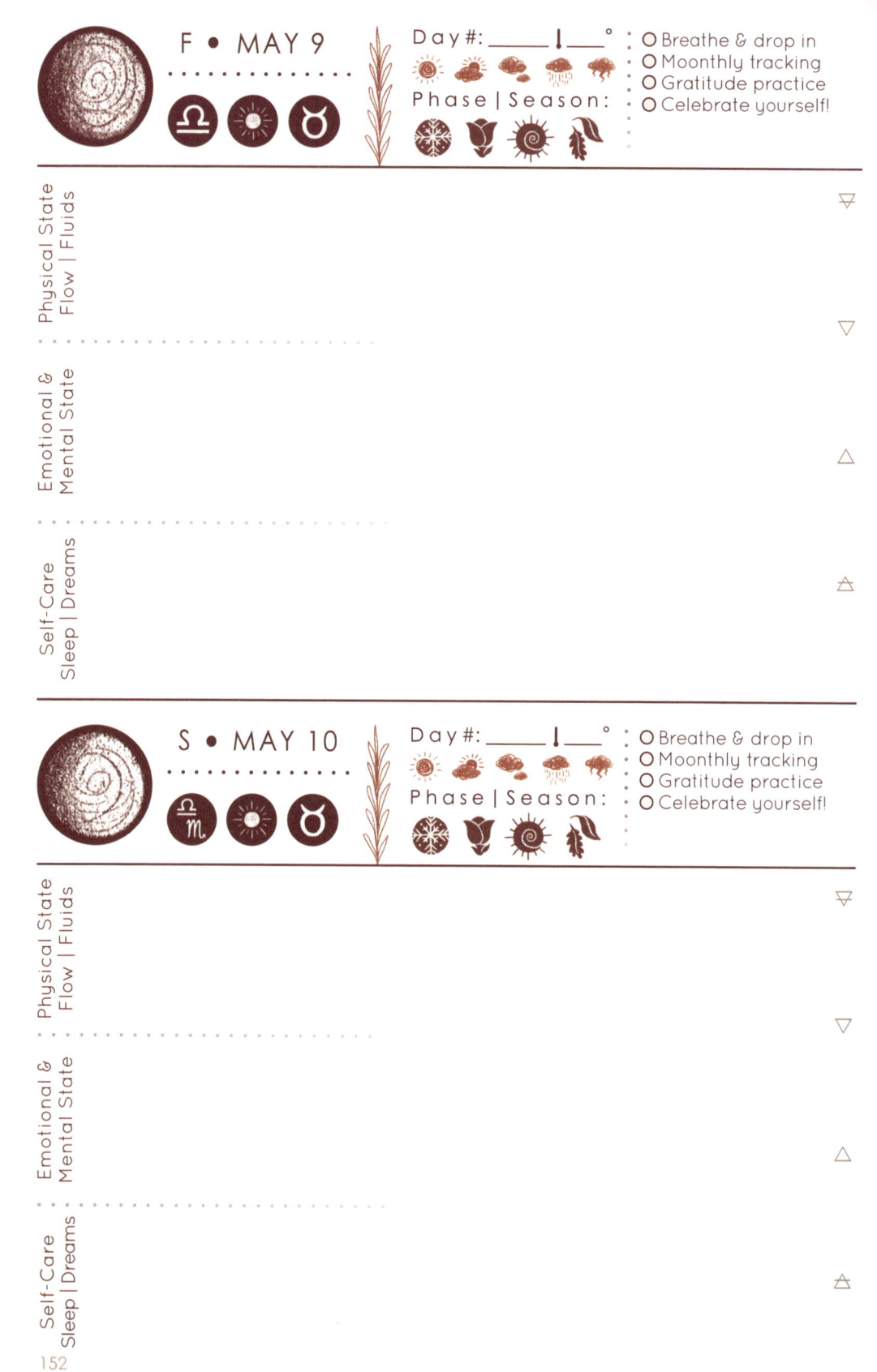

Day #: _____ | ____°

Phase | Season:

- O Breathe & drop in
- O Moonthly tracking
- O Gratitude practice
- O Celebrate yourself!

Physical State / Flow | Fluids

Emotional & Mental State

Self-Care / Sleep | Dreams

S • MAY 10

Day #: _____ | ____°

Phase | Season:

- O Breathe & drop in
- O Moonthly tracking
- O Gratitude practice
- O Celebrate yourself!

Physical State / Flow | Fluids

Emotional & Mental State

Self-Care / Sleep | Dreams

S • MAY 11

Day #: _____ | ___°

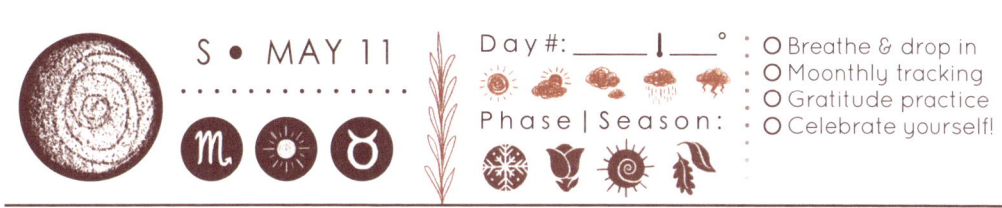

Phase | Season:

- Breathe & drop in
- Moonthly tracking
- Gratitude practice
- Celebrate yourself!

Physical State — Flow | Fluids

Emotional & Mental State

Self-Care — Sleep | Dreams

M • MAY 12

Day #: _____ | _____°

Phase | Season:

- Breathe & drop in
- Moonthly tracking
- Gratitude practice
- Celebrate yourself!

Physical State / Flow | Fluids

Emotional & Mental State

Self-Care / Sleep | Dreams

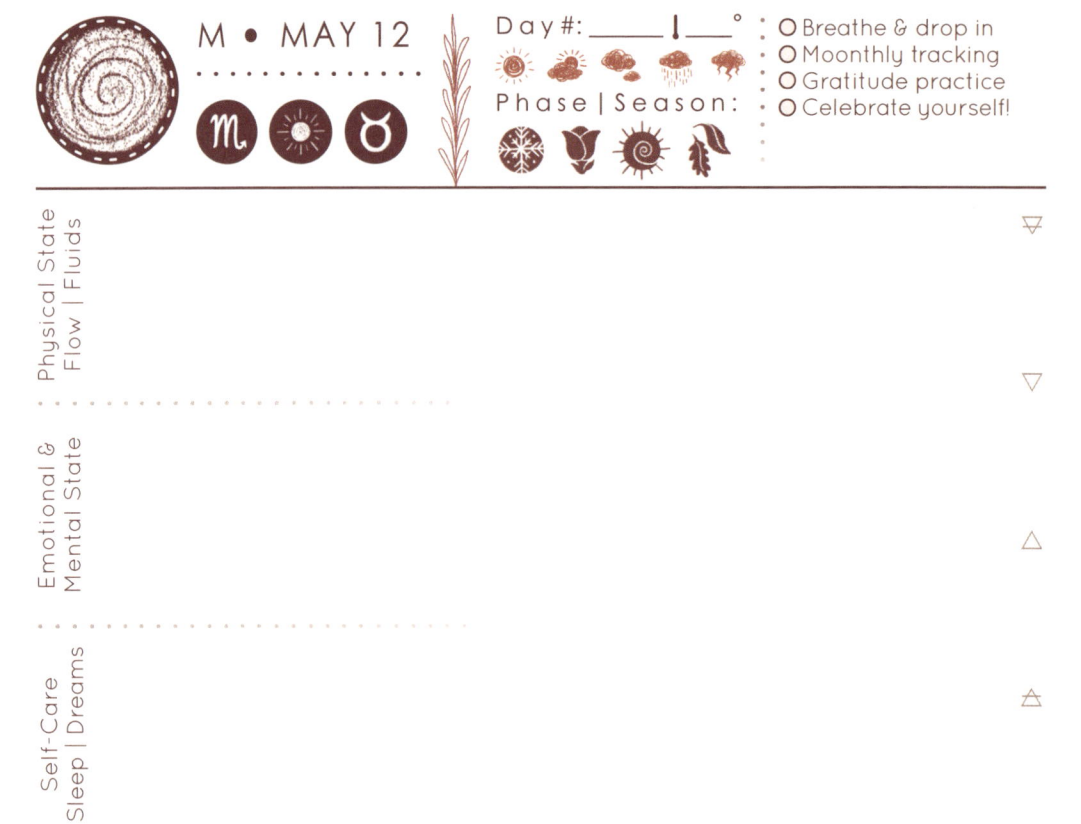

FULL MOON IN SCORPIO

Indulging in a deeper journey towards true pleasure

What is being illuminated?

I give gratitude for what is & what is becoming:

T • MAY 13

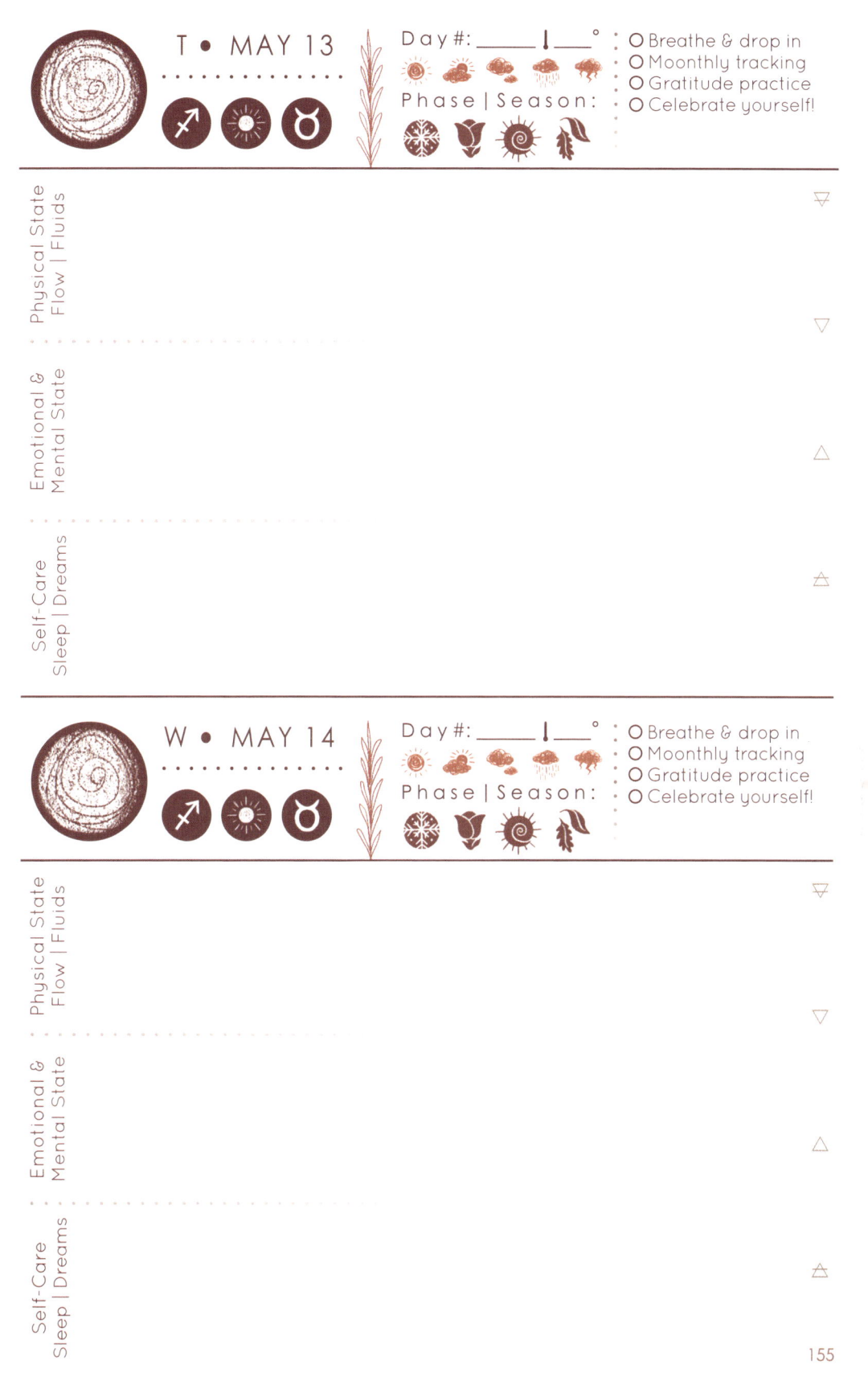

Day #: _____ | _____°

Phase | Season:

- ○ Breathe & drop in
- ○ Moonthly tracking
- ○ Gratitude practice
- ○ Celebrate yourself!

Physical State
Flow | Fluids

Emotional &
Mental State

Self-Care
Sleep | Dreams

W • MAY 14

Day #: _____ | _____°

Phase | Season:

- ○ Breathe & drop in
- ○ Moonthly tracking
- ○ Gratitude practice
- ○ Celebrate yourself!

Physical State
Flow | Fluids

Emotional &
Mental State

Self-Care
Sleep | Dreams

TH • MAY 15

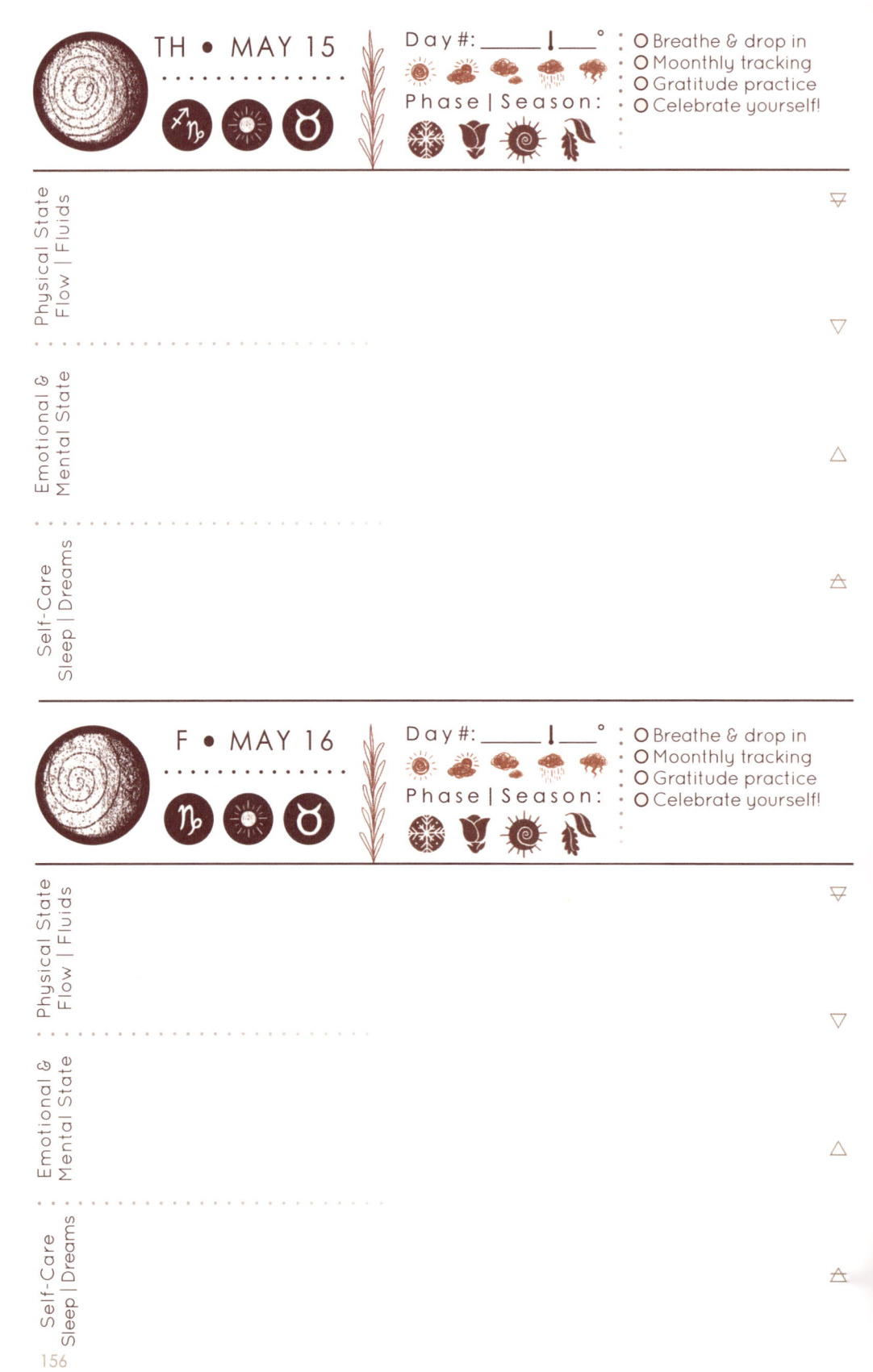

Day #: _____ | _____°

Phase | Season:

- ○ Breathe & drop in
- ○ Moonthly tracking
- ○ Gratitude practice
- ○ Celebrate yourself!

Physical State
Flow | Fluids

Emotional &
Mental State

Self-Care
Sleep | Dreams

F • MAY 16

Day #: _____ | _____°

Phase | Season:

- ○ Breathe & drop in
- ○ Moonthly tracking
- ○ Gratitude practice
- ○ Celebrate yourself!

Physical State
Flow | Fluids

Emotional &
Mental State

Self-Care
Sleep | Dreams

S • MAY 17

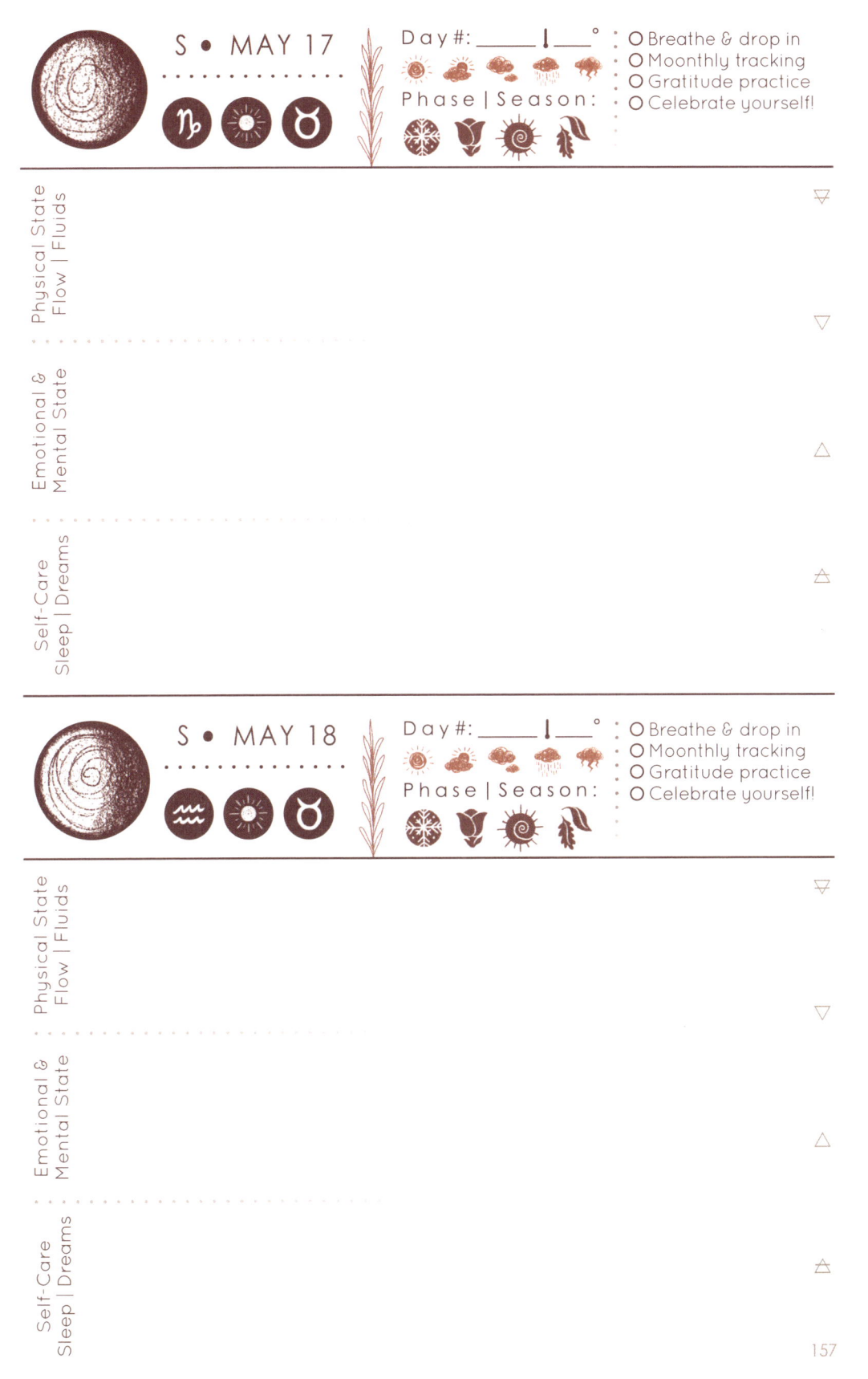

Day #: _____ | _____°

Phase | Season:

- ○ Breathe & drop in
- ○ Moonthly tracking
- ○ Gratitude practice
- ○ Celebrate yourself!

Physical State
Flow | Fluids

Emotional &
Mental State

Self-Care
Sleep | Dreams

S • MAY 18

Day #: _____ | _____°

Phase | Season:

- ○ Breathe & drop in
- ○ Moonthly tracking
- ○ Gratitude practice
- ○ Celebrate yourself!

Physical State
Flow | Fluids

Emotional &
Mental State

Self-Care
Sleep | Dreams

M • MAY 19

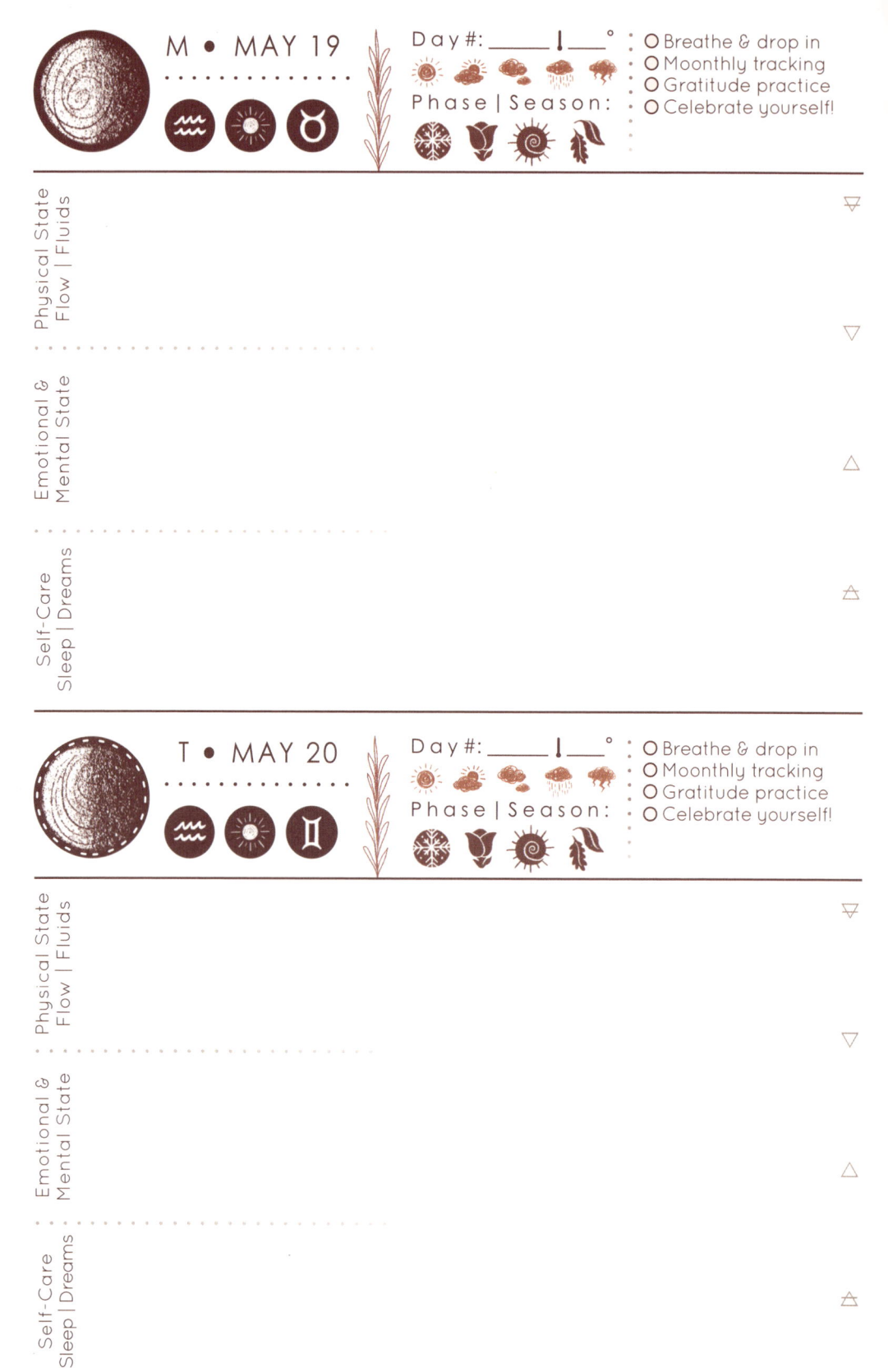

Day #: _____ | _____°

Phase | Season:

- Breathe & drop in
- Moonthly tracking
- Gratitude practice
- Celebrate yourself!

Physical State
Flow | Fluids

Emotional & Mental State

Self-Care
Sleep | Dreams

T • MAY 20

Day #: _____ | _____°

Phase | Season:

- Breathe & drop in
- Moonthly tracking
- Gratitude practice
- Celebrate yourself!

Physical State
Flow | Fluids

Emotional & Mental State

Self-Care
Sleep | Dreams

LAST QUARTER IN AQUARIUS

Releasing idealized situations that are not in alignment with higher truth

What am I leaving behind this lunar cycle?

Where can I make more space for reflection &/or integration?

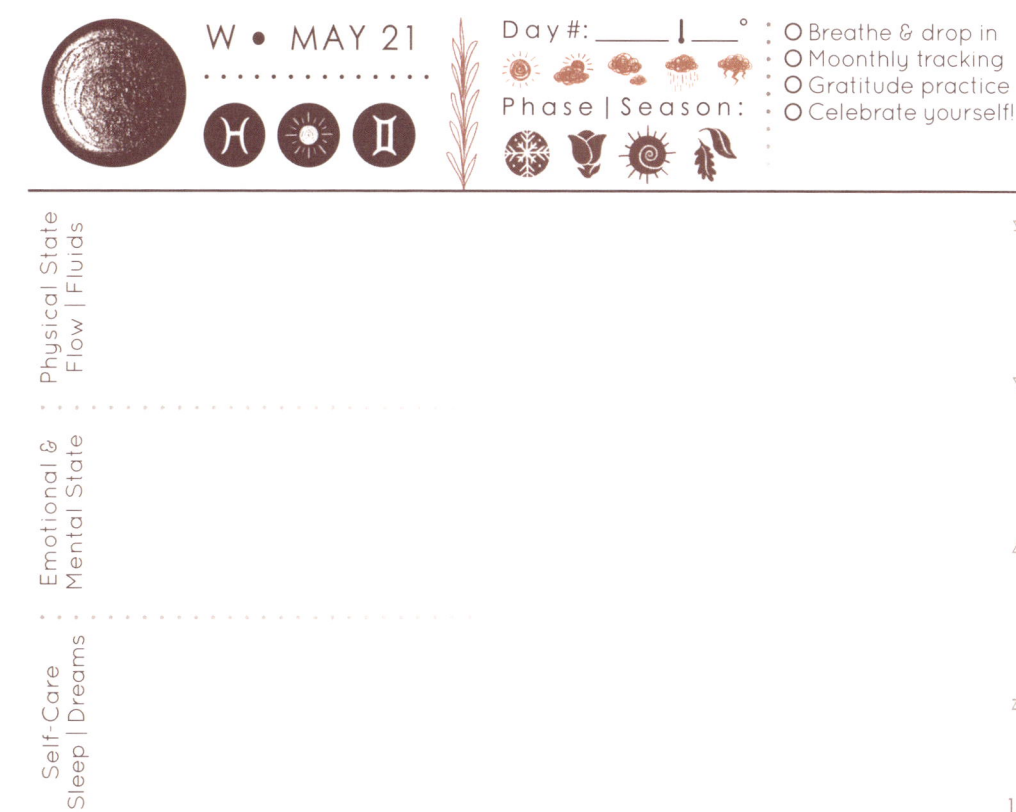

W • MAY 21

Day #: _____ | _____°
Phase | Season:

- ○ Breathe & drop in
- ○ Moonthly tracking
- ○ Gratitude practice
- ○ Celebrate yourself!

Physical State
Flow | Fluids

Emotional &
Mental State

Self-Care
Sleep | Dreams

TH • MAY 22

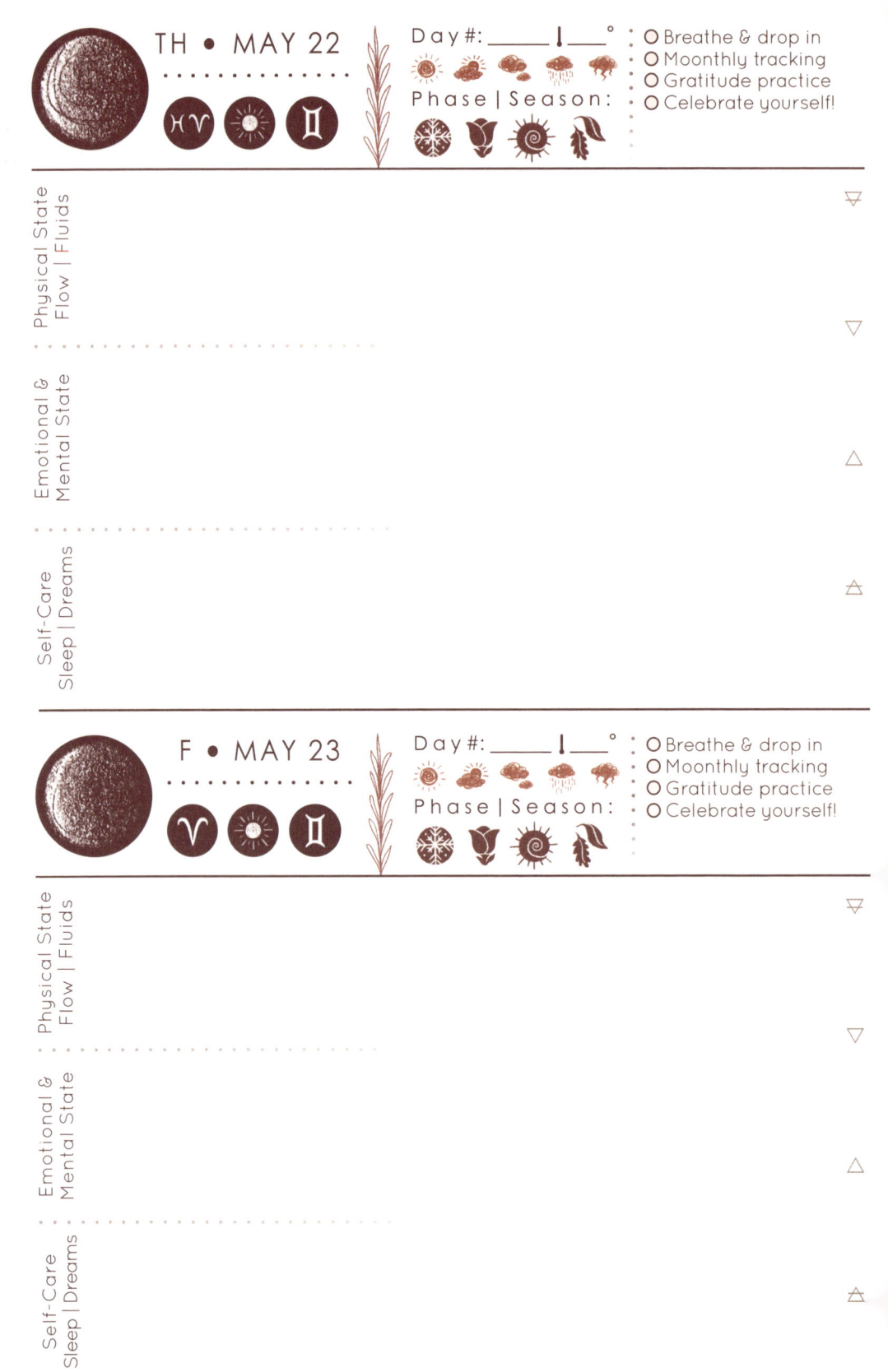

Day #: _____ | _____°

Phase | Season:

- ○ Breathe & drop in
- ○ Moonthly tracking
- ○ Gratitude practice
- ○ Celebrate yourself!

Physical State
Flow | Fluids

Emotional & Mental State

Self-Care
Sleep | Dreams

F • MAY 23

Day #: _____ | _____°

Phase | Season:

- ○ Breathe & drop in
- ○ Moonthly tracking
- ○ Gratitude practice
- ○ Celebrate yourself!

Physical State
Flow | Fluids

Emotional & Mental State

Self-Care
Sleep | Dreams

S • MAY 24

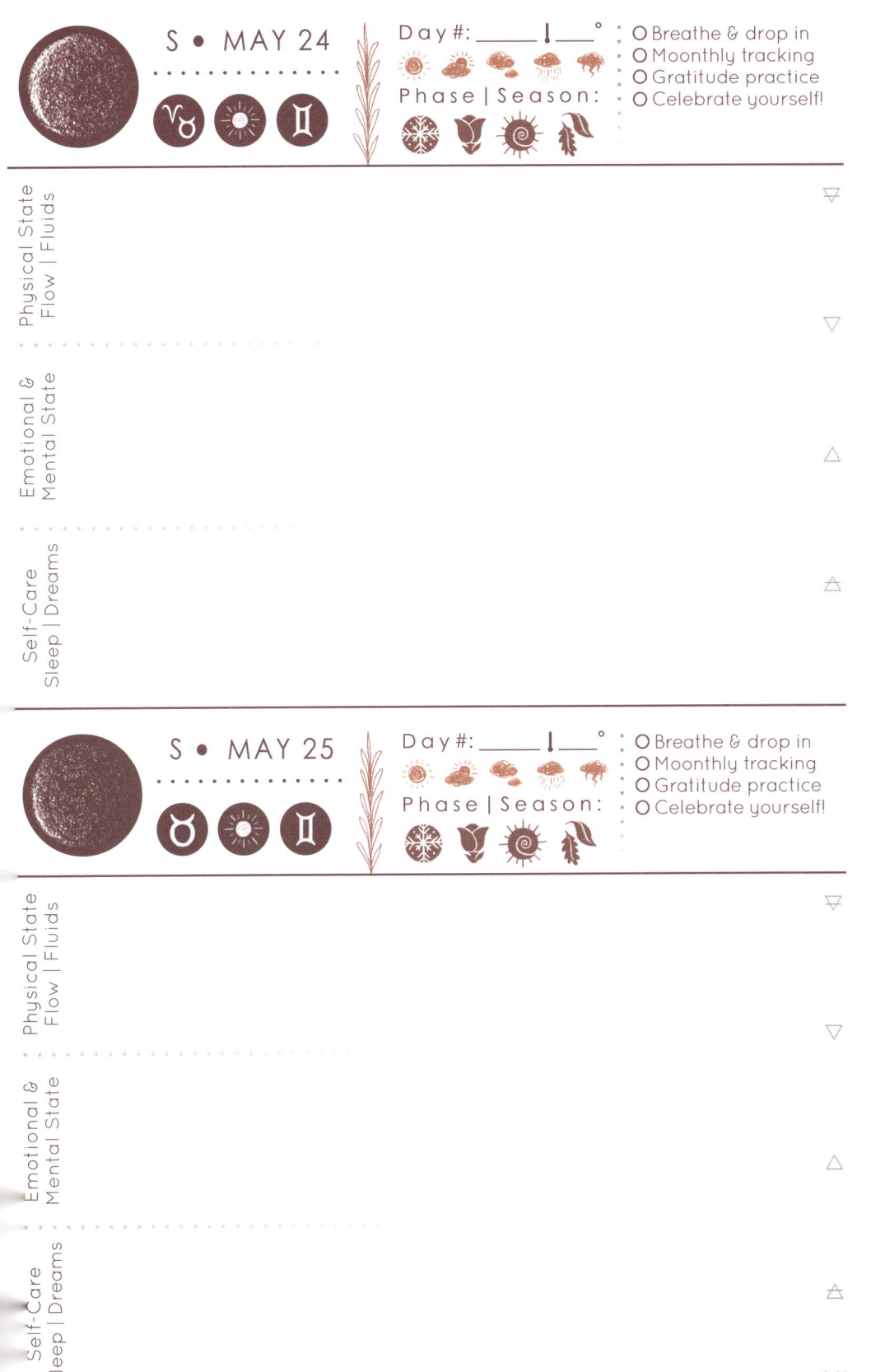

Day #: _____ | ____°

Phase | Season:

- Breathe & drop in
- Moonthly tracking
- Gratitude practice
- Celebrate yourself!

Physical State
Flow | Fluids

Emotional & Mental State

Self-Care
Sleep | Dreams

S • MAY 25

Day #: _____ | ____°

Phase | Season:

- Breathe & drop in
- Moonthly tracking
- Gratitude practice
- Celebrate yourself!

Physical State
Flow | Fluids

Emotional & Mental State

Self-Care
Sleep | Dreams

☾ 4th
04 | 27
05 | 25

CHECK IN & REFLECT

Last Cycle Day 1: _____

Last Cycle Length: _____

Circle the phase you bled near:

○ ☾ ☾ ☾ ● ● ● ● ☽ ☽ ☽ ○

Caution Days: (days I needed space) **Bliss Days:** (days I felt great)

Use this space to reflect on your experiences & findings from this ending lunar cycle or your last menstrual cycle. Use cycle day #s if you bleed, or moon phases if you don't.

SELF-CARE — What was helpful & nourishing?

OBSERVATIONS — Notice any changes or patterns?

DAYS TO NOTE — Which cycle days stood out?

162

PLAN & PREPARE

Next Predicted Cycle:
🩸 ☾ _____

CHECKLIST

Add the following to any other planners or calendars for your next cycle, then check it off.

- ☐ Predicted "days to note" _____
- ☐ Days to slow down (pre-bleed) _____
- ☐ Rest day(s) (next bleed) _____
- ☐ Date with yourself _____
- ☐ _____

- ☐ Self chest/breast exam
- ☐ Meal plan with cycle
- ☐ _____
- ☐ _____
- ☐ _____

OPEN SPACE

Use this space how you wish, or print out one of our free templates to paste here for BBT charting, dream tracking, or something else:

Embody your Ecosystems

by Rae (Rachael) Amber (they/she) • Intuitive Nature-Centric Channel & Artist • @rachael.amber • @embodiedecosystems • cyclicalroots.com •

We are beings of the Earthen elements – meaningful matter beyond magic. We are compilations and culminations of earth, water, firelight & air; states and phases of matter & spirit. We are here today because of these elements – that exist before us, within us, around us – and which connect us to all others. That of self, others, collective & spirit.

Slowly, through this realization, we remember our roots; we become less othered from and more unified with the planet we exist on and through. Without losing our centers, our essential individuality – the duality that must exist to transform beyond duality – we can embody the elements and rejoin our conscious selves to the ecosystems ever-present.

These are not separations or isolations, but starting points towards a wholeness that includes all. When we focus we have an anchor, and then the perceived separations can dissipate once we feel held.

The Elements of Our Ecosystems

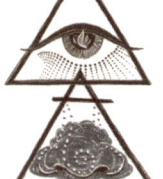

Firelight; our ocular systems; our vital vision, our insight and envisioned life force; reflected through the sunlight, warmth, energy & eyes.

Air; our nervous, auditory & respiratory systems; our atmosphere of awareness, the movement of mentality; reflected by sky, breath, thought, sound & scent.

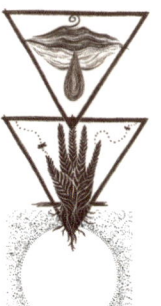

Water; our circulatory & digestive systems; our fluid forms, our felt sense and adaptability in functionality, and sensual emotion; reflected in water bodies, veins, vital organs, taste & digestion.

Earth; our musculoskeletal & skin systems; the meaning of matter, our primordial present body and tactile limbs; reflected by land, hands, sentient plants, soil & skin, feet & the touch of felt form.

Aether; our soul & spirit allies; our embodied archetypes; bodyscapes as a whole; sacred space & formlessness; interconnection.

Pick an element that resonates, or pull a card from your tarot deck. Let the element of its suit be your guide to which part of your inner ecosystem needs attention.

• Where do you feel this element in your body right now?

• What does it feel like? Can you connect it to an external environmental experience?

• How would the larger ecosystem naturally support this type of experience? (don't think it; feel it)

For more interconnective ecological somatics... check out the Embodied Ecosystems Tarot, guidebook, & practices.

Phasic Overview & In-Betweens

Use this space to focus on the phases of the moonth and the in-betweens of the peak lunations.

One way of using this space is to designate one column for your goal-planning, intention-setting or focus per phase/week. Use the other column for reflections, dream themes, nutrition tracking, cards pulls, etc!

M • MAY 26

Day #: _____ | _____°

Phase | Season:

- ○ Breathe & drop in
- ○ Moonthly tracking
- ○ Gratitude practice
- ○ Celebrate yourself!

Physical State / Flow | Fluids

Emotional & Mental State

Self-Care / Sleep | Dreams

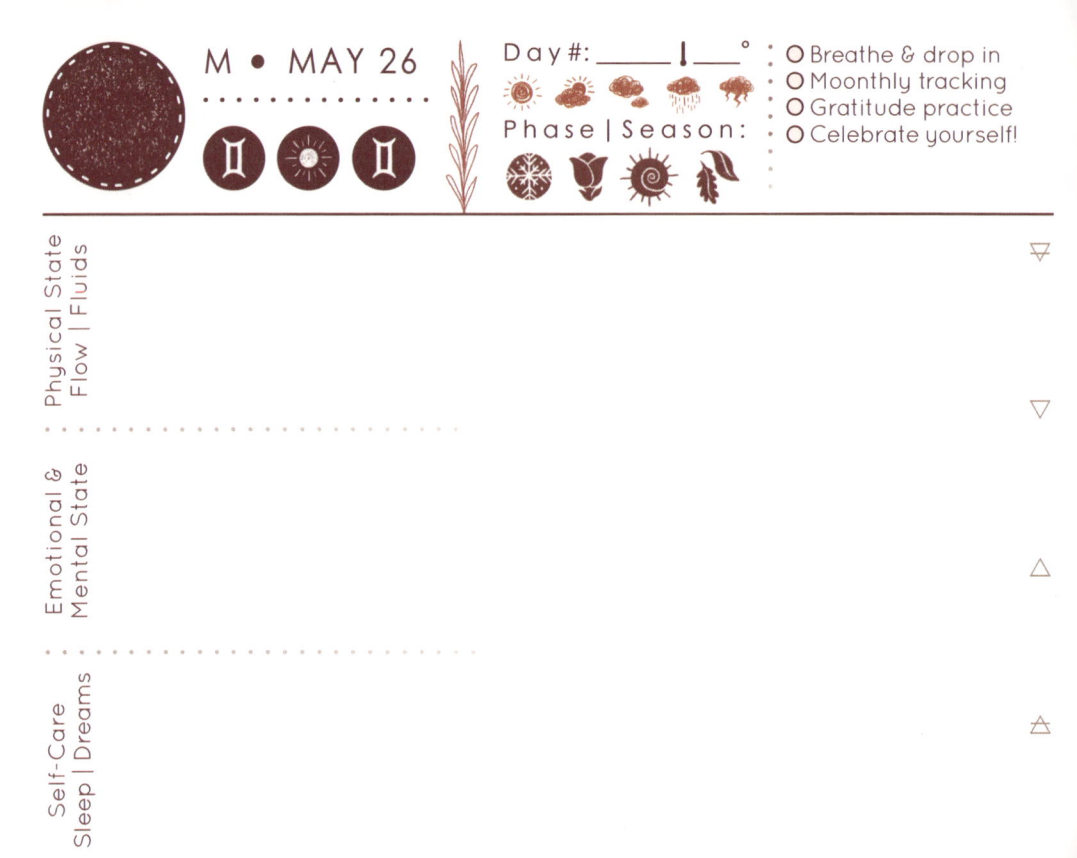

NEW MOON IN GEMINI

A renewed perspective of understanding & clarity

What do I want to grow & focus on during this lunar cycle?

How will I hold space for this?

T • MAY 27

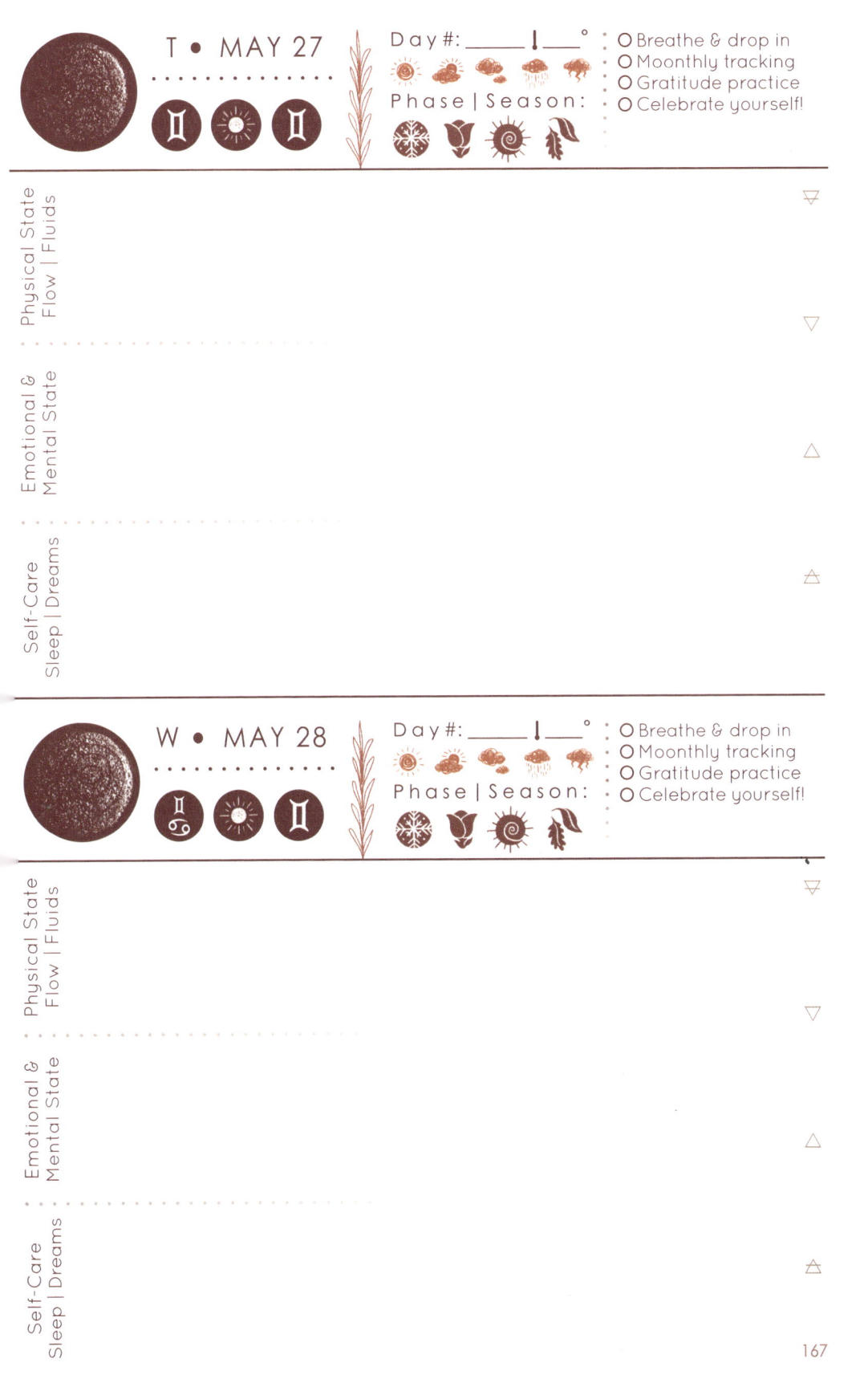

Day #: _____ | _____°

Phase | Season:

○ Breathe & drop in
○ Moonthly tracking
○ Gratitude practice
○ Celebrate yourself!

Physical State
Flow | Fluids

Emotional &
Mental State

Self-Care
Sleep | Dreams

W • MAY 28

Day #: _____ | _____°

Phase | Season:

○ Breathe & drop in
○ Moonthly tracking
○ Gratitude practice
○ Celebrate yourself!

Physical State
Flow | Fluids

Emotional &
Mental State

Self-Care
Sleep | Dreams

TH • MAY 29

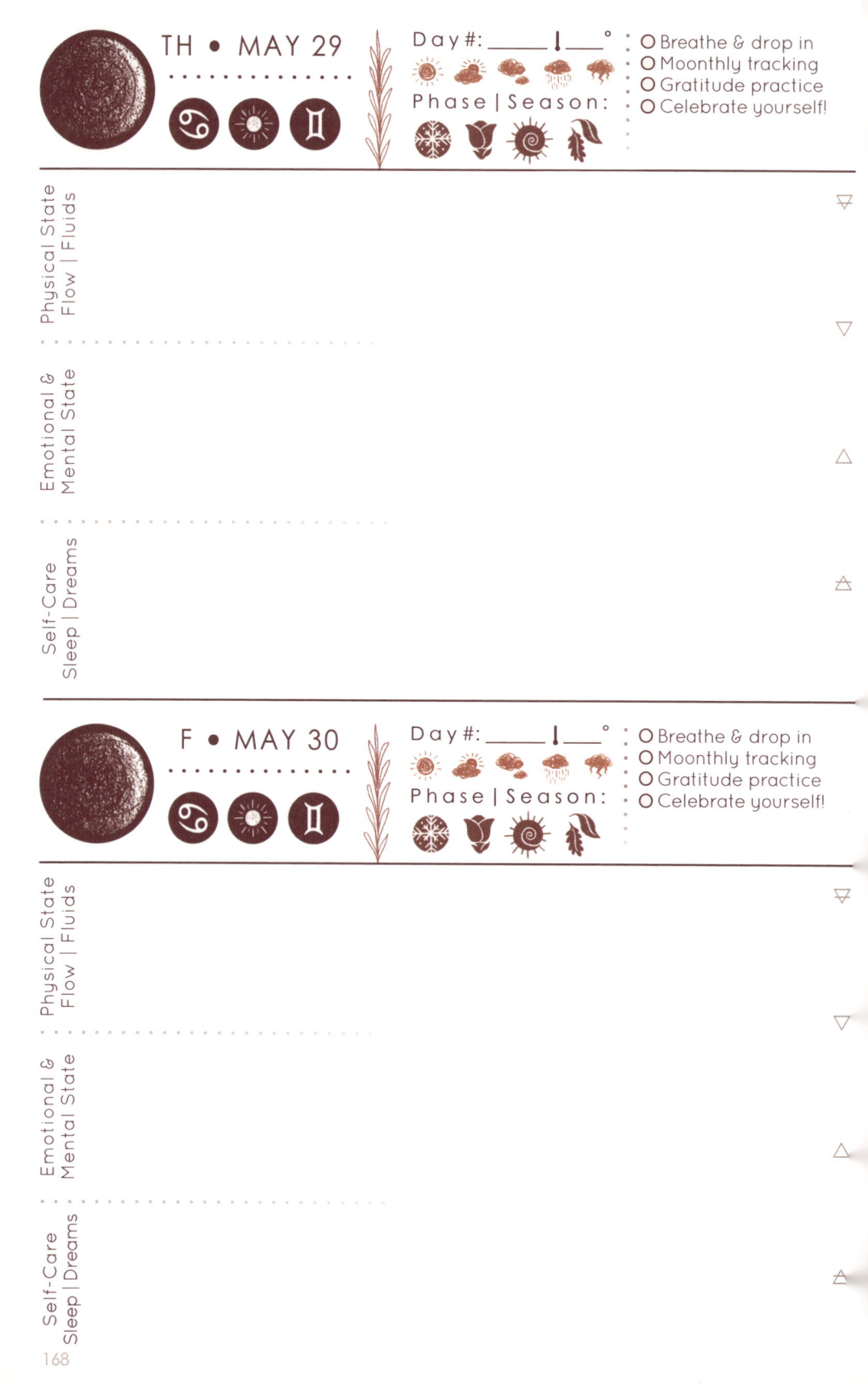

Day #: _____ | _____°

Phase | Season:

- ○ Breathe & drop in
- ○ Moonthly tracking
- ○ Gratitude practice
- ○ Celebrate yourself!

Physical State
Flow | Fluids

Emotional & Mental State

Self-Care
Sleep | Dreams

F • MAY 30

Day #: _____ | _____°

Phase | Season:

- ○ Breathe & drop in
- ○ Moonthly tracking
- ○ Gratitude practice
- ○ Celebrate yourself!

Physical State
Flow | Fluids

Emotional & Mental State

Self-Care
Sleep | Dreams

S • MAY 31

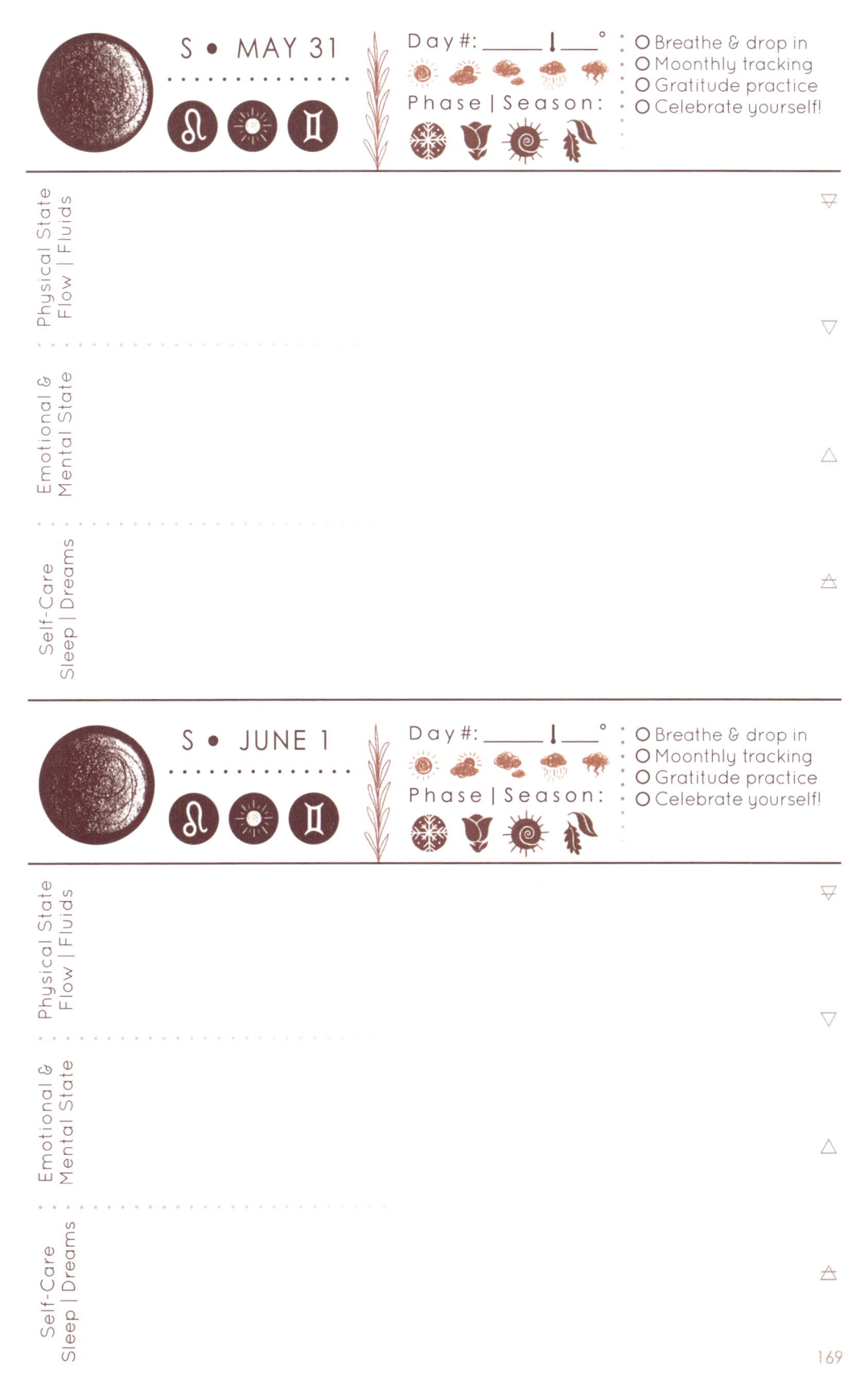

Day #: _____ | ___°

Phase | Season:

- ○ Breathe & drop in
- ○ Moonthly tracking
- ○ Gratitude practice
- ○ Celebrate yourself!

Physical State
Flow | Fluids

Emotional & Mental State

Self-Care
Sleep | Dreams

S • JUNE 1

Day #: _____ | ___°

Phase | Season:

- ○ Breathe & drop in
- ○ Moonthly tracking
- ○ Gratitude practice
- ○ Celebrate yourself!

Physical State
Flow | Fluids

Emotional & Mental State

Self-Care
Sleep | Dreams

M • JUNE 2

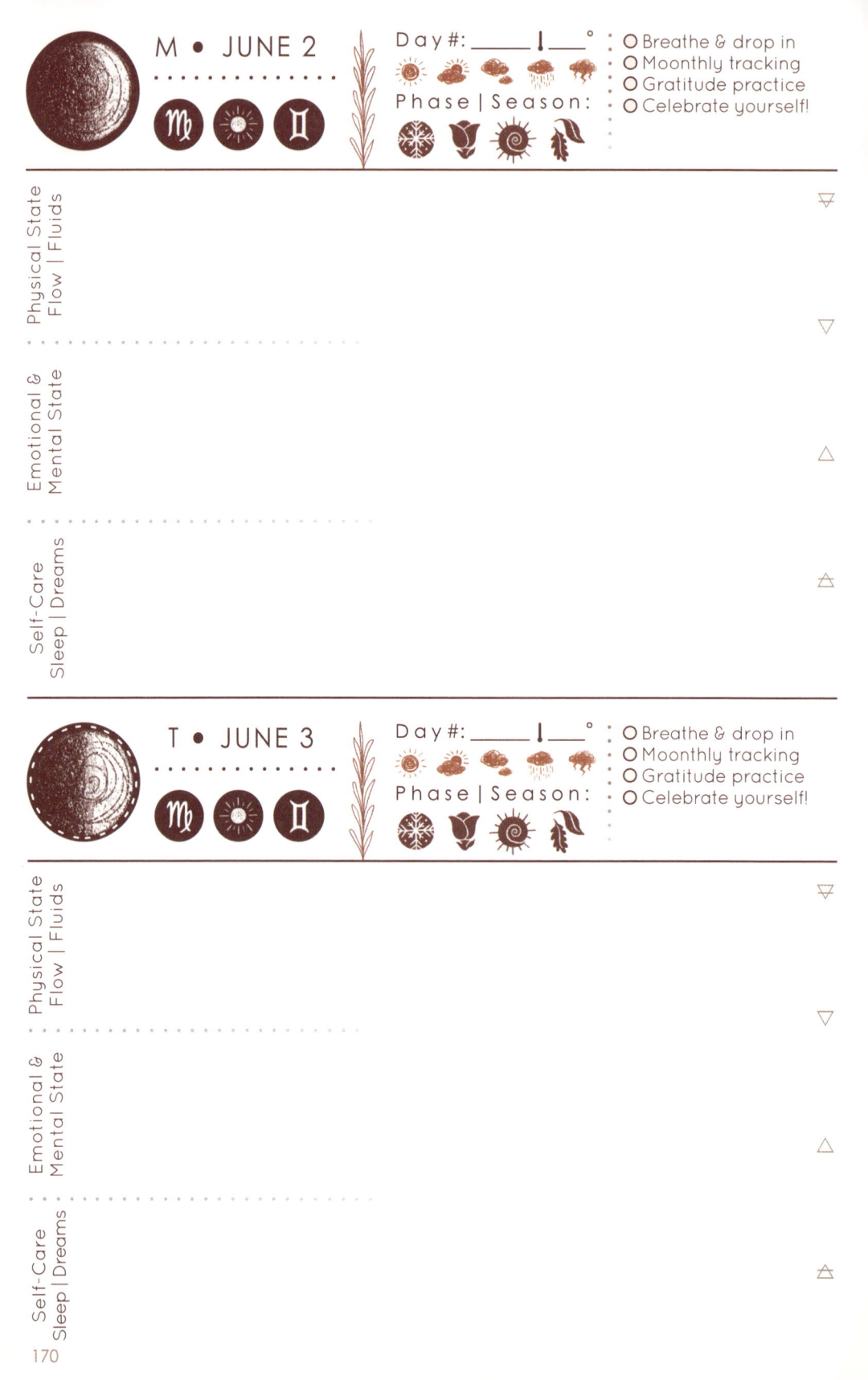

Day #: _____ | ___°

Phase | Season:

- ○ Breathe & drop in
- ○ Moonthly tracking
- ○ Gratitude practice
- ○ Celebrate yourself!

Physical State
Flow | Fluids

Emotional &
Mental State

Self-Care
Sleep | Dreams

T • JUNE 3

Day #: _____ | ___°

Phase | Season:

- ○ Breathe & drop in
- ○ Moonthly tracking
- ○ Gratitude practice
- ○ Celebrate yourself!

Physical State
Flow | Fluids

Emotional &
Mental State

Self-Care
Sleep | Dreams

FIRST QUARTER IN VIRGO

Unfolding into trusting, allowing & finding support

What is sprouting & coming into awareness?

What can I release to make space for further growth & grounding?

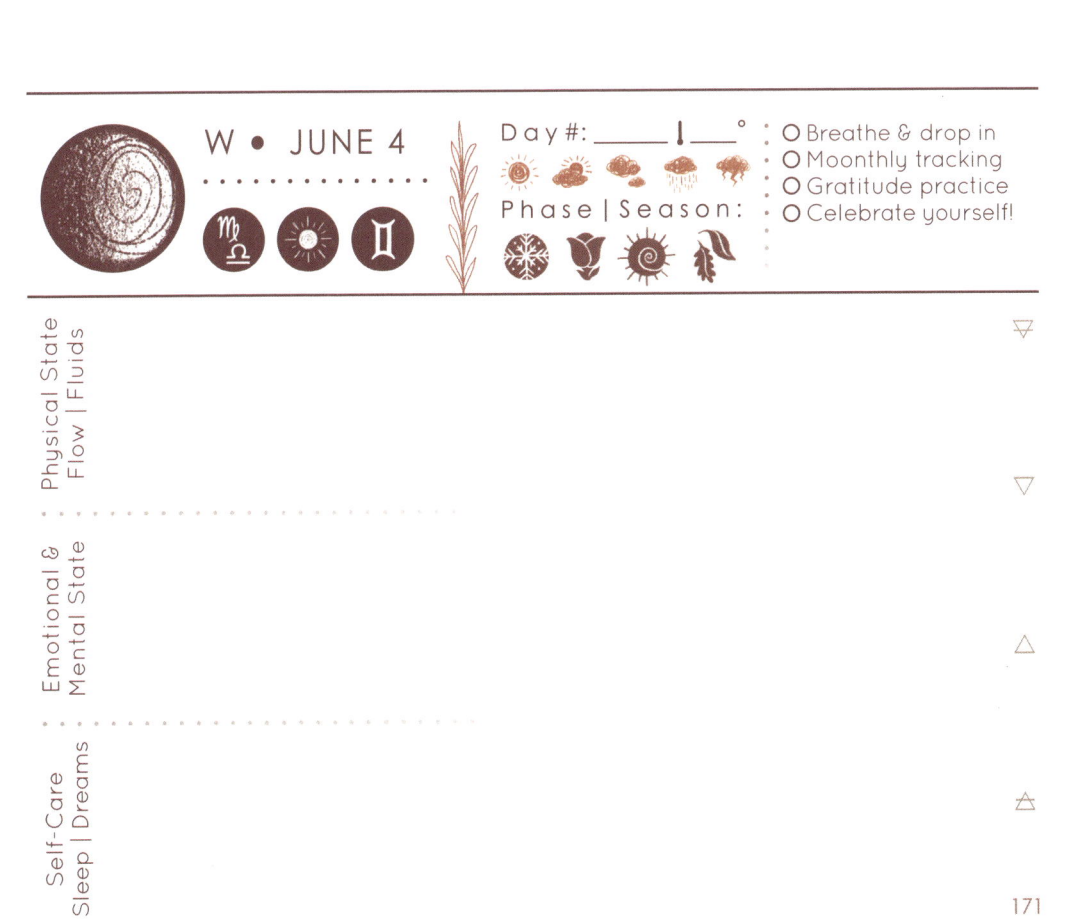

W • JUNE 4

Day #: _____ | _____°

Phase | Season:

○ Breathe & drop in
○ Moonthly tracking
○ Gratitude practice
○ Celebrate yourself!

Physical State
Flow | Fluids

Emotional &
Mental State

Self-Care
Sleep | Dreams

TH • JUNE 5

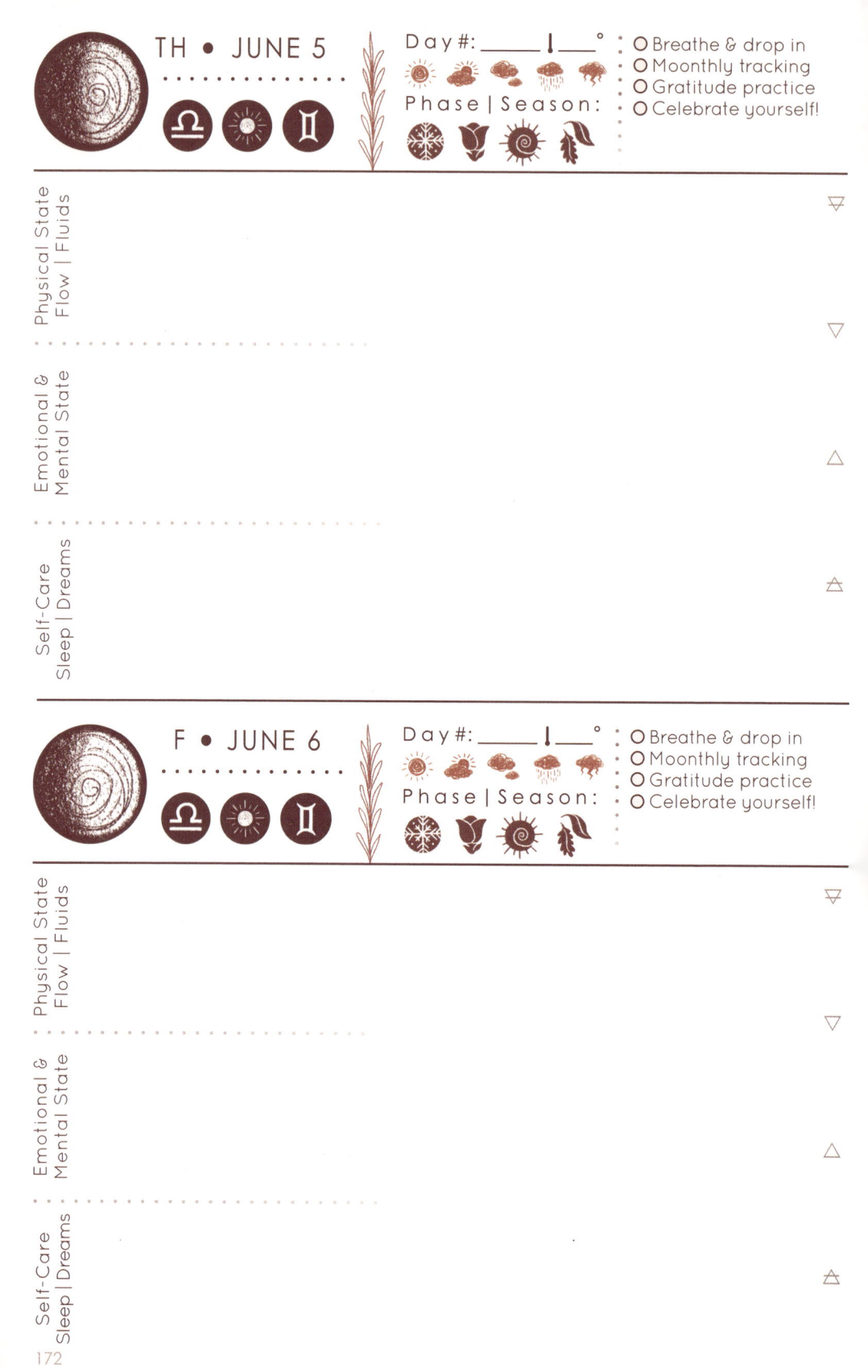

Day #: _____ | _____°

Phase | Season:

- ⚪ Breathe & drop in
- ⚪ Moonthly tracking
- ⚪ Gratitude practice
- ⚪ Celebrate yourself!

Physical State / Flow | Fluids

Emotional & Mental State

Self-Care / Sleep | Dreams

F • JUNE 6

Day #: _____ | _____°

Phase | Season:

- ⚪ Breathe & drop in
- ⚪ Moonthly tracking
- ⚪ Gratitude practice
- ⚪ Celebrate yourself!

Physical State / Flow | Fluids

Emotional & Mental State

Self-Care / Sleep | Dreams

S • JUNE 7

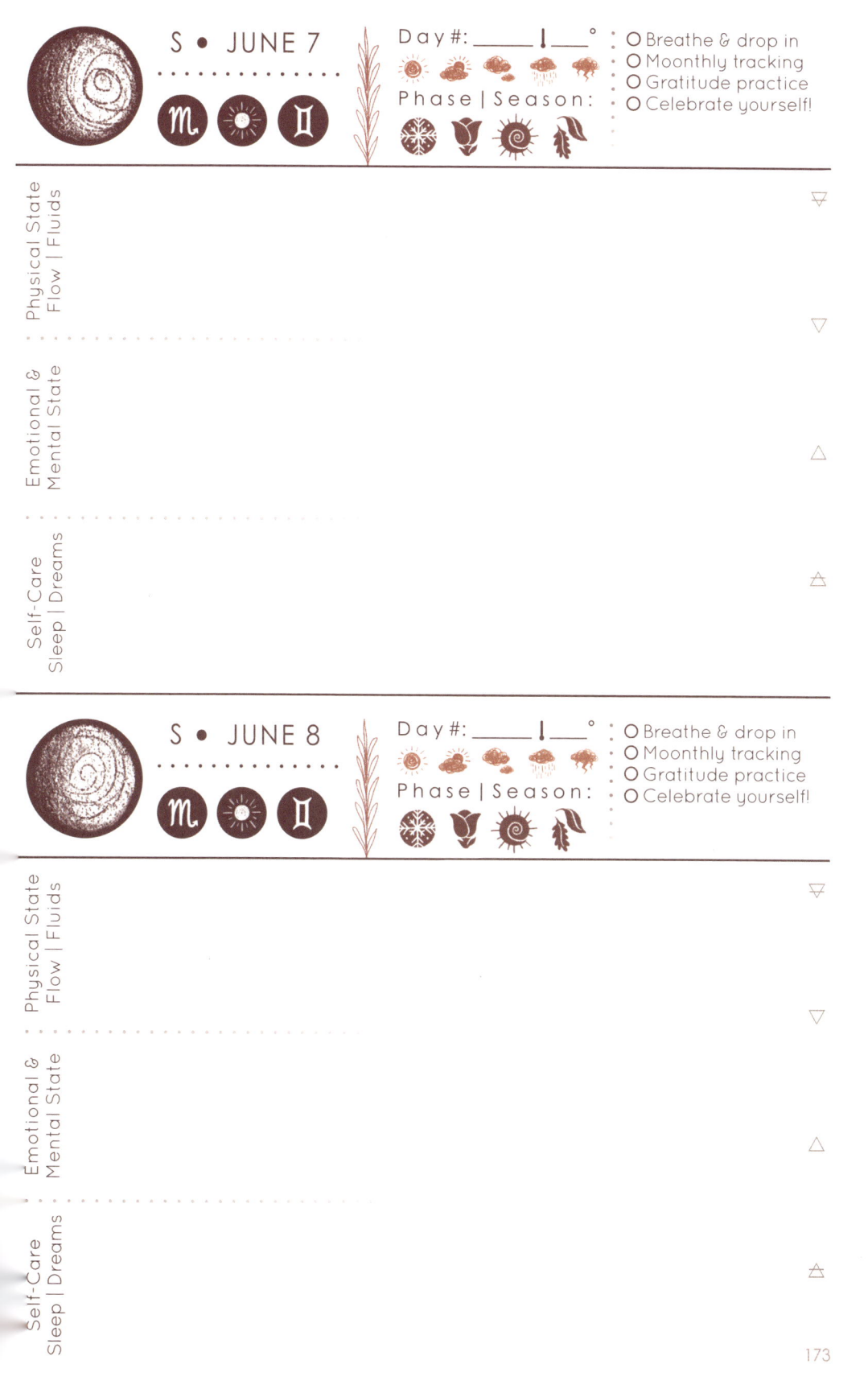

Day #: _____ | ___°

Phase | Season:

- ◯ Breathe & drop in
- ◯ Moonthly tracking
- ◯ Gratitude practice
- ◯ Celebrate yourself!

Physical State
Flow | Fluids

Emotional &
Mental State

Self-Care
Sleep | Dreams

S • JUNE 8

Day #: _____ | ___°

Phase | Season:

- ◯ Breathe & drop in
- ◯ Moonthly tracking
- ◯ Gratitude practice
- ◯ Celebrate yourself!

Physical State
Flow | Fluids

Emotional &
Mental State

Self-Care
Sleep | Dreams

M • JUNE 9

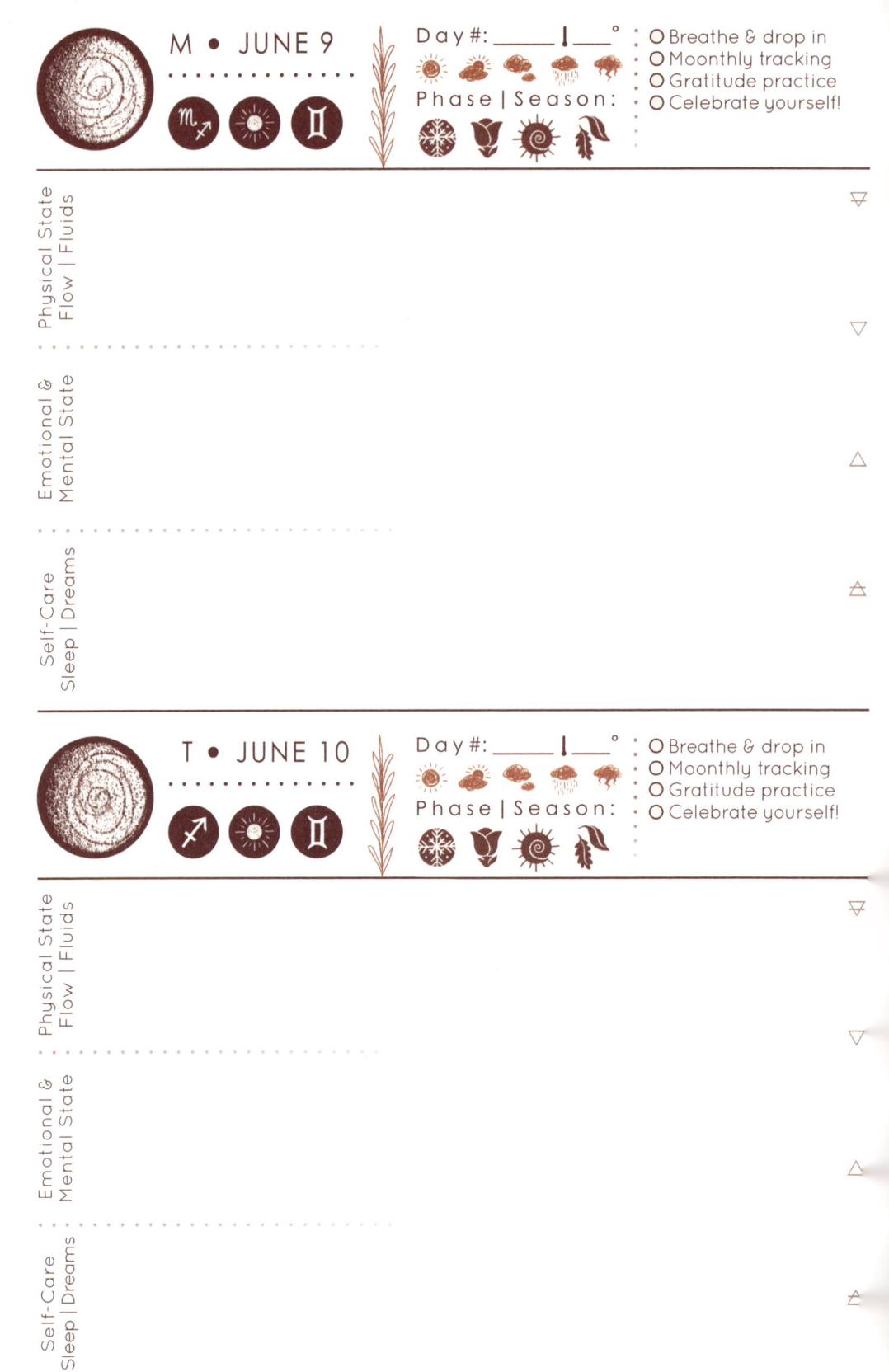

Day #: _____ | _____°
Phase | Season:

- ○ Breathe & drop in
- ○ Moonthly tracking
- ○ Gratitude practice
- ○ Celebrate yourself!

Physical State
Flow | Fluids

Emotional &
Mental State

Self-Care
Sleep | Dreams

T • JUNE 10

Day #: _____ | _____°
Phase | Season:

- ○ Breathe & drop in
- ○ Moonthly tracking
- ○ Gratitude practice
- ○ Celebrate yourself!

Physical State
Flow | Fluids

Emotional &
Mental State

Self-Care
Sleep | Dreams

174

W • JUNE 11

Day #: _____ | _____°

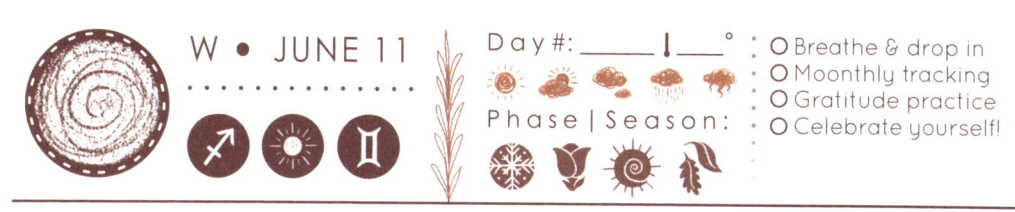

Phase | Season:

- ○ Breathe & drop in
- ○ Moonthly tracking
- ○ Gratitude practice
- ○ Celebrate yourself!

Physical State / Flow | Fluids

Emotional & Mental State

Self-Care / Sleep | Dreams

FULL MOON IN SAGITTARIUS

Expanding into curiosity & exploration for a higher purpose

What is being illuminated?

I give gratitude for what is & what is becoming:

TH • JUNE 12

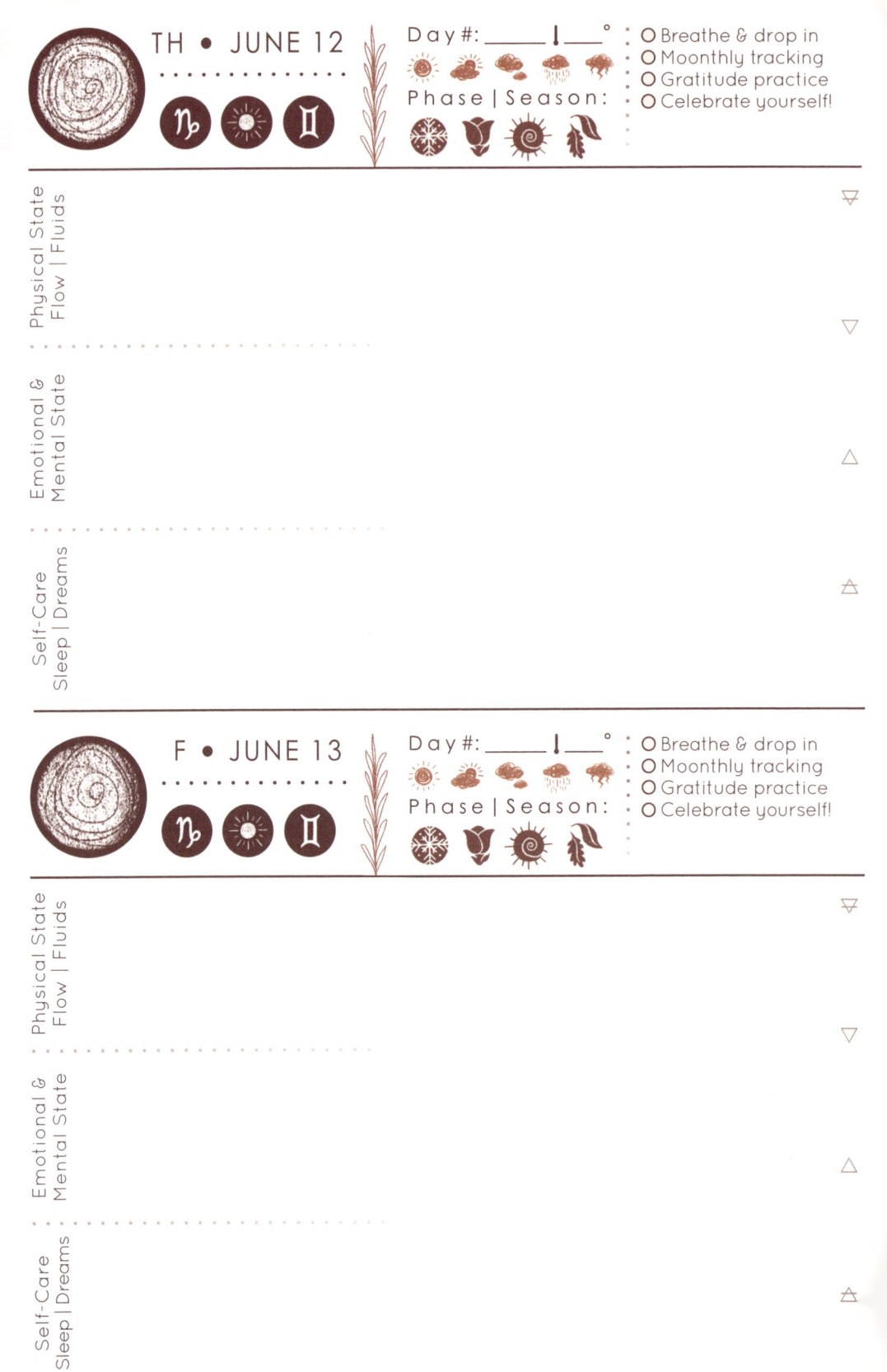

Day #: _____ | _____°

Phase | Season:

- ○ Breathe & drop in
- ○ Moonthly tracking
- ○ Gratitude practice
- ○ Celebrate yourself!

Physical State / Flow | Fluids

Emotional & Mental State

Self-Care / Sleep | Dreams

F • JUNE 13

Day #: _____ | _____°

Phase | Season:

- ○ Breathe & drop in
- ○ Moonthly tracking
- ○ Gratitude practice
- ○ Celebrate yourself!

Physical State / Flow | Fluids

Emotional & Mental State

Self-Care / Sleep | Dreams

S • JUNE 14

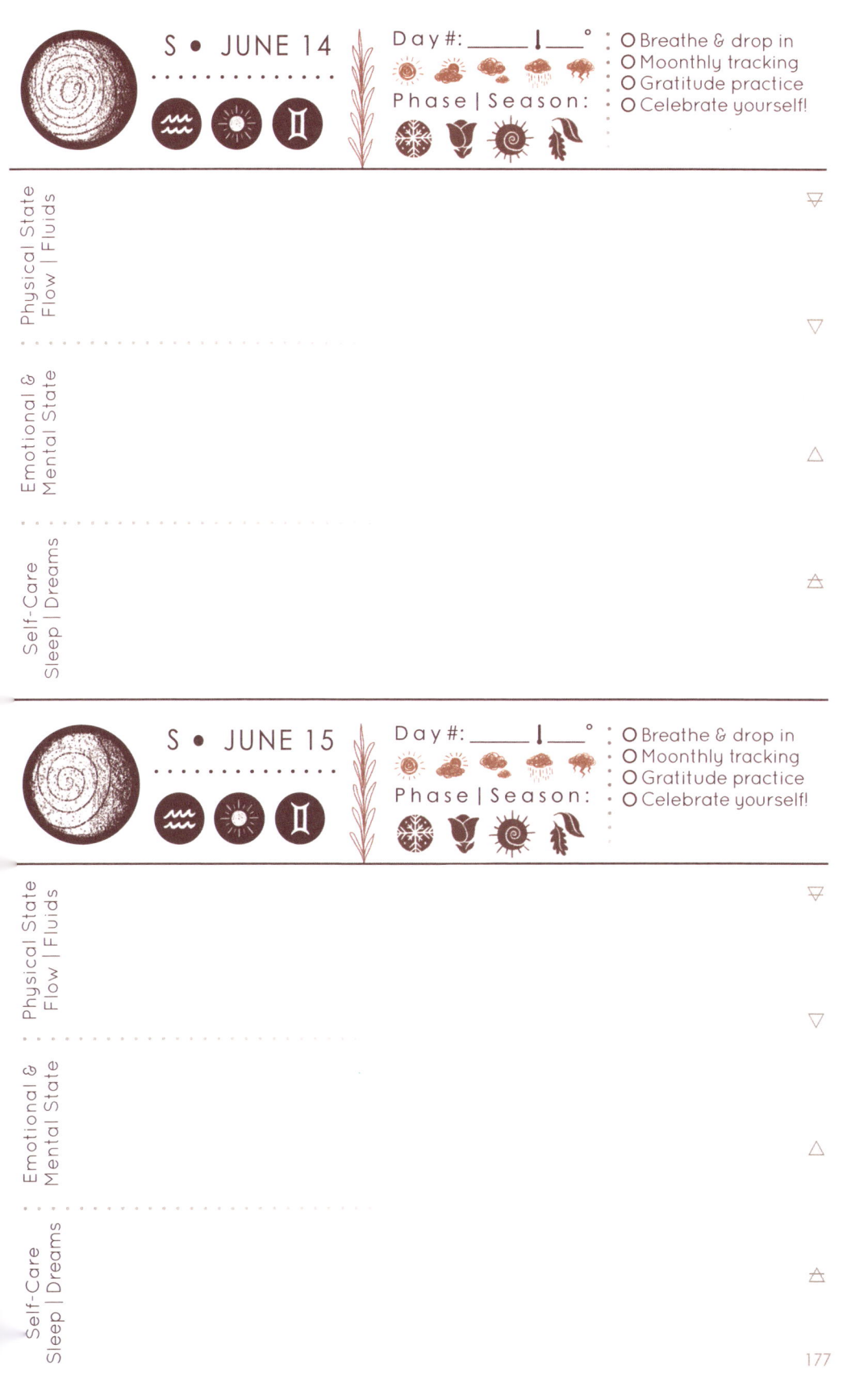

Day #: _____ | _____°

Phase | Season:

- ○ Breathe & drop in
- ○ Moonthly tracking
- ○ Gratitude practice
- ○ Celebrate yourself!

Physical State / Flow | Fluids

Emotional & Mental State

Self-Care / Sleep | Dreams

S • JUNE 15

Day #: _____ | _____°

Phase | Season:

- ○ Breathe & drop in
- ○ Moonthly tracking
- ○ Gratitude practice
- ○ Celebrate yourself!

Physical State / Flow | Fluids

Emotional & Mental State

Self-Care / Sleep | Dreams

M • JUNE 16

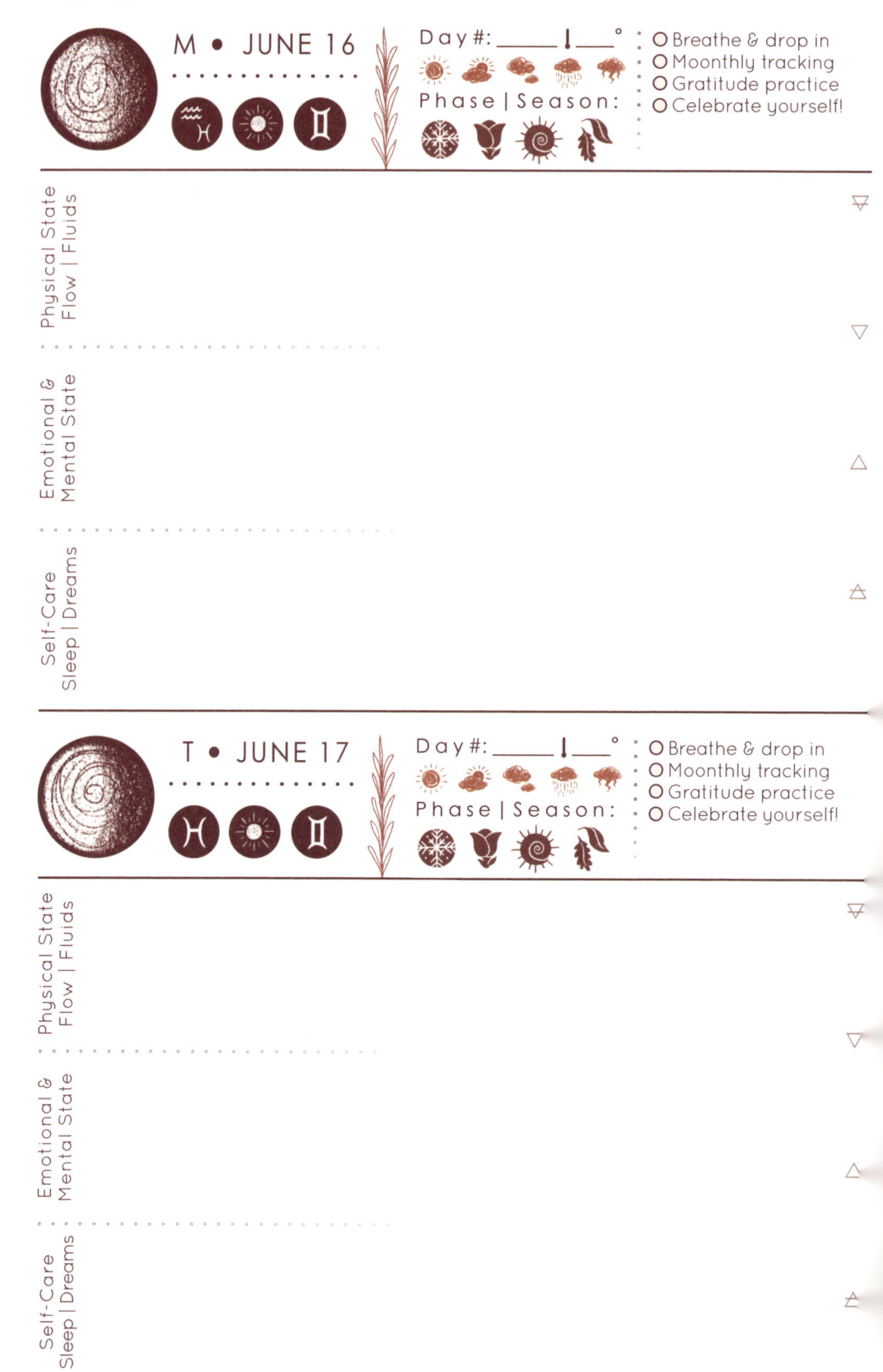

Day #: _____ | ___°

Phase | Season:

- ○ Breathe & drop in
- ○ Moonthly tracking
- ○ Gratitude practice
- ○ Celebrate yourself!

Physical State / Flow | Fluids

Emotional & Mental State

Self-Care / Sleep | Dreams

T • JUNE 17

Day #: _____ | ___°

Phase | Season:

- ○ Breathe & drop in
- ○ Moonthly tracking
- ○ Gratitude practice
- ○ Celebrate yourself!

Physical State / Flow | Fluids

Emotional & Mental State

Self-Care / Sleep | Dreams

W • JUNE 18

Day #: _____ | ___°

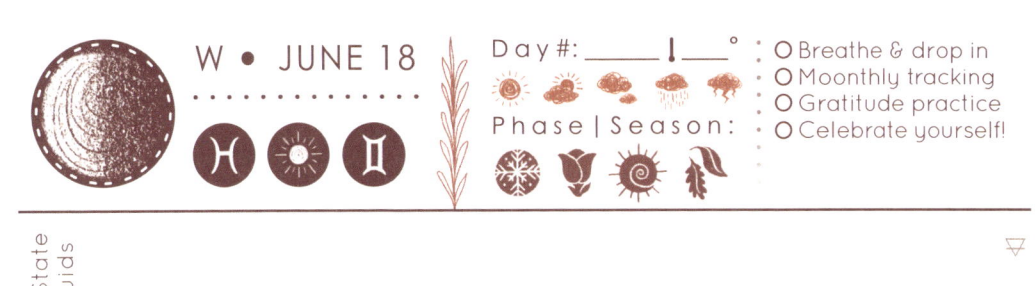

Phase | Season:

- ○ Breathe & drop in
- ○ Moonthly tracking
- ○ Gratitude practice
- ○ Celebrate yourself!

Physical State
Flow | Fluids

Emotional &
Mental State

Self-Care
Sleep | Dreams

LAST QUARTER IN PISCES

Cleansing any energetic debris in the way of true feeling

What am I leaving behind this lunar cycle?

Where can I make more space for reflection &/or integration?

TH • JUNE 19

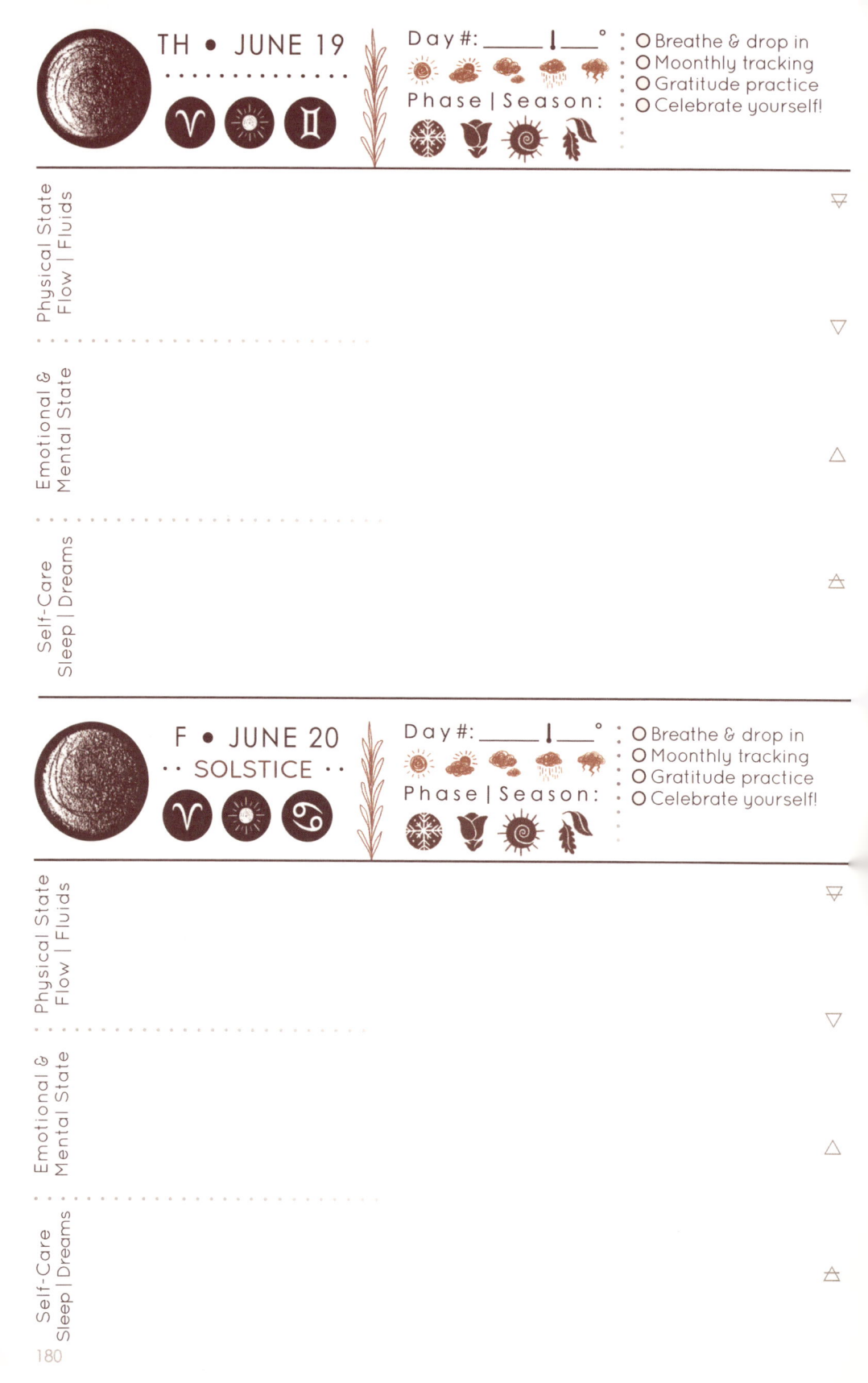

Day #: _____ | ___°
Phase | Season:

- O Breathe & drop in
- O Moonthly tracking
- O Gratitude practice
- O Celebrate yourself!

Physical State
Flow | Fluids

Emotional &
Mental State

Self-Care
Sleep | Dreams

F • JUNE 20
·· SOLSTICE ··

Day #: _____ | ___°
Phase | Season:

- O Breathe & drop in
- O Moonthly tracking
- O Gratitude practice
- O Celebrate yourself!

Physical State
Flow | Fluids

Emotional &
Mental State

Self-Care
Sleep | Dreams

S • JUNE 21

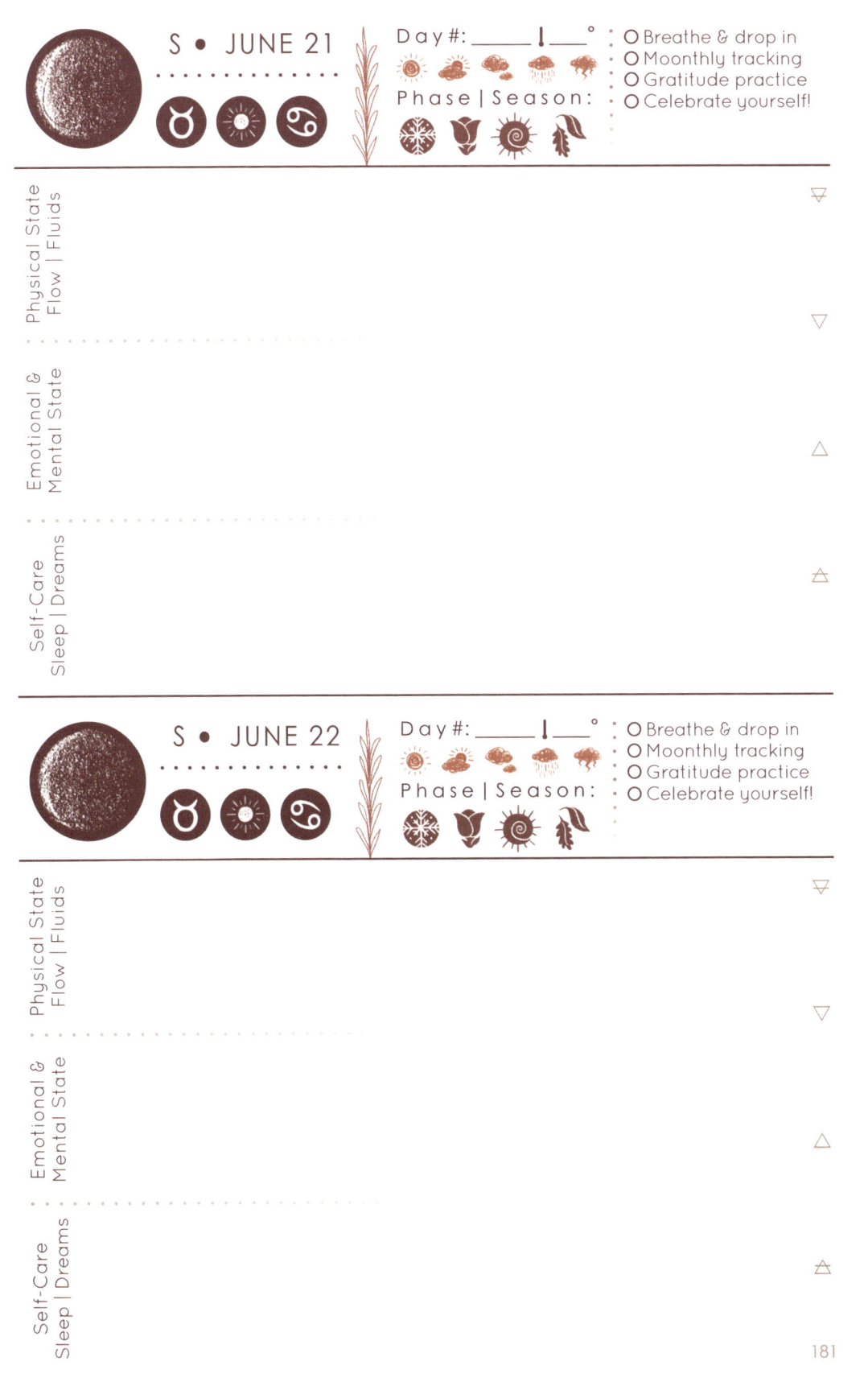

Day #: _____ | _____°

Phase | Season:

- ○ Breathe & drop in
- ○ Moonthly tracking
- ○ Gratitude practice
- ○ Celebrate yourself!

Physical State
Flow | Fluids

Emotional & Mental State

Self-Care
Sleep | Dreams

S • JUNE 22

Day #: _____ | _____°

Phase | Season:

- ○ Breathe & drop in
- ○ Moonthly tracking
- ○ Gratitude practice
- ○ Celebrate yourself!

Physical State
Flow | Fluids

Emotional & Mental State

Self-Care
Sleep | Dreams

☾ 5th
05 | 26
06 | 24

CHECK IN & REFLECT

Use this space to reflect on your experiences & findings from this ending lunar cycle or your last menstrual cycle. Use cycle day #s if you bleed, or moon phases if you don't.

Last Cycle Day 1: _____

Last Cycle Length: _____

Circle the phase you bled near:

○ ☾ ☾ ☾ ● ● ● ● ☽ ☽ ☽ ○

Caution Days: (days I needed space)

Bliss Days: (days I felt great)

—— DAYS TO NOTE —— Which cycle days stood out?

—— OBSERVATIONS —— Notice any changes or patterns?

—— SELF-CARE —— What was helpful & nourishing?

PLAN & PREPARE

Next Predicted Cycle:
🩸 ☾ _____

CHECKLIST

Add the following to any other planners or calendars for your next cycle, then check it off.

- ☐ Predicted "days to note" _____
- ☐ Days to slow down (pre-bleed) _____
- ☐ Rest day(s) (next bleed) _____
- ☐ Date with yourself _____
- ☐ _____

- ☐ Self chest/breast exam
- ☐ Meal plan with cycle
- ☐ _____
- ☐ _____
- ☐ _____

OPEN SPACE

Use this space how you wish, or print out one of our free templates to paste here for BBT charting, dream tracking, or something else:

Using Cannabliss for Your Cycles

by Hope Milagro Aguilera (she/her/they/them) of Luna Xochitl • Cannabis extractor, herbalist, artist, + educator • @lunaxochitl_ • lunaxochitl.com •

The Cannabis plant is believed to be on one of the very first plants that humans domesticated. Working with the cannabis plant is one of the most ancient bonds between humans and plants.

We can't mention Cannabis without mentioning the fact that black and brown people continue to be disproportionately arrested and targeted for its racist prohibition and stigma, and we must continue to advocate.

Cannabis has been my biggest ally for menstrual pain. I want more uterus bearers to know – cannabis helps cycle pain and can be taken vaginally since you have endocannabinoid receptors in your uterus. Our endocannabinoid system is specifically designed to receive cannabinoids to regulate our systems - we are designed to consume cannabis!

Not everyone enjoys the psychoactive effects of THC, so you can also try its non-psychoactive but relaxing sibling, CBD hemp. They are the same plant, just bred differently to express either THC or CBD as the major cannabinoid.

How to use canna for cycle relief:

* Use a tbsp of flower for tea for pain or anxiety relief

* Try a tincture orally – we recommend a FULL SPECTRUM organic tincture, ideally locally/handmade

* Make your own CBD SALVE! All you need is flower, organic oil, and beeswax

* Use a topical oil or salve over your womb space

* Try a tincture oil vaginally! Use a FULL SPECTRUM, organic OIL-based tincture – NOT ALCOHOL-based for this. Suppositories are a super medicinal way to take in cannabis either anally or vaginally. It is very important to know your own body and tolerance for this. Full Spectrum CBD will have minuscule amounts of THC as well so be careful by starting with a low low dose, not driving after, and monitoring your reaction. Keep your oil bacteria free by keeping it clean. Source from a trusted herbalist that makes a concentrated extract. You can rub oil on your labia externally or squirt onto your menstrual cup/product used internally.

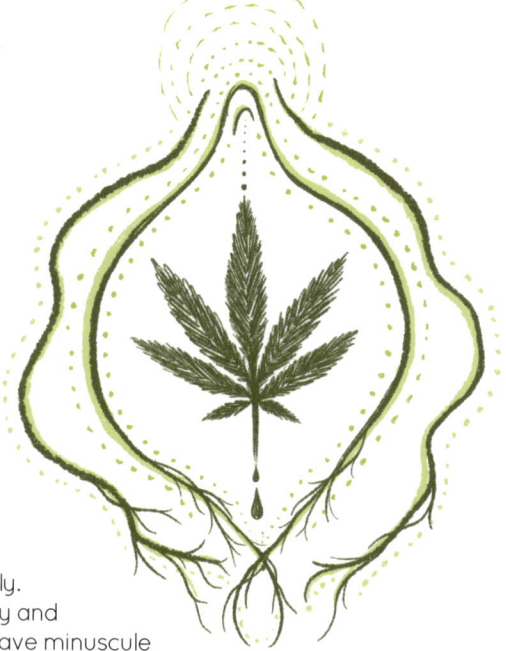

Phasic Overview & In-Betweens

Use this space to focus on the phases of the moonth and the in-betweens of the peak lunations.

One way of using this space is to designate one column for your goal-planning, intention-setting or focus per phase/week. Use the other column for reflections, dream themes, nutrition tracking, cards pulls, etc!

M • JUNE 23

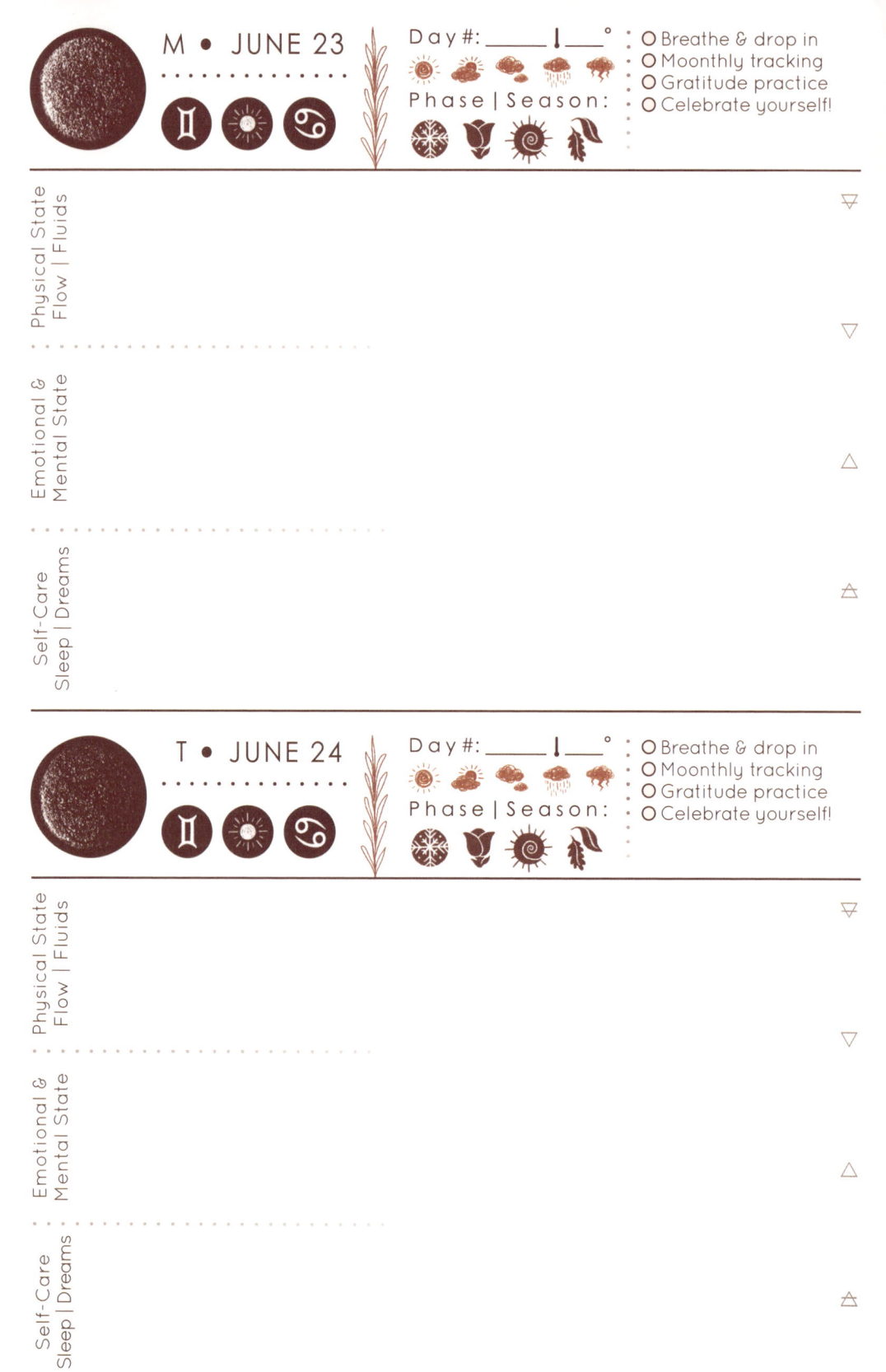

Day #: _____ | _____°

Phase | Season:

- ○ Breathe & drop in
- ○ Moonthly tracking
- ○ Gratitude practice
- ○ Celebrate yourself!

Physical State | Flow | Fluids

Emotional & Mental State

Self-Care | Sleep | Dreams

T • JUNE 24

Day #: _____ | _____°

Phase | Season:

- ○ Breathe & drop in
- ○ Moonthly tracking
- ○ Gratitude practice
- ○ Celebrate yourself!

Physical State | Flow | Fluids

Emotional & Mental State

Self-Care | Sleep | Dreams

W • JUNE 25

Day #: _____ | _____°

Phase | Season:

- ○ Breathe & drop in
- ○ Moonthly tracking
- ○ Gratitude practice
- ○ Celebrate yourself!

Physical State — Flow | Fluids

Emotional & Mental State

Self-Care — Sleep | Dreams

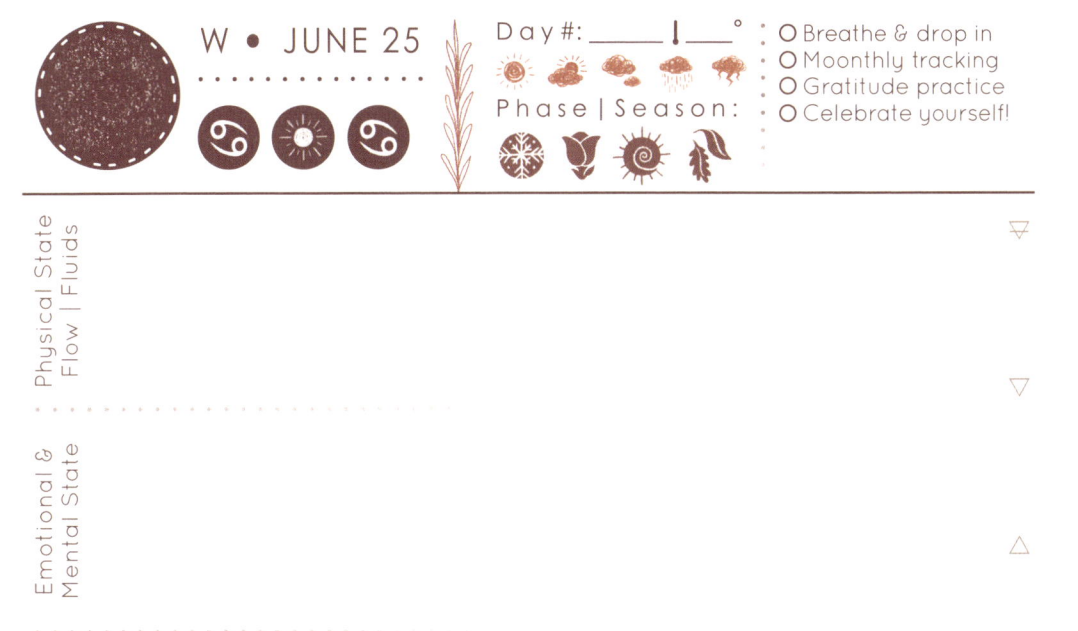

NEW MOON IN CANCER

Inviting familiarity into new spaces of evolving comfort

What do I want to grow & focus on during this lunar cycle?

How will I hold space for this?

TH • JUNE 26

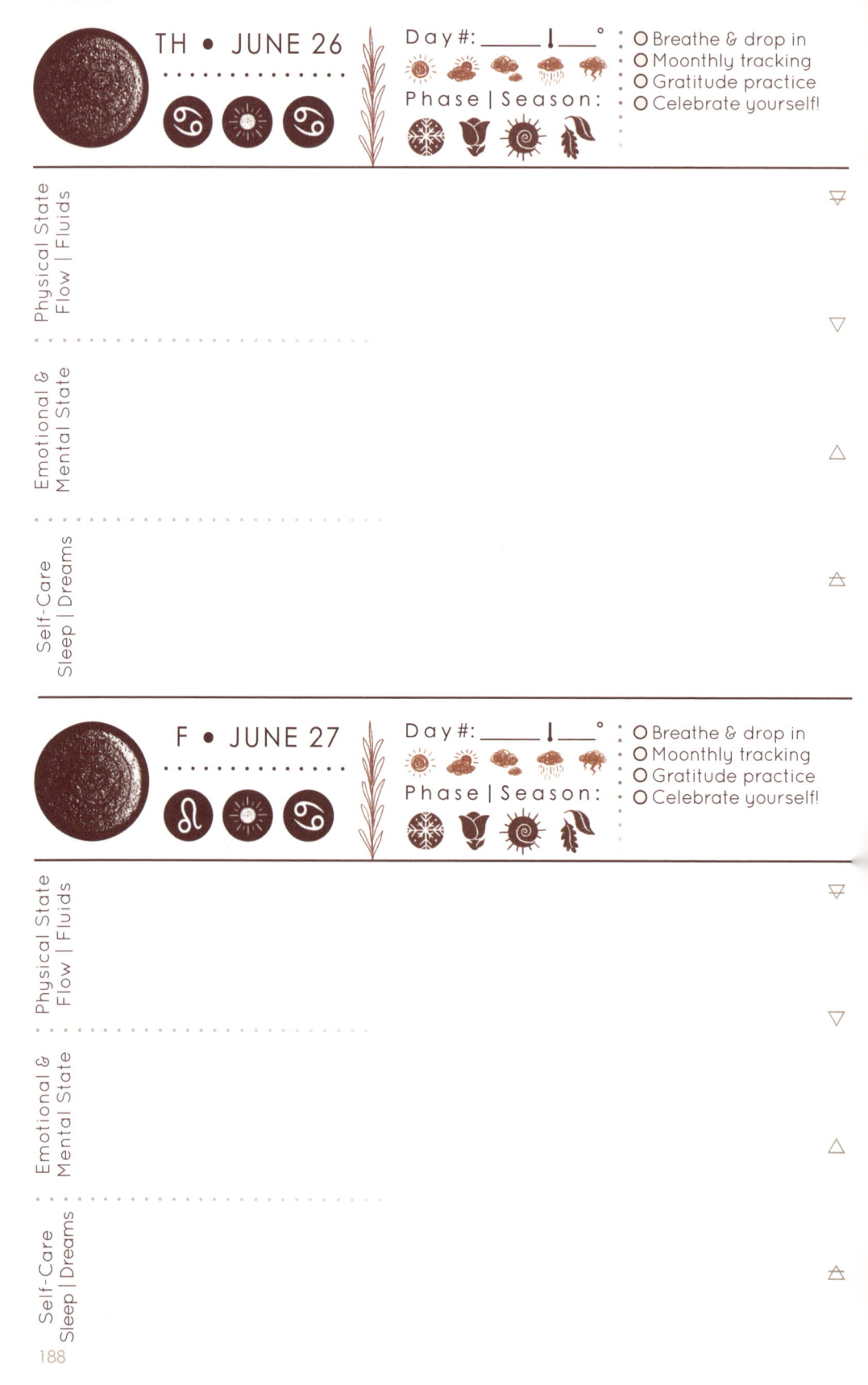

Day #: _____ | _____°

Phase | Season:

- ◯ Breathe & drop in
- ◯ Moonthly tracking
- ◯ Gratitude practice
- ◯ Celebrate yourself!

Physical State
Flow | Fluids

Emotional &
Mental State

Self-Care
Sleep | Dreams

F • JUNE 27

Day #: _____ | _____°

Phase | Season:

- ◯ Breathe & drop in
- ◯ Moonthly tracking
- ◯ Gratitude practice
- ◯ Celebrate yourself!

Physical State
Flow | Fluids

Emotional &
Mental State

Self-Care
Sleep | Dreams

S • JUNE 28

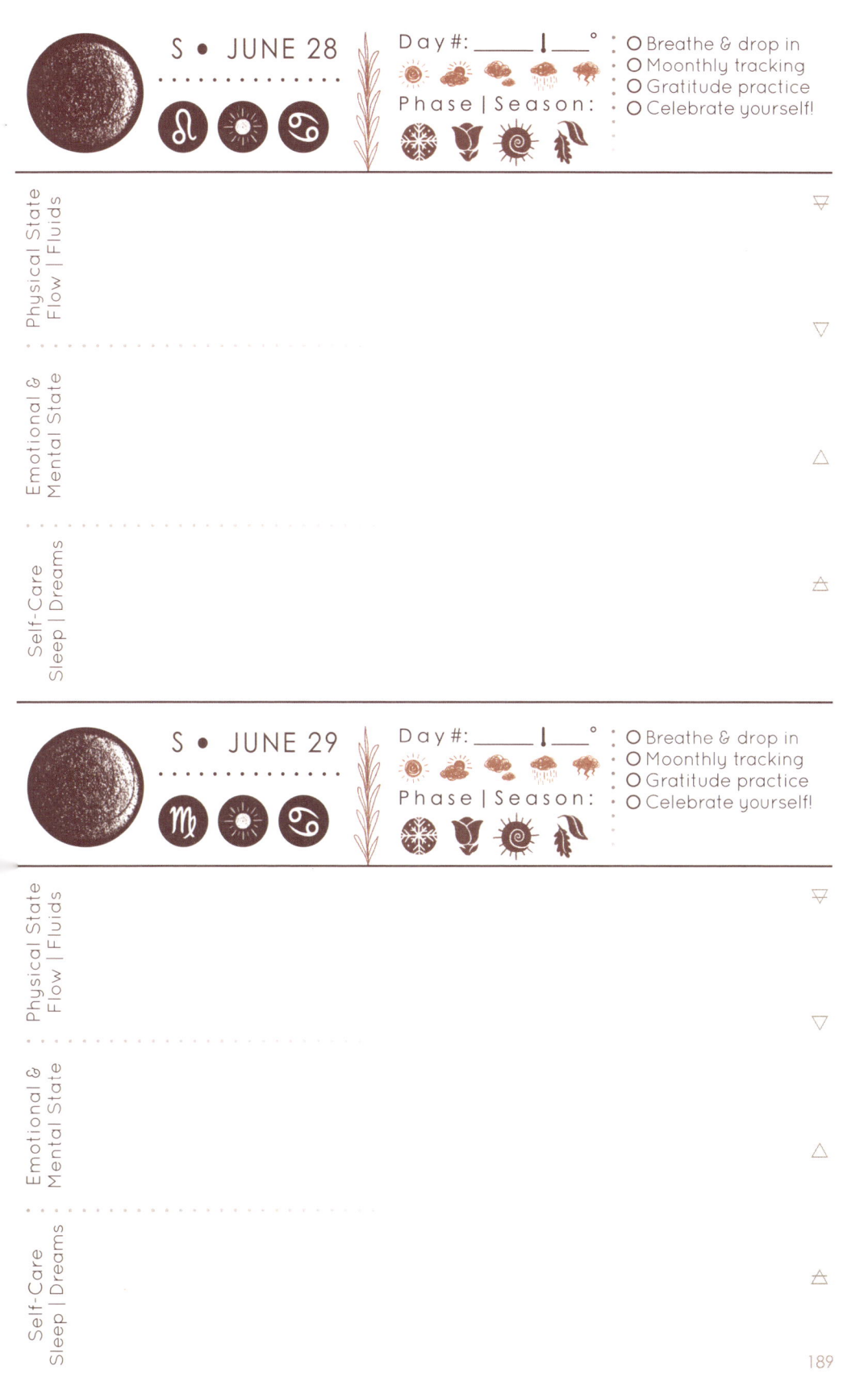

Day #: _____ | _____°

Phase | Season:

- Breathe & drop in
- Moonthly tracking
- Gratitude practice
- Celebrate yourself!

Physical State
Flow | Fluids

Emotional & Mental State

Self-Care
Sleep | Dreams

S • JUNE 29

Day #: _____ | _____°

Phase | Season:

- Breathe & drop in
- Moonthly tracking
- Gratitude practice
- Celebrate yourself!

Physical State
Flow | Fluids

Emotional & Mental State

Self-Care
Sleep | Dreams

M • JUNE 30

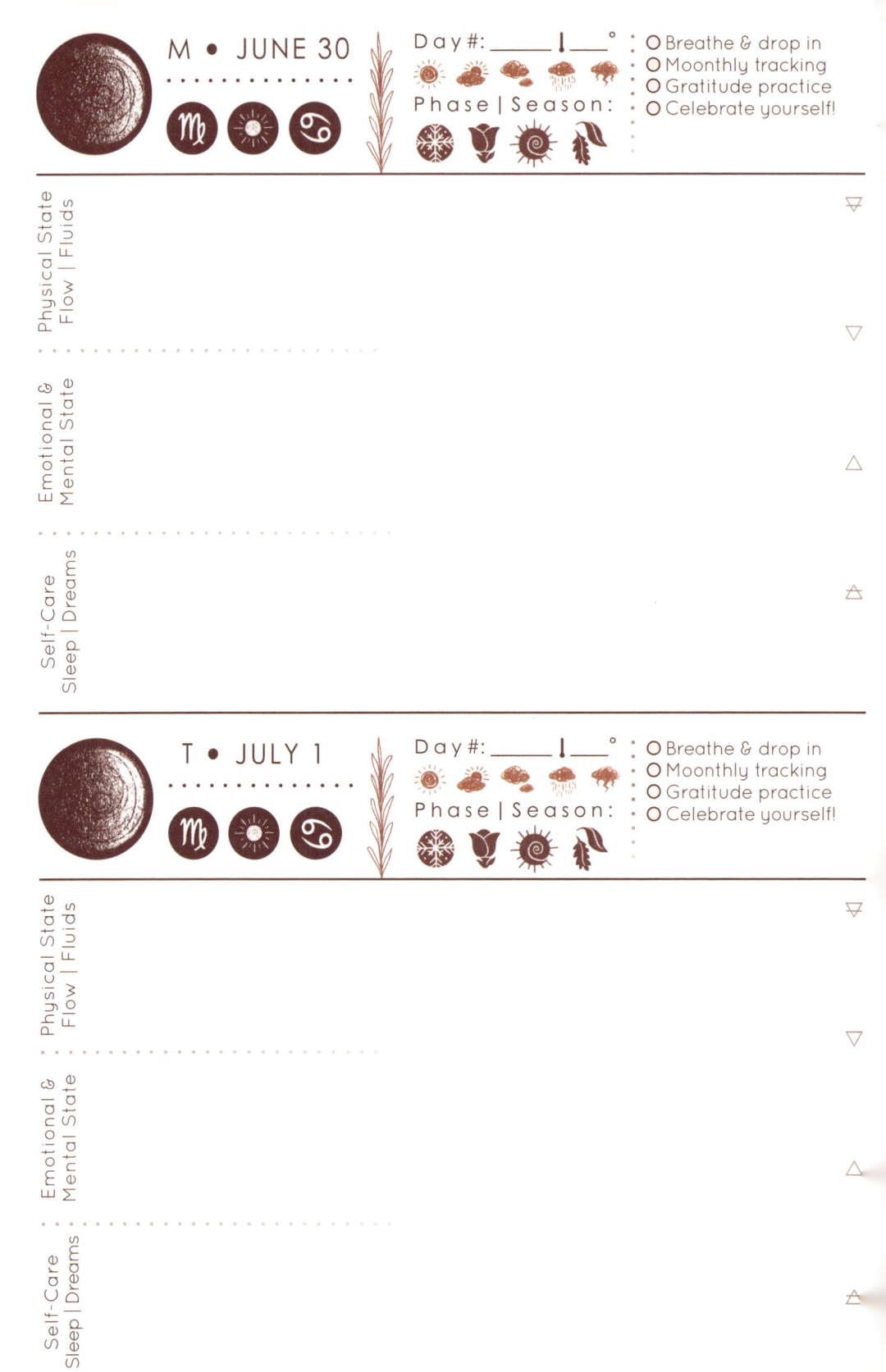

Day #: _____ | _____°

Phase | Season:

- ○ Breathe & drop in
- ○ Moonthly tracking
- ○ Gratitude practice
- ○ Celebrate yourself!

Physical State
Flow | Fluids

**Emotional &
Mental State**

Self-Care
Sleep | Dreams

T • JULY 1

Day #: _____ | _____°

Phase | Season:

- ○ Breathe & drop in
- ○ Moonthly tracking
- ○ Gratitude practice
- ○ Celebrate yourself!

Physical State
Flow | Fluids

**Emotional &
Mental State**

Self-Care
Sleep | Dreams

W • JULY 2

Day #: _____ | _____°

Phase | Season:

- ○ Breathe & drop in
- ○ Moonthly tracking
- ○ Gratitude practice
- ○ Celebrate yourself!

Physical State Flow | Fluids

Emotional & Mental State

Self-Care Sleep | Dreams

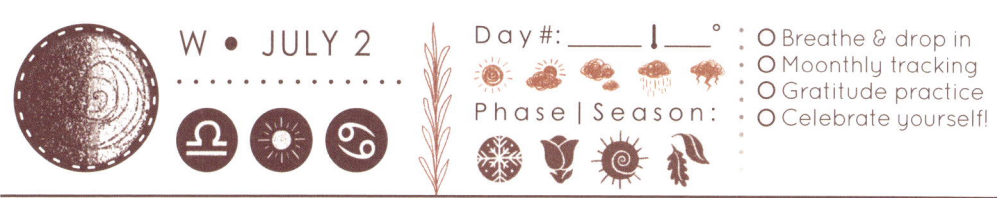

FIRST QUARTER IN LIBRA

Deciding on boundaries to balance open space

What is sprouting & coming into awareness?

What can I release to make space for further growth & grounding?

TH • JULY 3

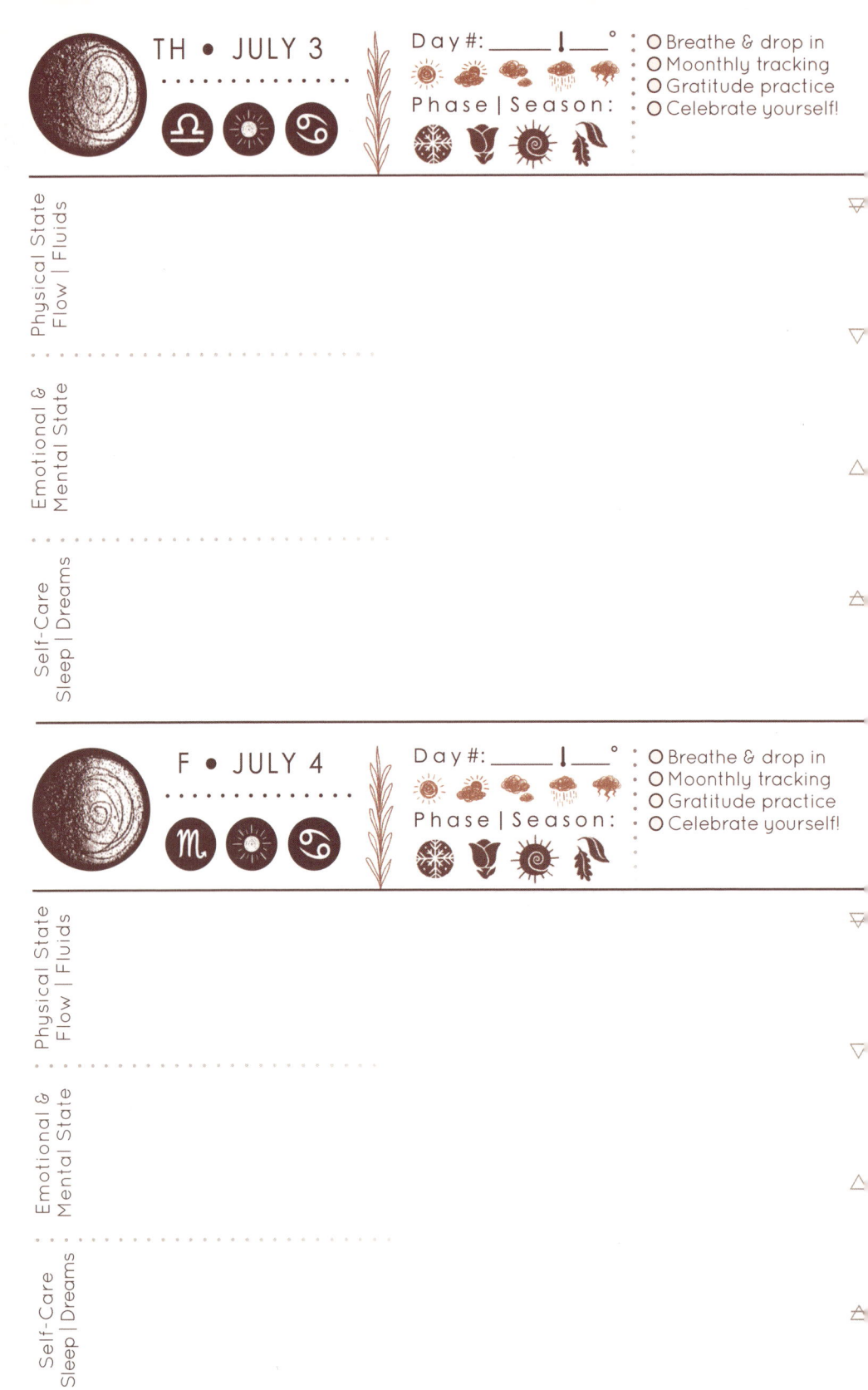

Day #: _____ | _____°

Phase | Season:

- ○ Breathe & drop in
- ○ Moonthly tracking
- ○ Gratitude practice
- ○ Celebrate yourself!

Physical State / Flow | Fluids

Emotional & Mental State

Self-Care / Sleep | Dreams

F • JULY 4

Day #: _____ | _____°

Phase | Season:

- ○ Breathe & drop in
- ○ Moonthly tracking
- ○ Gratitude practice
- ○ Celebrate yourself!

Physical State / Flow | Fluids

Emotional & Mental State

Self-Care / Sleep | Dreams

S • JULY 5

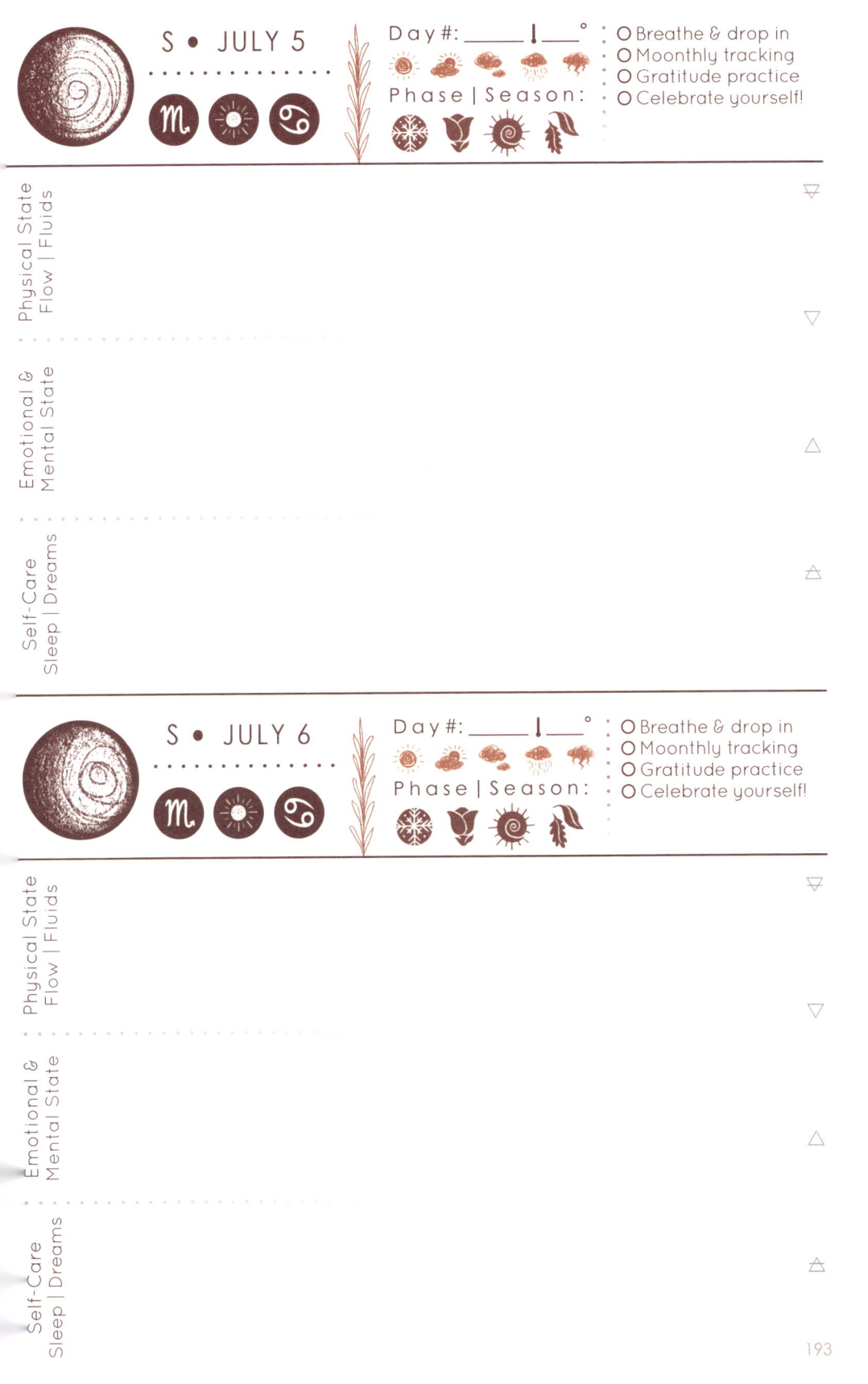

Day #: _____ | _____°

Phase | Season:

- ○ Breathe & drop in
- ○ Moonthly tracking
- ○ Gratitude practice
- ○ Celebrate yourself!

Physical State / Flow | Fluids

Emotional & Mental State

Self-Care / Sleep | Dreams

S • JULY 6

Day #: _____ | _____°

Phase | Season:

- ○ Breathe & drop in
- ○ Moonthly tracking
- ○ Gratitude practice
- ○ Celebrate yourself!

Physical State / Flow | Fluids

Emotional & Mental State

Self-Care / Sleep | Dreams

M • JULY 7

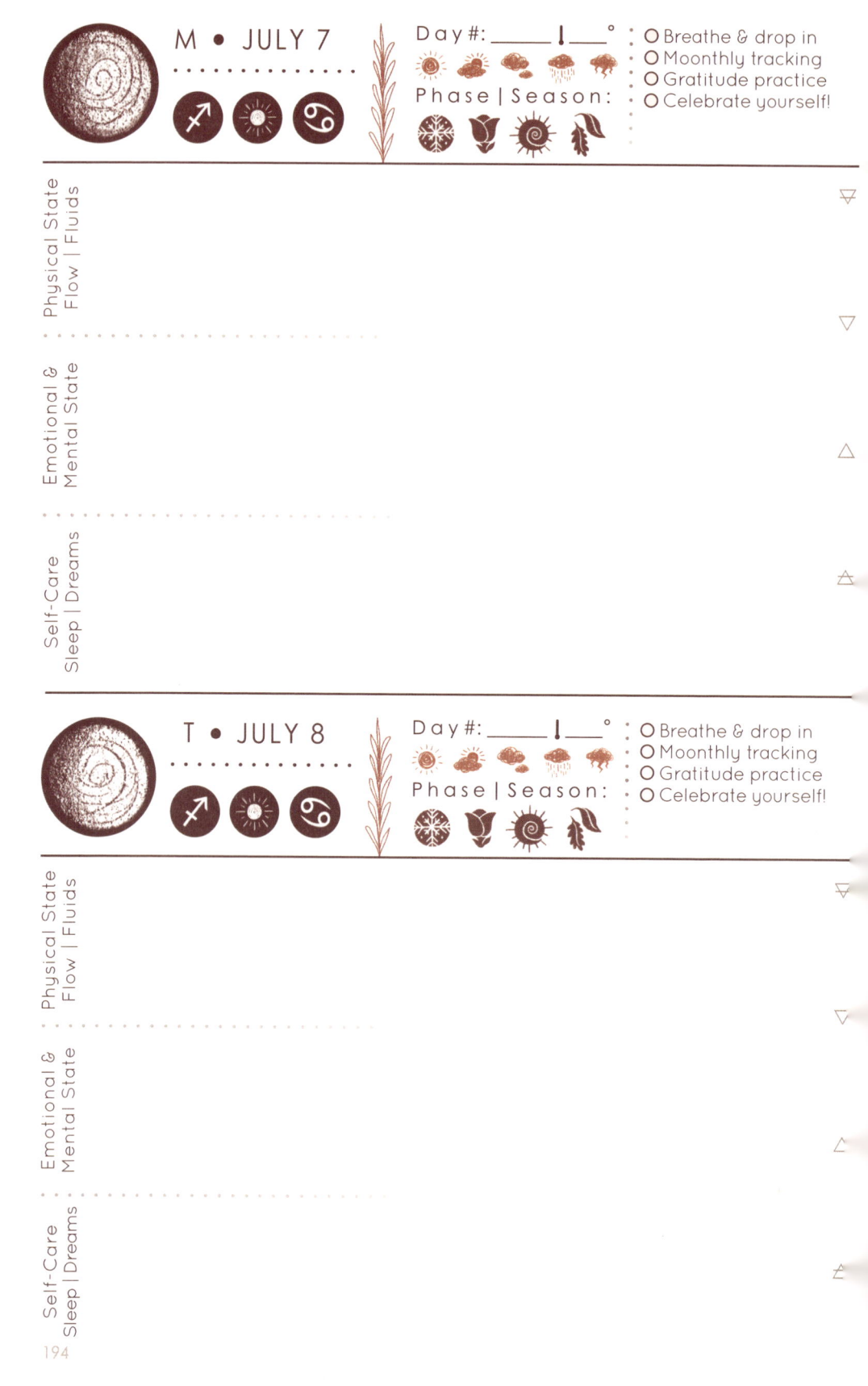

Day #: _____ | _____°

Phase | Season:

- ○ Breathe & drop in
- ○ Moonthly tracking
- ○ Gratitude practice
- ○ Celebrate yourself!

Physical State / Flow | Fluids

Emotional & Mental State

Self-Care / Sleep | Dreams

T • JULY 8

Day #: _____ | _____°

Phase | Season:

- ○ Breathe & drop in
- ○ Moonthly tracking
- ○ Gratitude practice
- ○ Celebrate yourself!

Physical State / Flow | Fluids

Emotional & Mental State

Self-Care / Sleep | Dreams

194

W • JULY 9

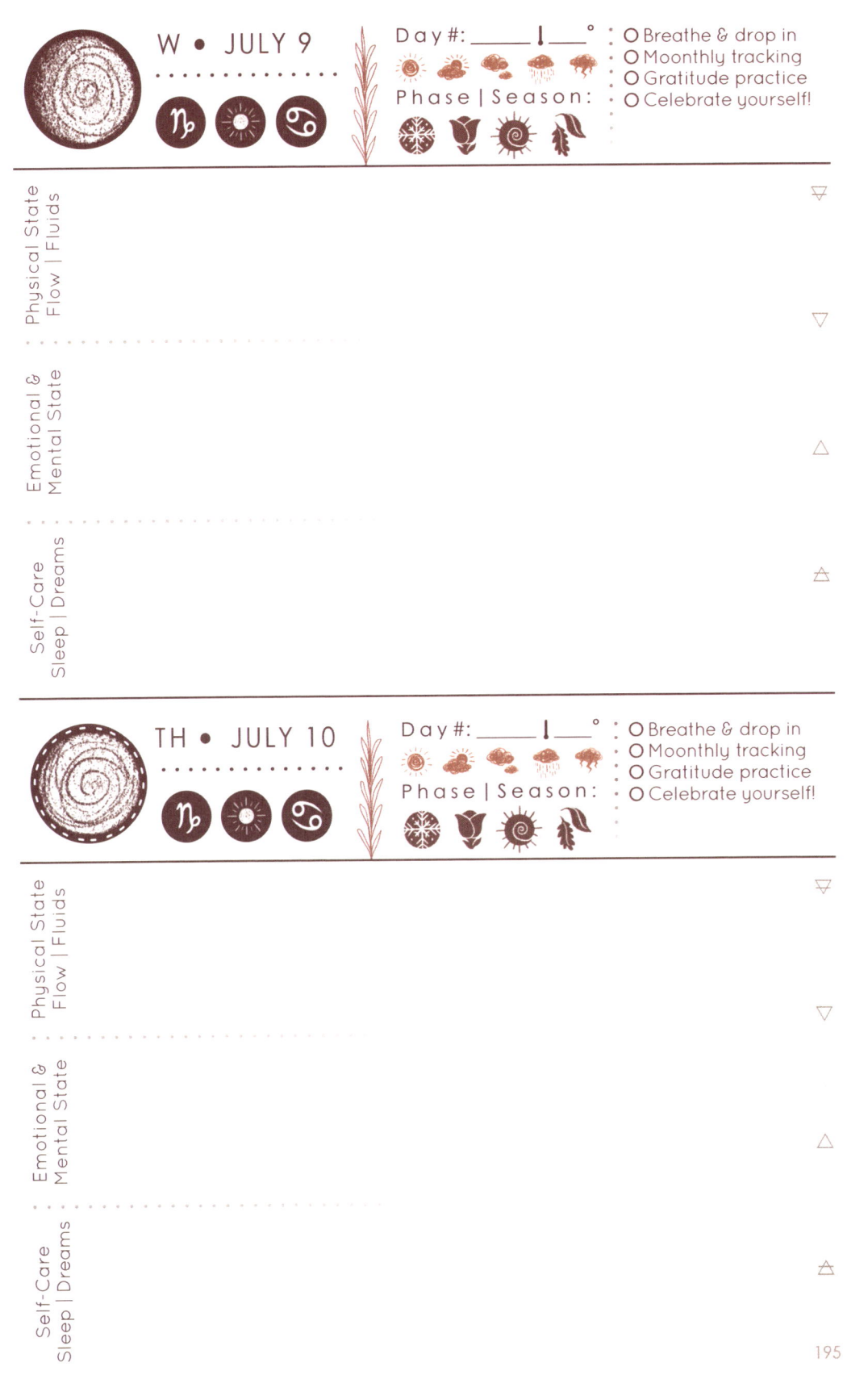

Day #: _____ | ___°

Phase | Season:

- Breathe & drop in
- Moonthly tracking
- Gratitude practice
- Celebrate yourself!

Physical State
Flow | Fluids

Emotional &
Mental State

Self-Care
Sleep | Dreams

TH • JULY 10

Day #: _____ | ___°

Phase | Season:

- Breathe & drop in
- Moonthly tracking
- Gratitude practice
- Celebrate yourself!

Physical State
Flow | Fluids

Emotional &
Mental State

Self-Care
Sleep | Dreams

FULL MOON IN CAPRICORN

Finding enoughness in every moment of physical presence

What is being illuminated?

I give gratitude for what is & what is becoming:

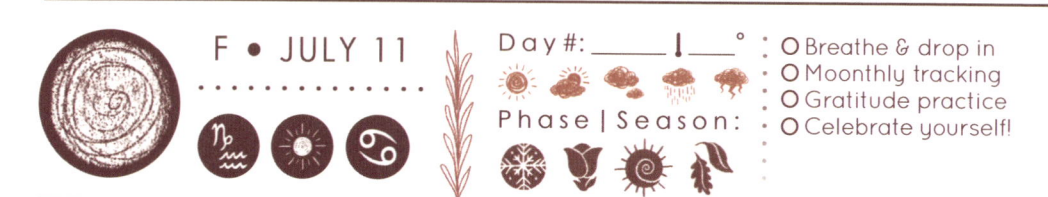

F • JULY 11

Day #: _____ | ____°

Phase | Season:

- O Breathe & drop in
- O Moonthly tracking
- O Gratitude practice
- O Celebrate yourself!

Physical State / Flow | Fluids

Emotional & Mental State

Self-Care / Sleep | Dreams

S • JULY 12

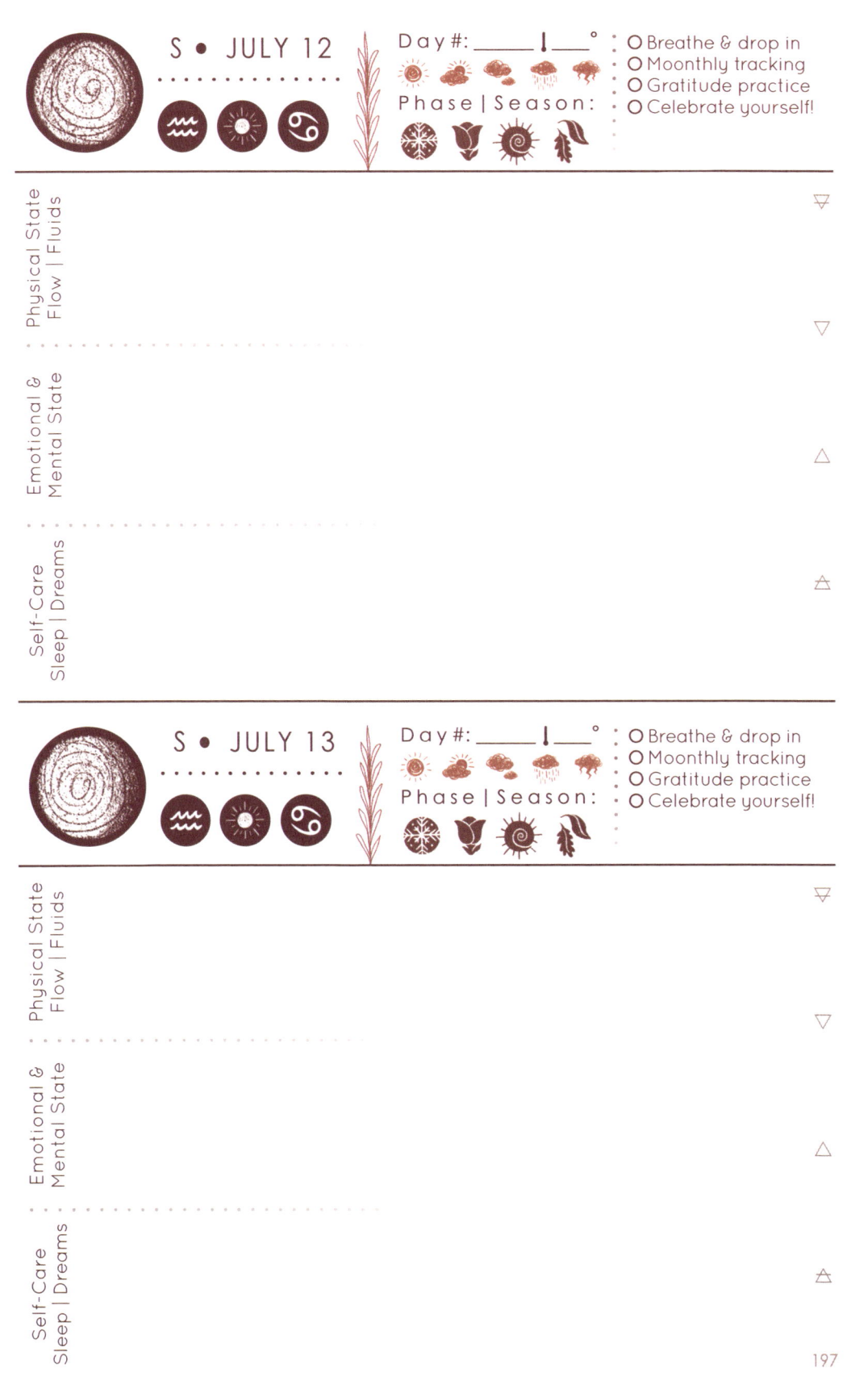

Day #: _____ | _____°

Phase | Season:

- ○ Breathe & drop in
- ○ Moonthly tracking
- ○ Gratitude practice
- ○ Celebrate yourself!

Physical State
Flow | Fluids

Emotional &
Mental State

Self-Care
Sleep | Dreams

S • JULY 13

Day #: _____ | _____°

Phase | Season:

- ○ Breathe & drop in
- ○ Moonthly tracking
- ○ Gratitude practice
- ○ Celebrate yourself!

Physical State
Flow | Fluids

Emotional &
Mental State

Self-Care
Sleep | Dreams

M • JULY 14

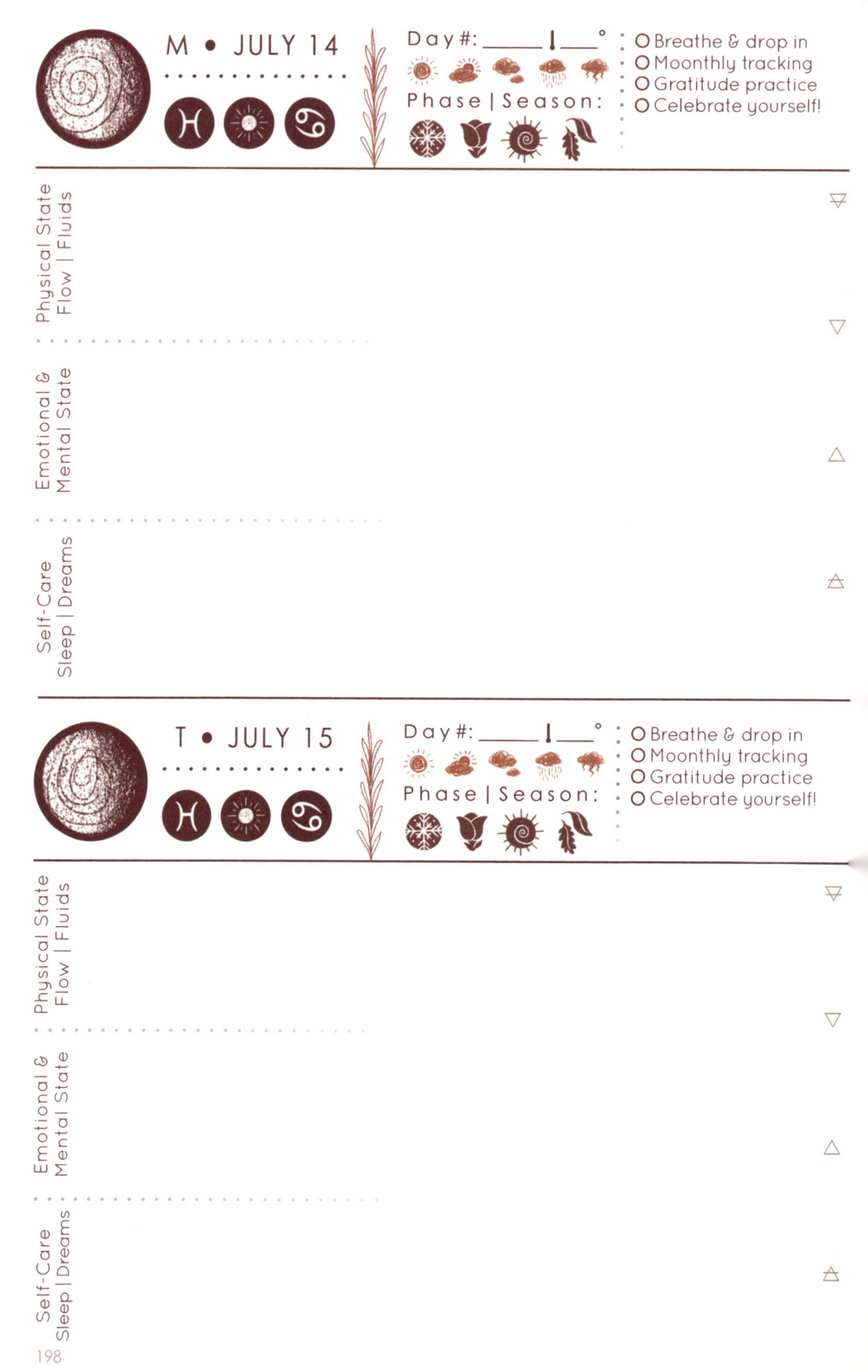

Day #: _____ | _____°

Phase | Season:

- ○ Breathe & drop in
- ○ Moonthly tracking
- ○ Gratitude practice
- ○ Celebrate yourself!

Physical State / Flow | Fluids

Emotional & Mental State

Self-Care / Sleep | Dreams

T • JULY 15

Day #: _____ | _____°

Phase | Season:

- ○ Breathe & drop in
- ○ Moonthly tracking
- ○ Gratitude practice
- ○ Celebrate yourself!

Physical State / Flow | Fluids

Emotional & Mental State

Self-Care / Sleep | Dreams

W • JULY 16

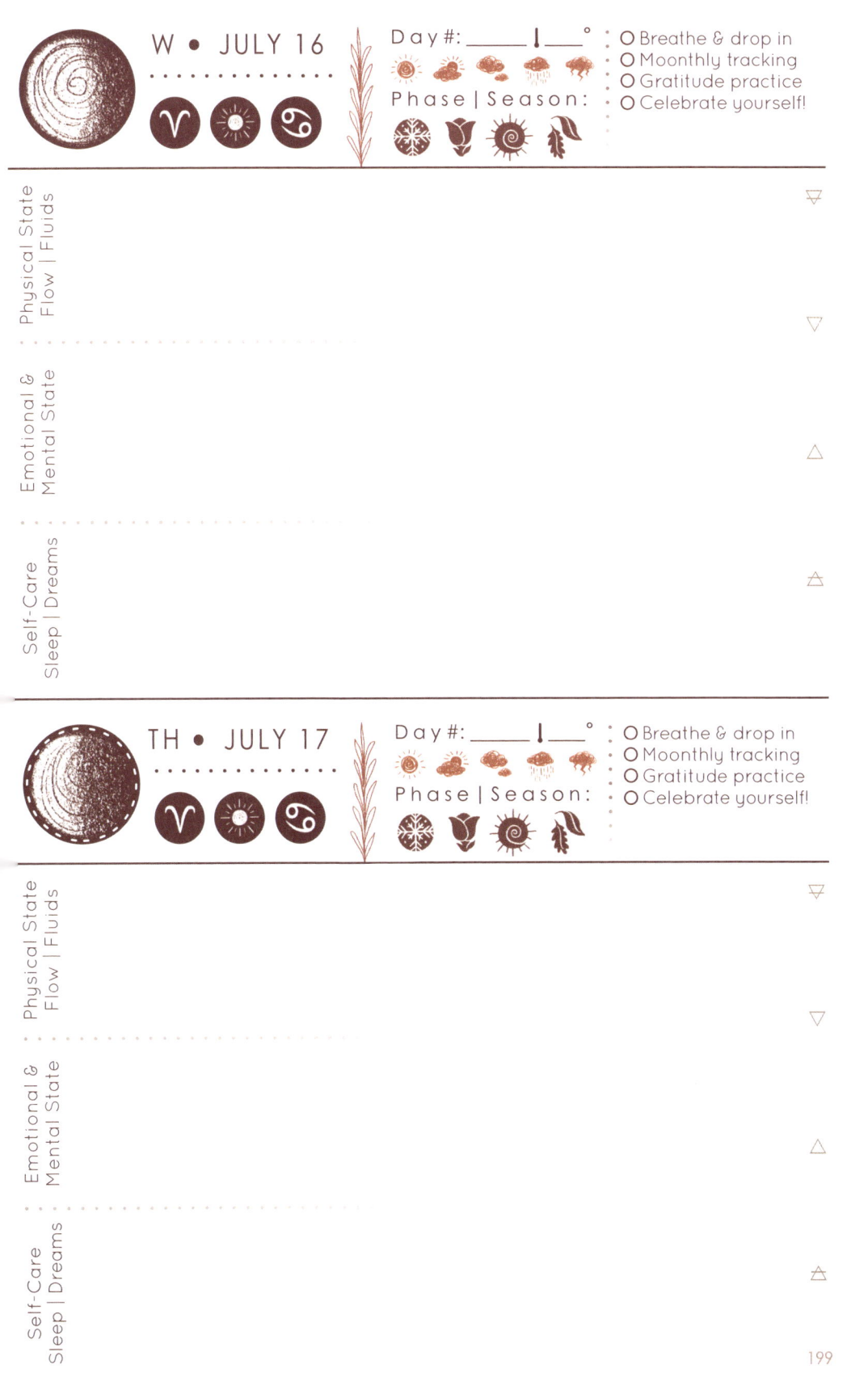

♈ ☉ ♋

Day #: _____ | _____°

Phase | Season:

- Breathe & drop in
- Moonthly tracking
- Gratitude practice
- Celebrate yourself!

Physical State / Flow | Fluids

Emotional & Mental State

Self-Care / Sleep | Dreams

TH • JULY 17

♈ ☉ ♋

Day #: _____ | _____°

Phase | Season:

- Breathe & drop in
- Moonthly tracking
- Gratitude practice
- Celebrate yourself!

Physical State / Flow | Fluids

Emotional & Mental State

Self-Care / Sleep | Dreams

LAST QUARTER IN ARIES

Unleashing restraints from core desires & ambitions

What am I leaving behind this lunar cycle?

Where can I make more space for reflection &/or integration?

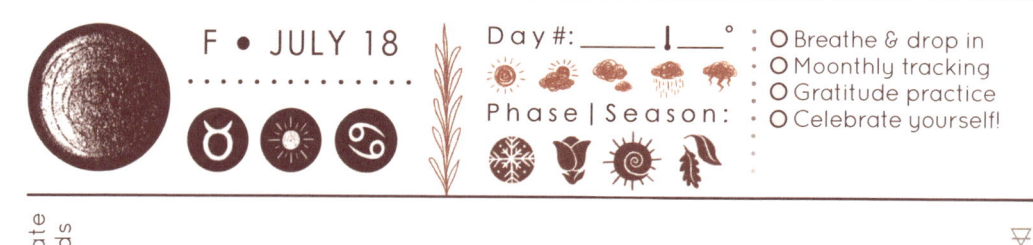

F • JULY 18

Day #: _____ | ___°
Phase | Season:

○ Breathe & drop in
○ Moonthly tracking
○ Gratitude practice
○ Celebrate yourself!

Physical State
Flow | Fluids

Emotional &
Mental State

Self-Care
Sleep | Dreams

S • JULY 19

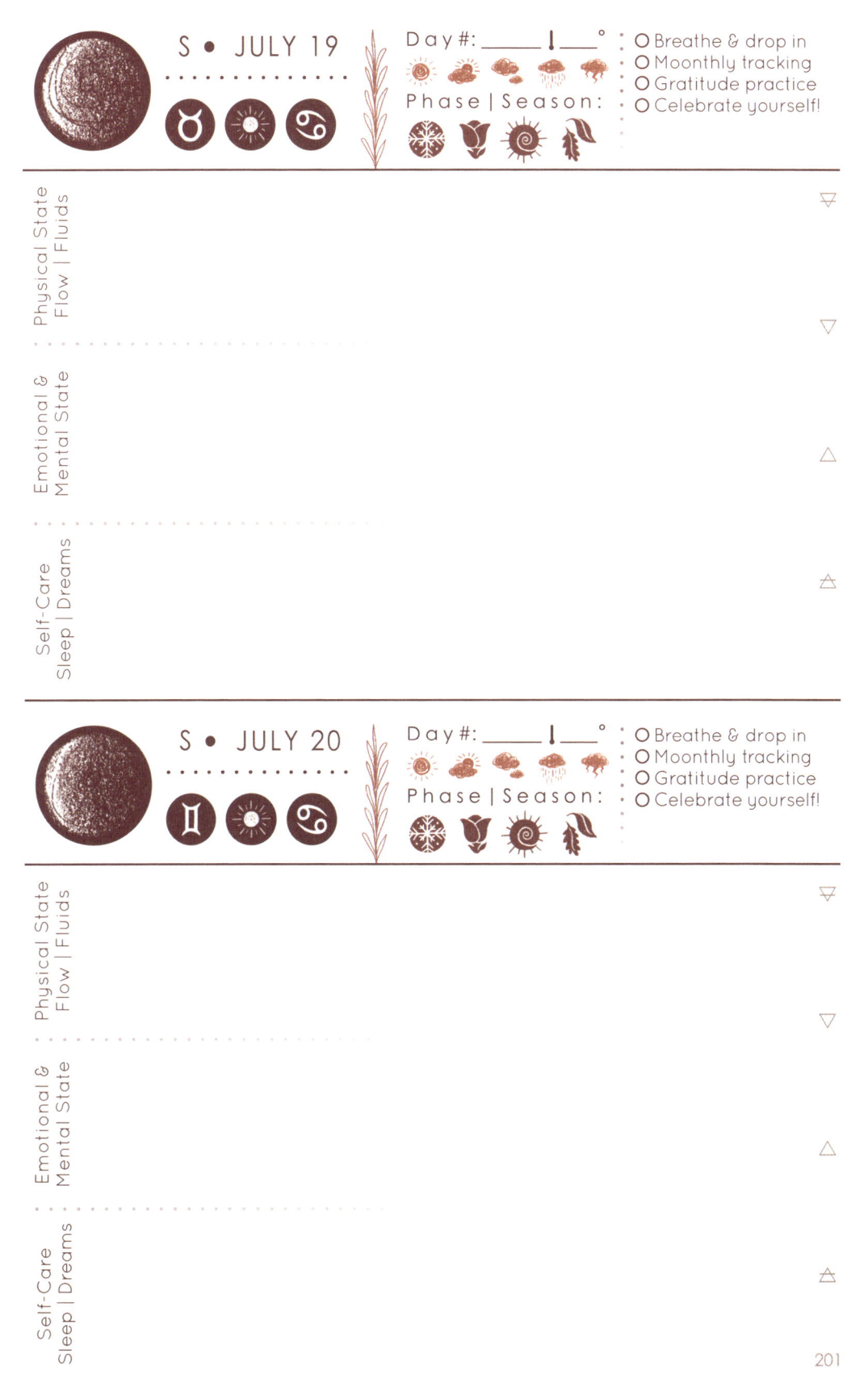

Day #: _____ | _____°
Phase | Season:

- ○ Breathe & drop in
- ○ Moonthly tracking
- ○ Gratitude practice
- ○ Celebrate yourself!

Physical State
Flow | Fluids

Emotional &
Mental State

Self-Care
Sleep | Dreams

S • JULY 20

Day #: _____ | _____°
Phase | Season:

- ○ Breathe & drop in
- ○ Moonthly tracking
- ○ Gratitude practice
- ○ Celebrate yourself!

Physical State
Flow | Fluids

Emotional &
Mental State

Self-Care
Sleep | Dreams

☾ 6th
06 | 25
07 | 23

CHECK IN & REFLECT

Use this space to reflect on your experiences & findings from this ending lunar cycle or your last menstrual cycle. Use cycle day #s if you bleed, or moon phases if you don't.

Last Cycle Day 1: _____

Last Cycle Length: _____

Circle the phase you bled near:

○ ☾ ☾ ☾ ● ● ● ● ● ● ☽ ☽ ☽ ○

Caution Days: (days I needed space)

Bliss Days: (days I felt great)

DAYS TO NOTE — Which cycle days stood out?

OBSERVATIONS — Notice any changes or patterns?

SELF-CARE — What was helpful & nourishing?

PLAN & PREPARE

Next Predicted Cycle:
🩸 ☾ _____

CHECKLIST

Add the following to any other planners or calendars for your next cycle, then check it off.

- ☐ Predicted "days to note" _____
- ☐ Days to slow down (pre-bleed) _____
- ☐ Rest day(s) (next bleed) _____
- ☐ Date with yourself _____
- ☐ _____

- ☐ Self chest/breast exam
- ☐ Meal plan with cycle
- ☐ _____
- ☐ _____
- ☐ _____

OPEN SPACE

Use this space how you wish, or print out one of our free templates to paste here for BBT charting, dream tracking, or something else:

The Xero's/SHEro's Journey of the Womb Cycle

by Josephina Loha (she/her) • Somatic Intimacy Coach and Eros Priestess • @templeofloha • cur8chicago.com •

Understanding the Womb Cycle as the SHEro's / Xero's journey is an illuminating and powerful way for us connect with our menstrual cycle, as a gateway to intuitive gnosis, embodied exploration and creative expansion.

Day 1 of our cycle is the Menstrual Phase (or new moon if you don't bleed), as we descend into the Underworld, the subconscious realms of our psyche. Here we meet our Shadow and embrace our inner Shamanika / Wytch. We journey into the Darkness, embracing the depths of ourselves in stillness, comfort, and potentially isolation; we go into the cave or the Womb Tomb, to release all that no longer serves us in our highest frequency.

As we shift out of this phase of "winter" we move into the Follicular phase which takes all this wisdom gleaned from the shedding of the layers and the releasing of what no longer serves us, embracing our inner mystical capacities and we awaken our inner Wild One as well as the Rebel Muse, the Siren and the Sacred Disruptor – here to play with all of life in our inner Spring of the Follicular Phase.

In the Ovulatory Phase, our sensuality comes more online and we can unite with our inner Beloved; our sacred life force energy is activated to create, to share our gifts and talents with the world. Our energetic fields are more open, and this is the best time to launch a new offering or business.

We codify our power in the Luteal Phase as we step into our Embodied Exaltedness – we celebrate the harvest of our creation in this autumnal season, as we then prepare to enter the cycle of letting go, once again.

This map is a re-wiring of Joseph Campbell's "Hero's Journey" and could happen every month and/ or attuned to the moon cycles.

Phasic Overview & In-Betweens

Use this space to focus on the phases of the moonth and the in-betweens of the peak lunations.

One way of using this space is to designate one column for your goal-planning, intention-setting or focus per phase/week. Use the other column for reflections, dream themes, nutrition tracking, cards pulls, etc!

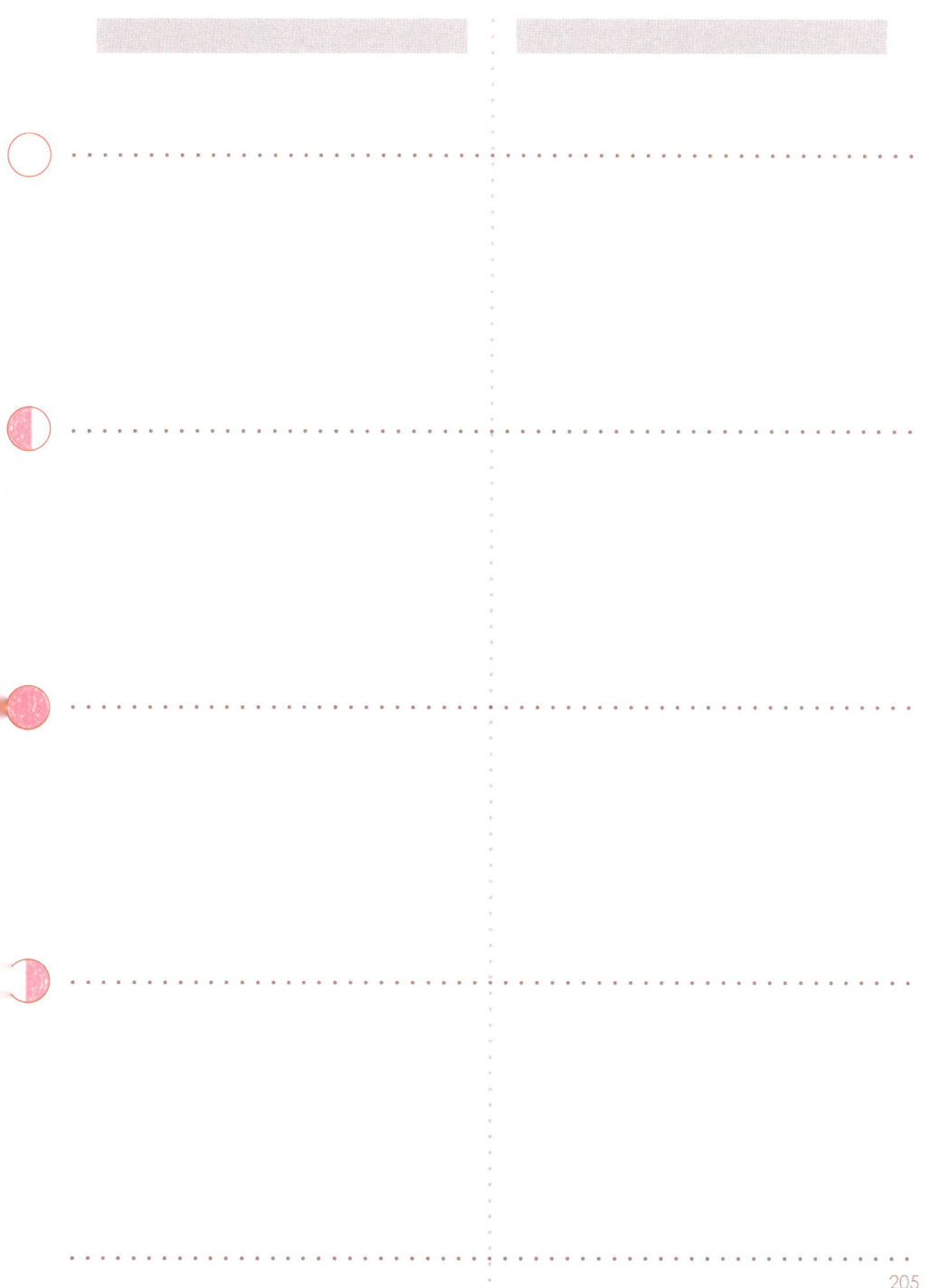

M • JULY 21

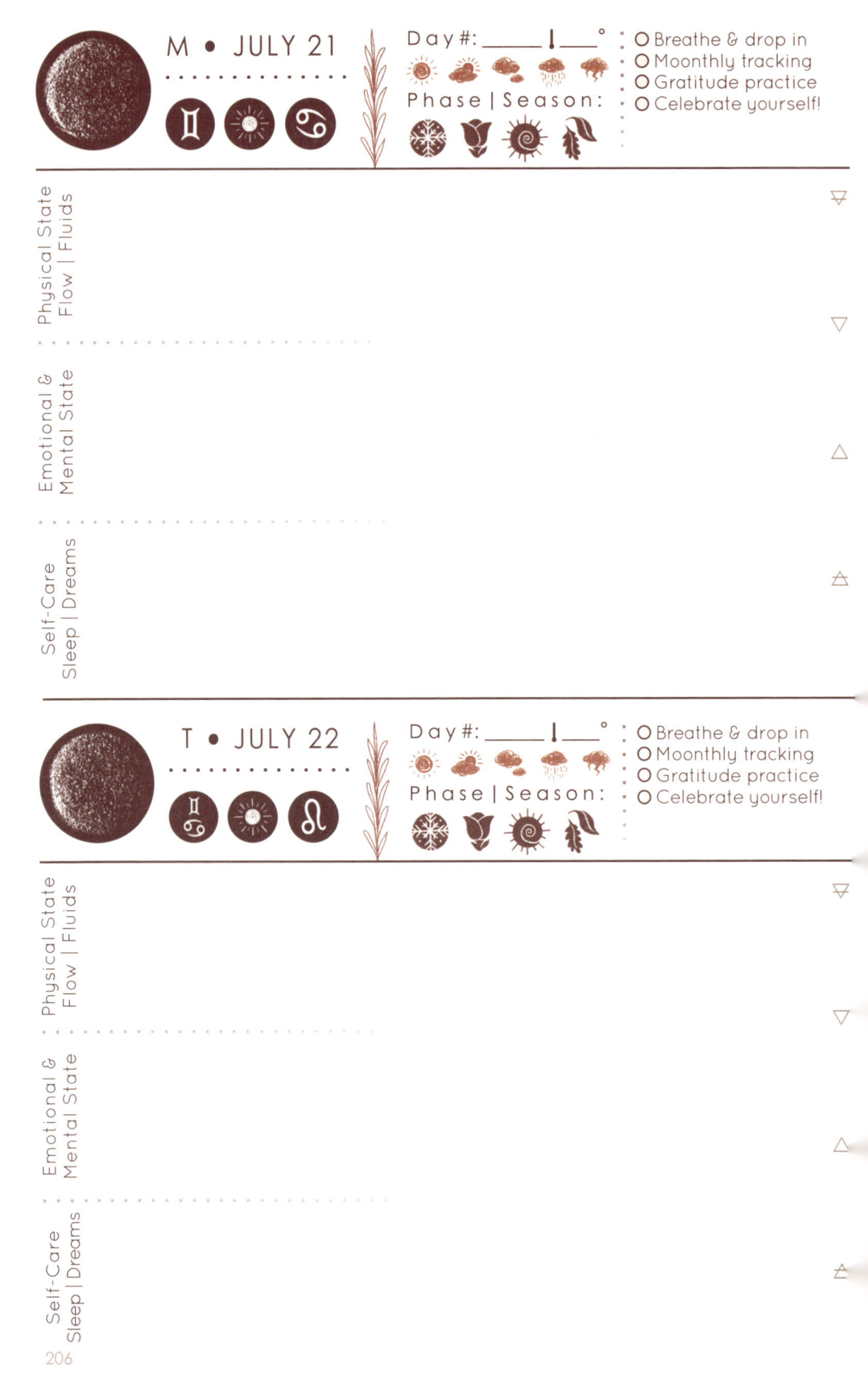

Day #: _____ | ___°

Phase | Season:

- O Breathe & drop in
- O Moonthly tracking
- O Gratitude practice
- O Celebrate yourself!

Physical State
Flow | Fluids

Emotional & Mental State

Self-Care
Sleep | Dreams

T • JULY 22

Day #: _____ | ___°

Phase | Season:

- O Breathe & drop in
- O Moonthly tracking
- O Gratitude practice
- O Celebrate yourself!

Physical State
Flow | Fluids

Emotional & Mental State

Self-Care
Sleep | Dreams

W • JULY 23

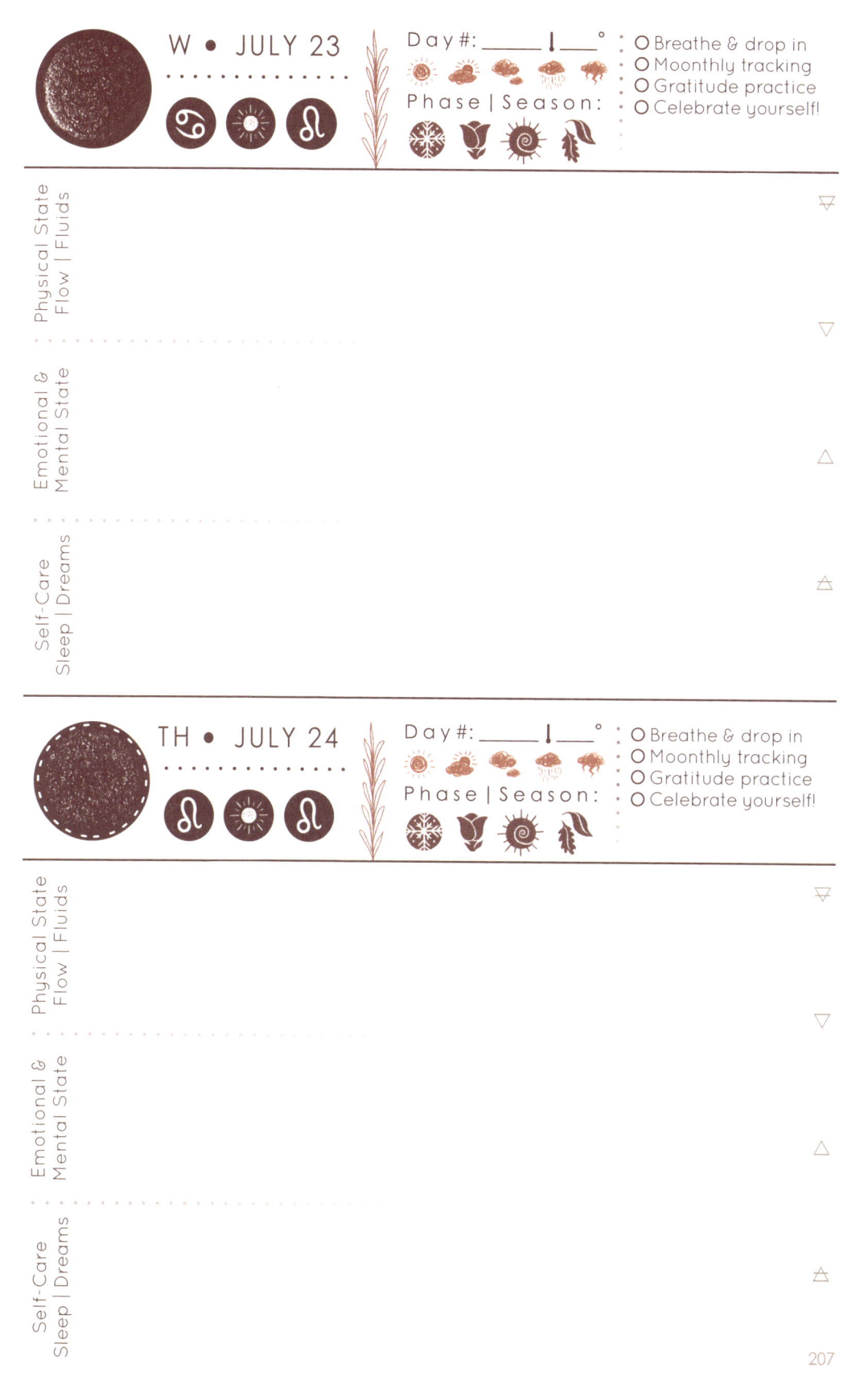

Day #: _____ | ____°

Phase | Season:

- Breathe & drop in
- Moonthly tracking
- Gratitude practice
- Celebrate yourself!

Physical State
Flow | Fluids

Emotional &
Mental State

Self-Care
Sleep | Dreams

TH • JULY 24

Day #: _____ | ____°

Phase | Season:

- Breathe & drop in
- Moonthly tracking
- Gratitude practice
- Celebrate yourself!

Physical State
Flow | Fluids

Emotional &
Mental State

Self-Care
Sleep | Dreams

NEW MOON IN LEO

A renewed spark of energy & inspiration emerging

What do I want to grow & focus on during this lunar cycle?

How will I hold space for this?

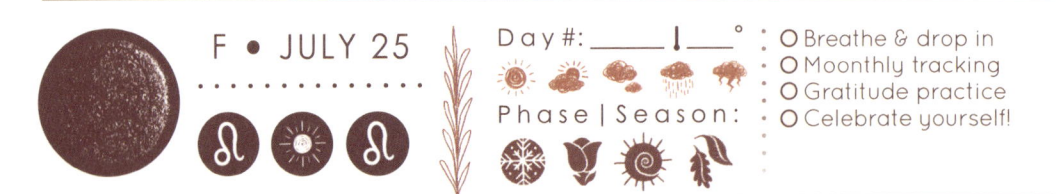

F • JULY 25

Day #: _____ | _____°

Phase | Season:

- Breathe & drop in
- Monthly tracking
- Gratitude practice
- Celebrate yourself!

Physical State
Flow | Fluids

Emotional &
Mental State

Self-Care
Sleep | Dreams

S • JULY 26

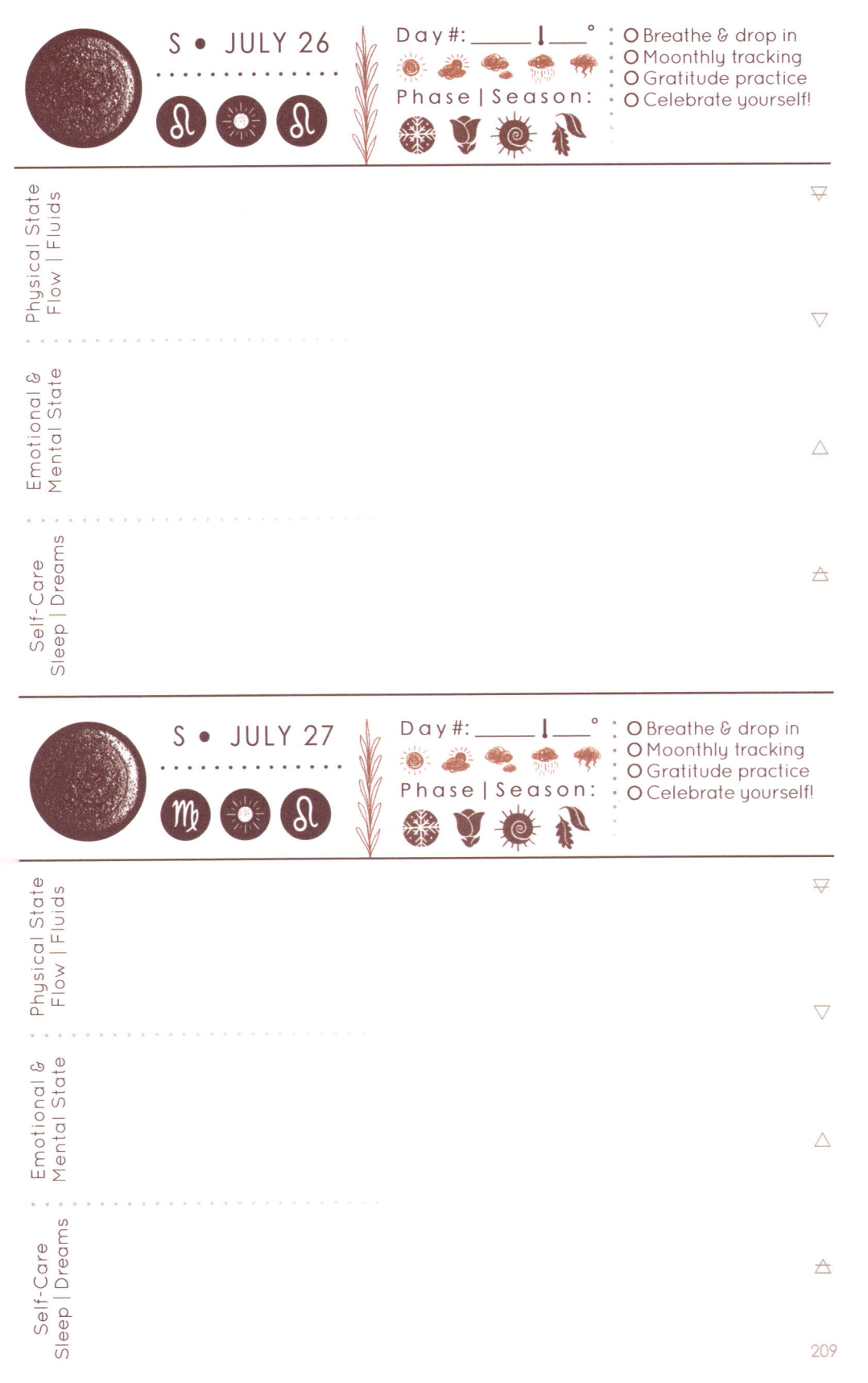

Day #: _____ | ___°

Phase | Season:

- ○ Breathe & drop in
- ○ Moonthly tracking
- ○ Gratitude practice
- ○ Celebrate yourself!

Physical State / Flow | Fluids

Emotional & Mental State

Self-Care / Sleep | Dreams

S • JULY 27

Day #: _____ | ___°

Phase | Season:

- ○ Breathe & drop in
- ○ Moonthly tracking
- ○ Gratitude practice
- ○ Celebrate yourself!

Physical State / Flow | Fluids

Emotional & Mental State

Self-Care / Sleep | Dreams

M • JULY 28

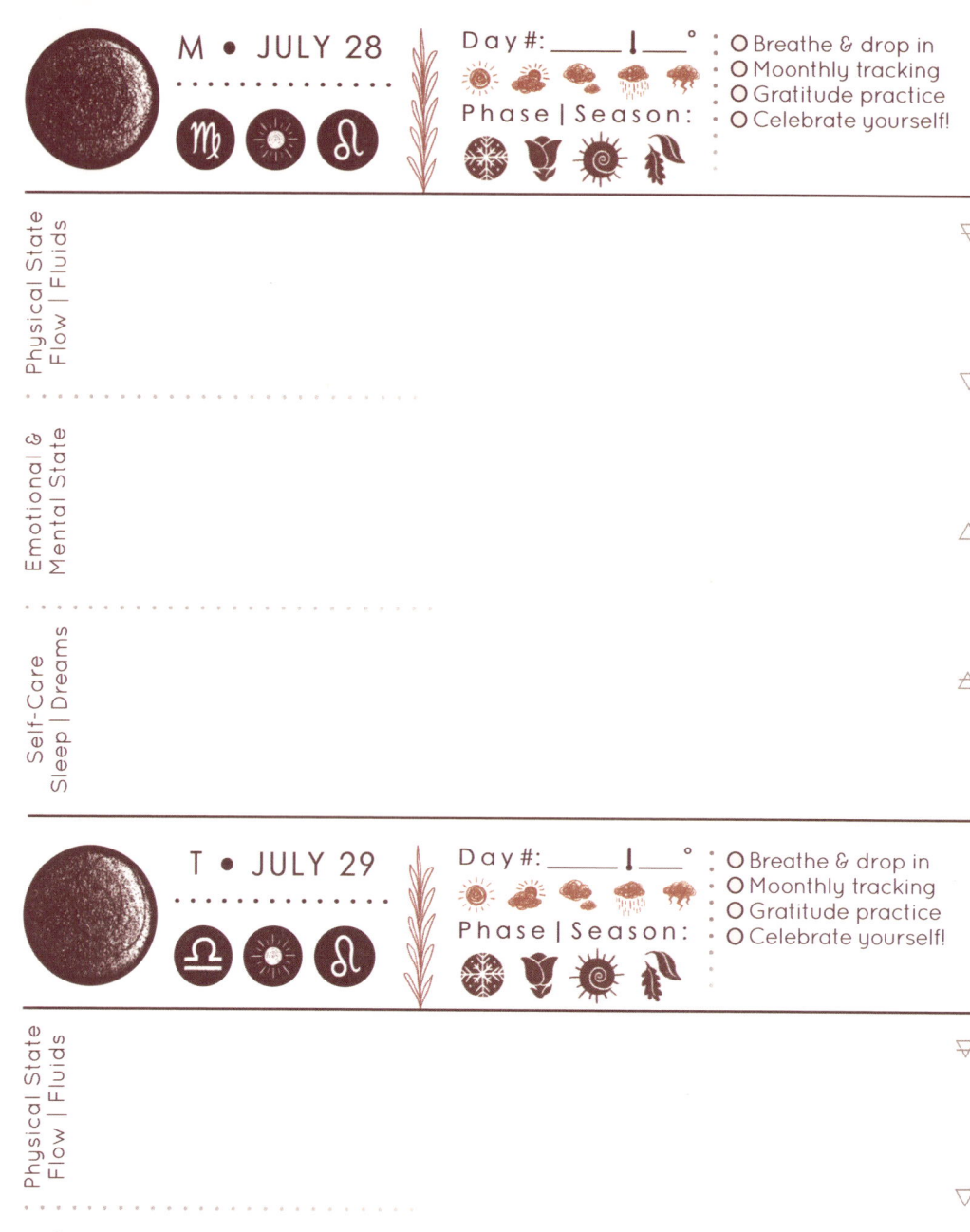

Day #: _____ | ___°

Phase | Season:

- ○ Breathe & drop in
- ○ Moonthly tracking
- ○ Gratitude practice
- ○ Celebrate yourself!

Physical State / Flow | Fluids

Emotional & Mental State

Self-Care / Sleep | Dreams

T • JULY 29

Day #: _____ | ___°

Phase | Season:

- ○ Breathe & drop in
- ○ Moonthly tracking
- ○ Gratitude practice
- ○ Celebrate yourself!

Physical State / Flow | Fluids

Emotional & Mental State

Self-Care / Sleep | Dreams

W • JULY 30

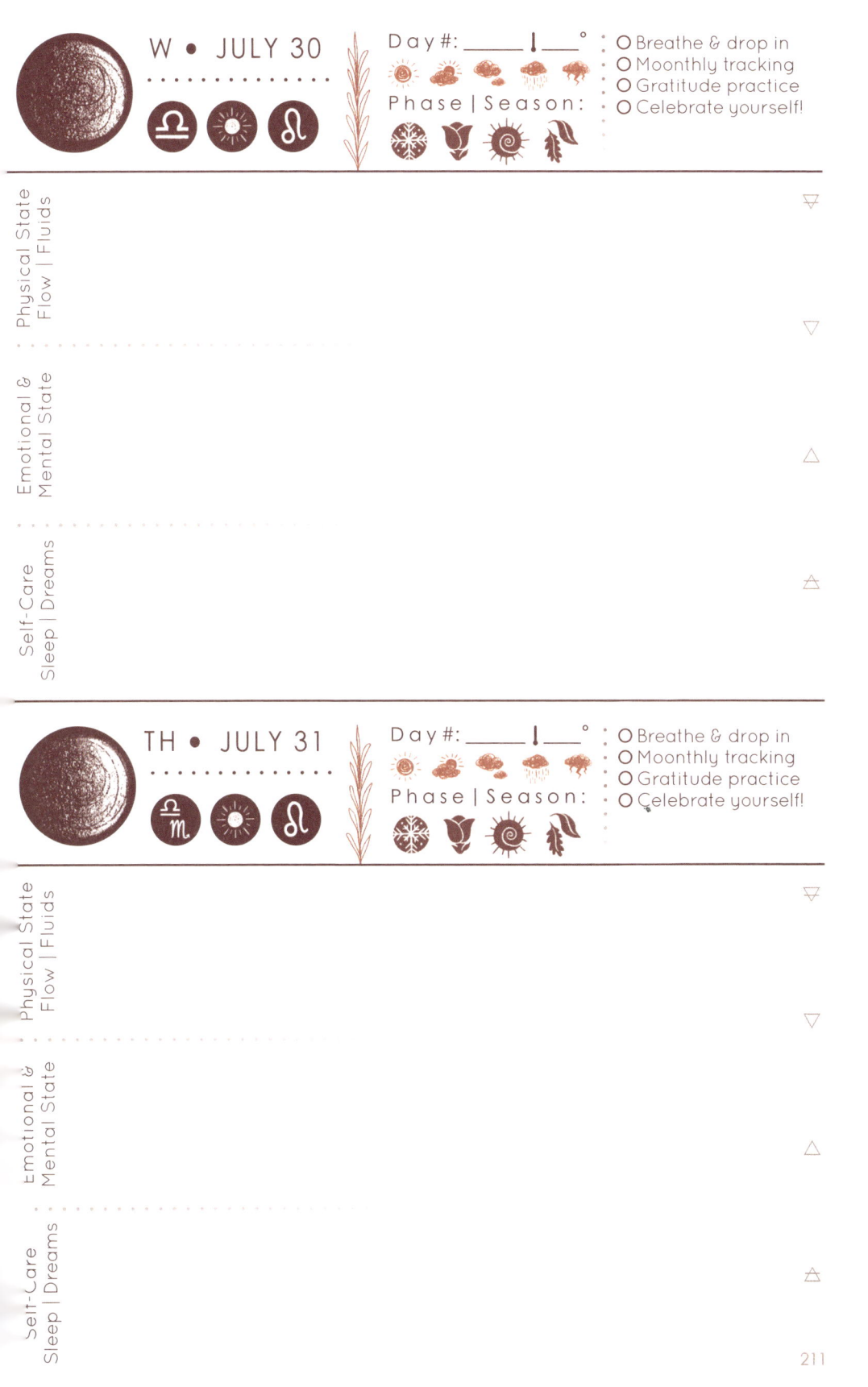

Day #: _____ | _____°

Phase | Season:

- ○ Breathe & drop in
- ○ Moonthly tracking
- ○ Gratitude practice
- ○ Celebrate yourself!

Physical State / Flow | Fluids

Emotional & Mental State

Self-Care / Sleep | Dreams

TH • JULY 31

Day #: _____ | _____°

Phase | Season:

- ○ Breathe & drop in
- ○ Moonthly tracking
- ○ Gratitude practice
- ○ Celebrate yourself!

Physical State / Flow | Fluids

Emotional & Mental State

Self-Care / Sleep | Dreams

F • AUG 1

Day #: _____ | ___°

Phase | Season:

- ○ Breathe & drop in
- ○ Moonthly tracking
- ○ Gratitude practice
- ○ Celebrate yourself!

Physical State
Flow | Fluids

Emotional & Mental State

Self-Care
Sleep | Dreams

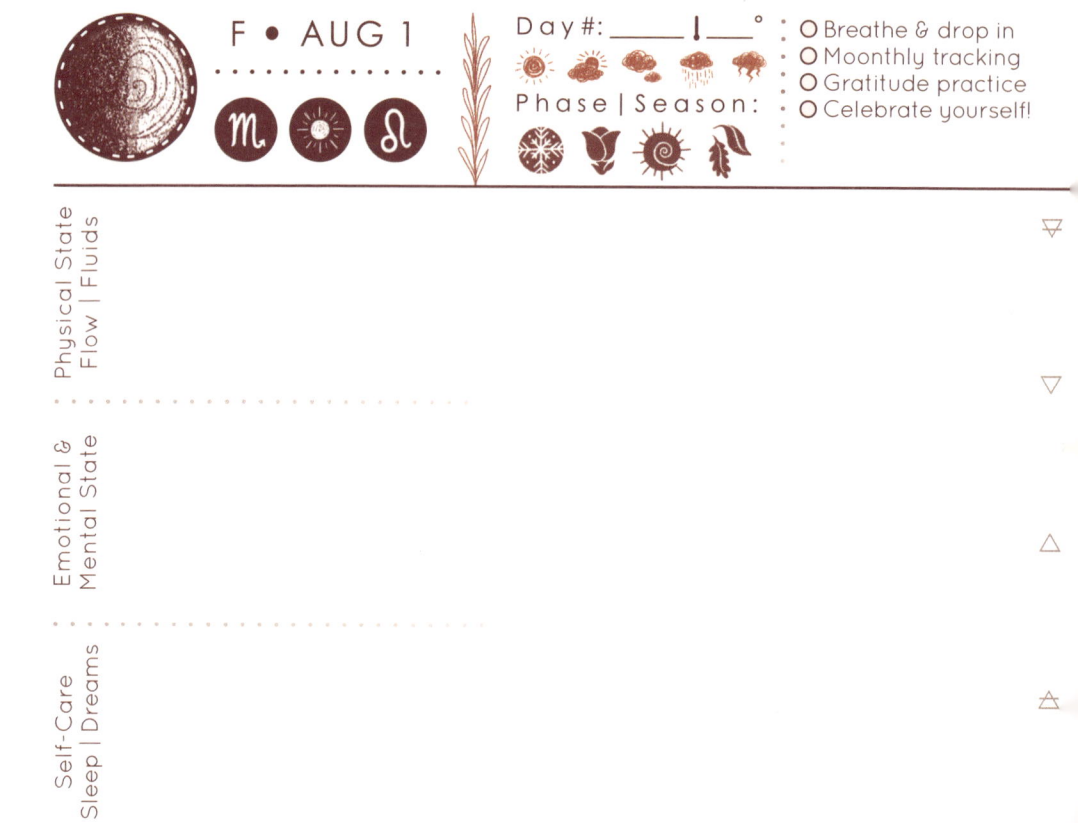

FIRST QUARTER IN SCORPIO

Awakening to the realm of spiritual possibility

What is sprouting & coming into awareness?

What can I release to make space for further growth & grounding?

S • AUG 2

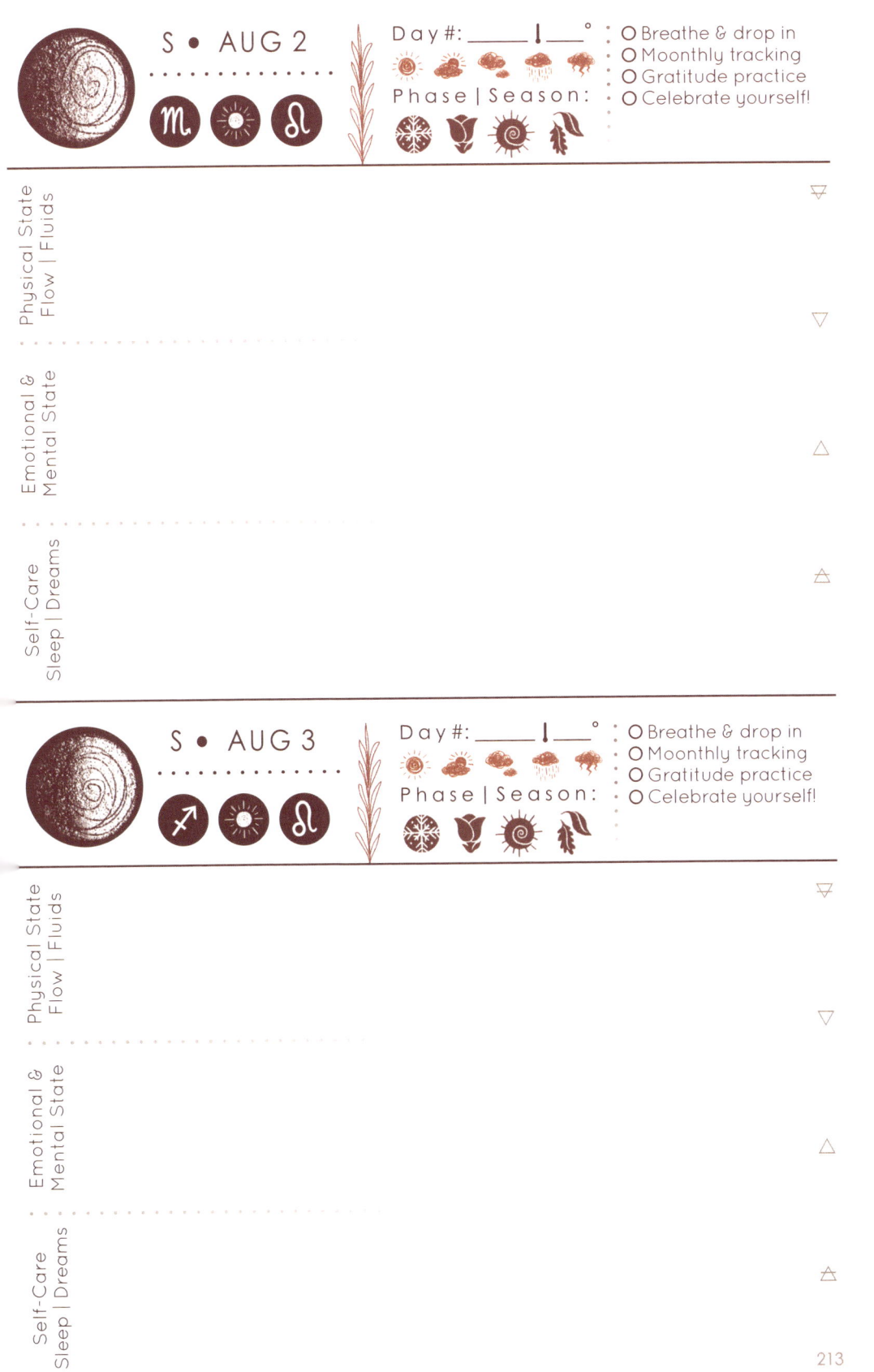

♏ ☀ ♌

Day #: ____ | ____°

Phase | Season:

- ○ Breathe & drop in
- ○ Moonthly tracking
- ○ Gratitude practice
- ○ Celebrate yourself!

Physical State / Flow | Fluids

Emotional & Mental State

Self-Care / Sleep | Dreams

S • AUG 3

♐ ☀ ♌

Day #: ____ | ____°

Phase | Season:

- ○ Breathe & drop in
- ○ Moonthly tracking
- ○ Gratitude practice
- ○ Celebrate yourself!

Physical State / Flow | Fluids

Emotional & Mental State

Self-Care / Sleep | Dreams

M • AUG 4

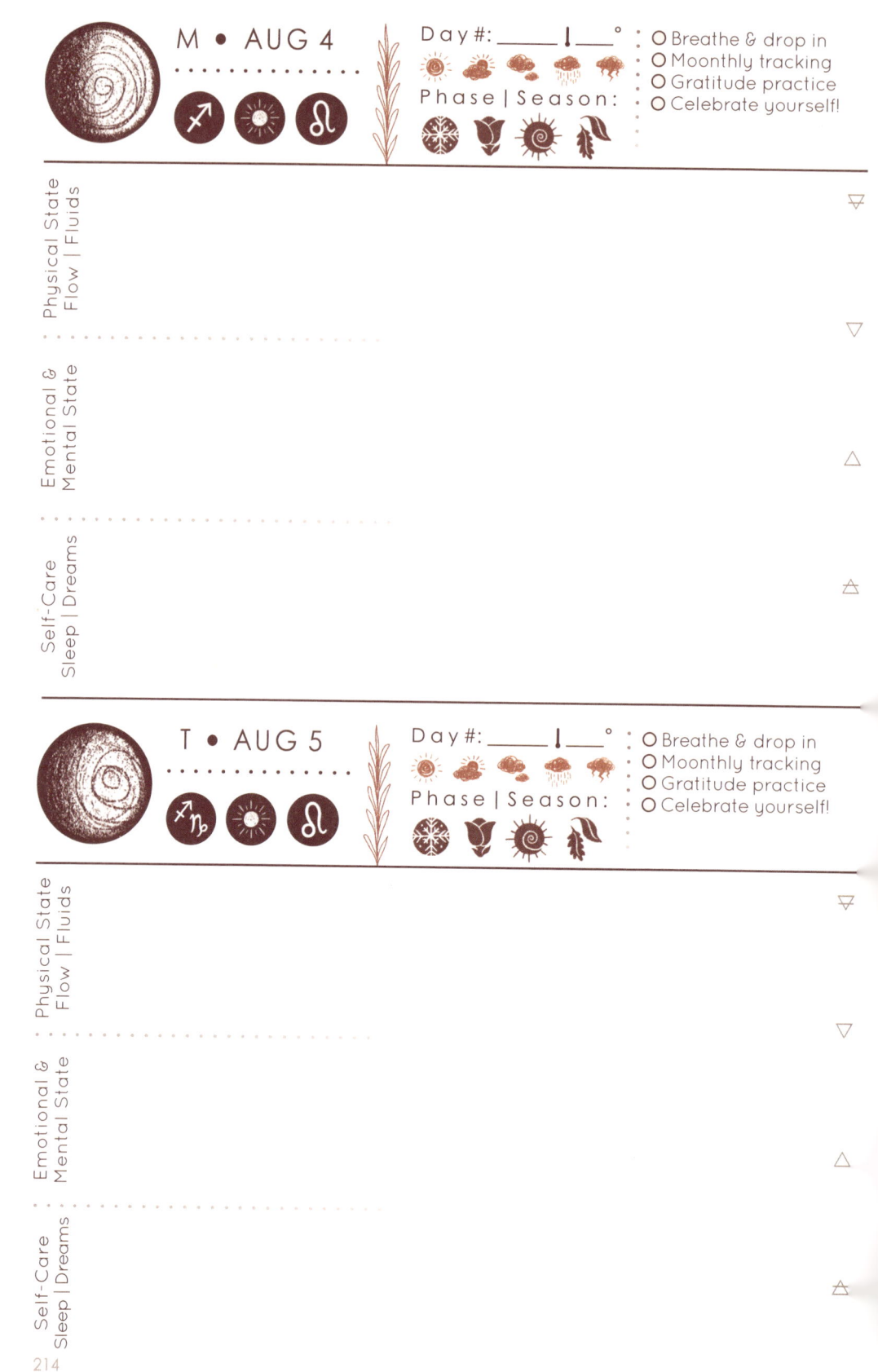

Day #: _____ | _____°

Phase | Season:

- ○ Breathe & drop in
- ○ Moonthly tracking
- ○ Gratitude practice
- ○ Celebrate yourself!

Physical State / Flow | Fluids

Emotional & Mental State

Self-Care / Sleep | Dreams

T • AUG 5

Day #: _____ | _____°

Phase | Season:

- ○ Breathe & drop in
- ○ Moonthly tracking
- ○ Gratitude practice
- ○ Celebrate yourself!

Physical State / Flow | Fluids

Emotional & Mental State

Self-Care / Sleep | Dreams

W • AUG 6

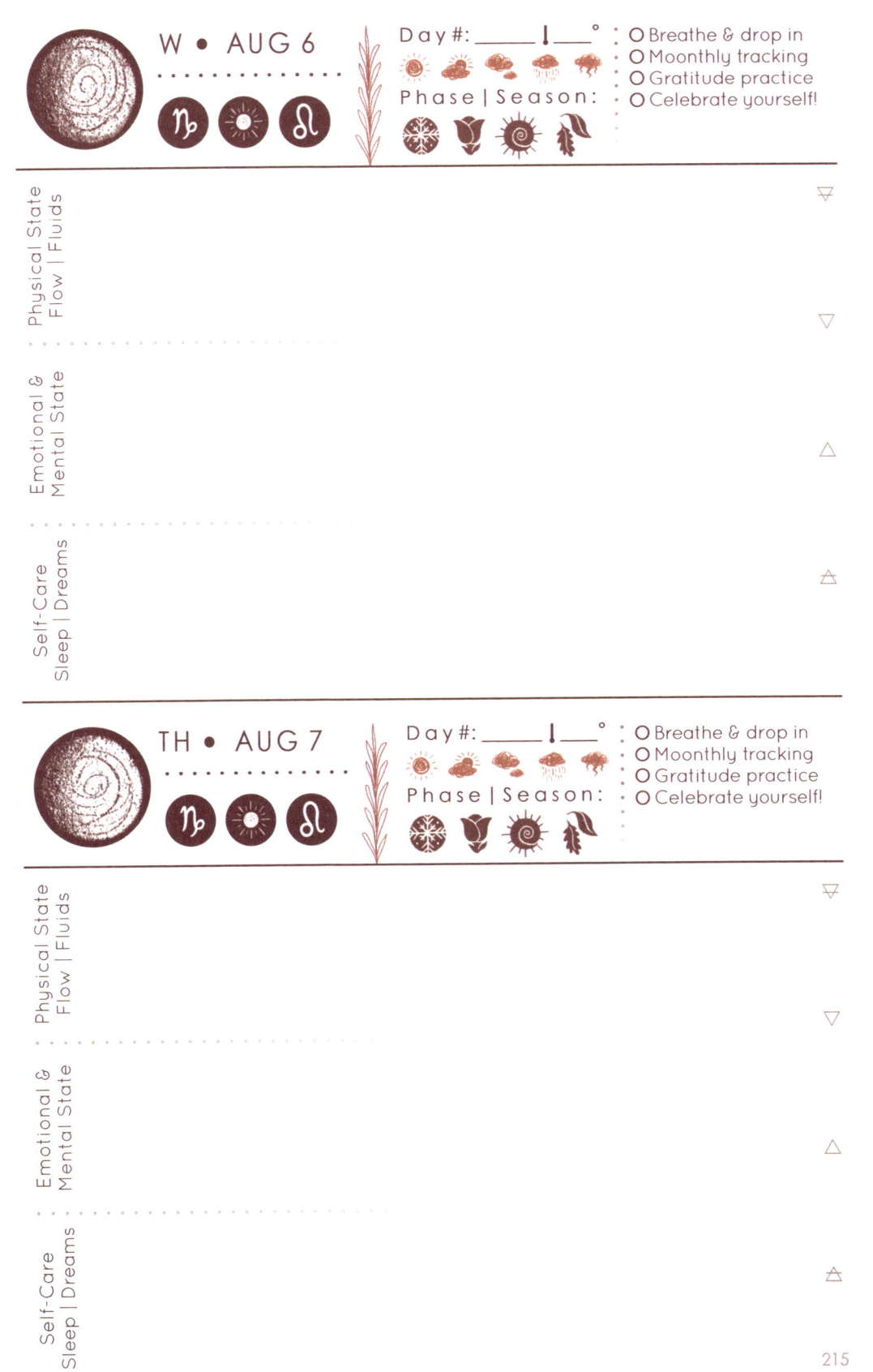

♑ ☉ ♌

Day #: _____ | _____°

Phase | Season:

- ○ Breathe & drop in
- ○ Moonthly tracking
- ○ Gratitude practice
- ○ Celebrate yourself!

Physical State / Flow | Fluids

Emotional & Mental State

Self-Care / Sleep | Dreams

TH • AUG 7

♑ ☉ ♌

Day #: _____ | _____°

Phase | Season:

- ○ Breathe & drop in
- ○ Moonthly tracking
- ○ Gratitude practice
- ○ Celebrate yourself!

Physical State / Flow | Fluids

Emotional & Mental State

Self-Care / Sleep | Dreams

F • AUG 8

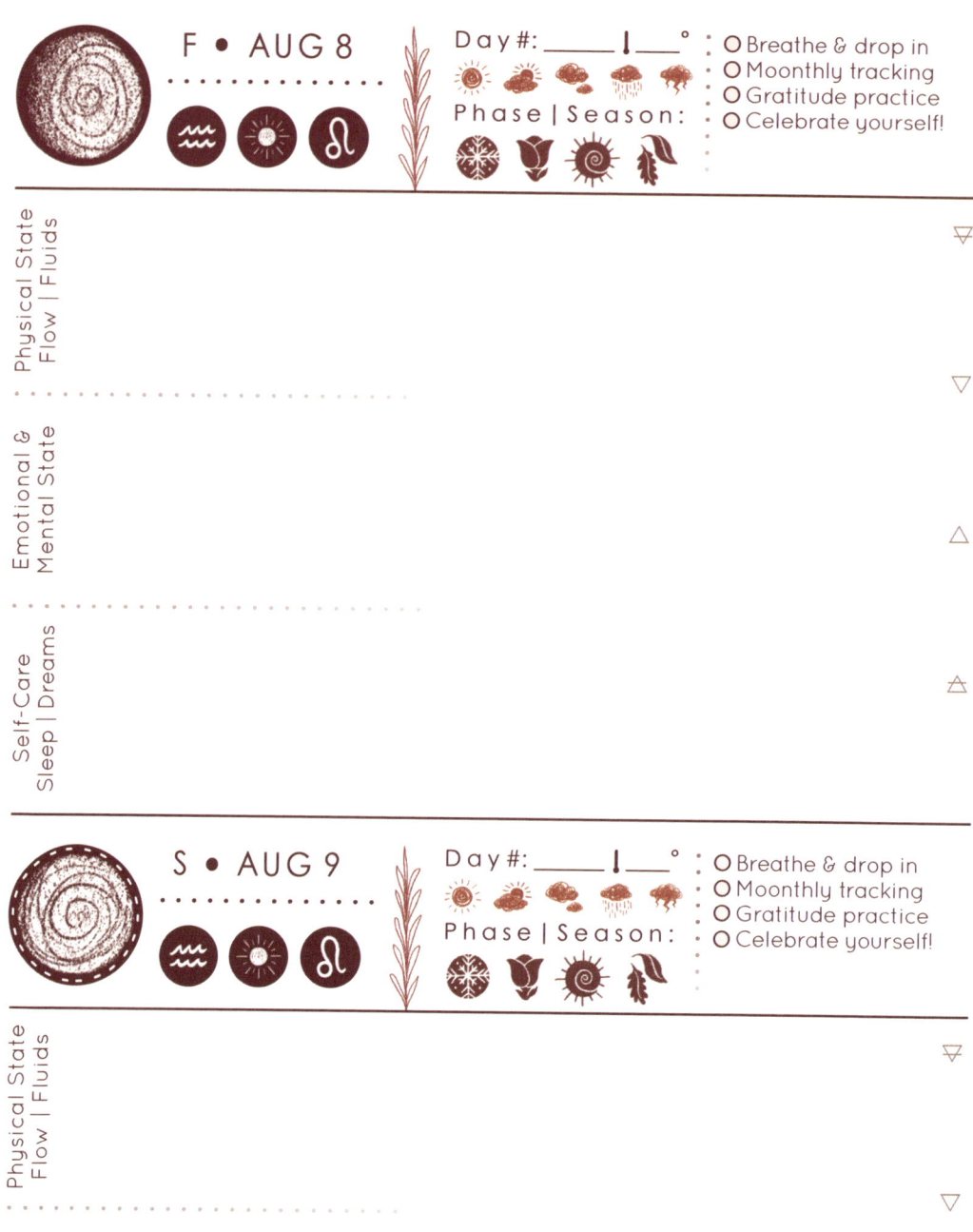

Day #: _____ | _____°

Phase | Season:

- ○ Breathe & drop in
- ○ Moonthly tracking
- ○ Gratitude practice
- ○ Celebrate yourself!

Physical State / Flow | Fluids

Emotional & Mental State

Self-Care / Sleep | Dreams

S • AUG 9

Day #: _____ | _____°

Phase | Season:

- ○ Breathe & drop in
- ○ Moonthly tracking
- ○ Gratitude practice
- ○ Celebrate yourself!

Physical State / Flow | Fluids

Emotional & Mental State

Self-Care / Sleep | Dreams

FULL MOON IN AQUARIUS

Embracing experimentation & allowing open interpretation of all discoveries

What is being illuminated?

I give gratitude for what is & what is becoming:

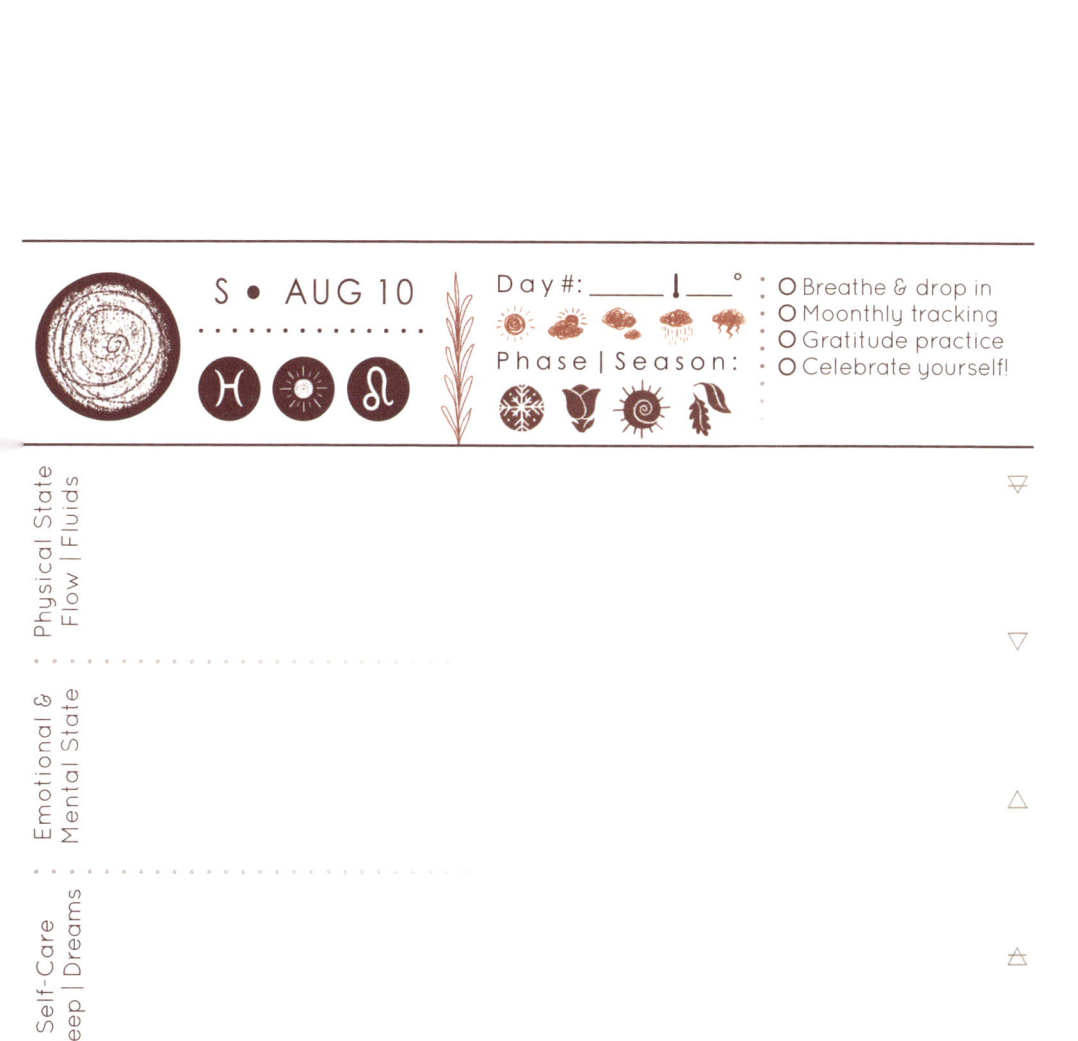

S • AUG 10

Day #: _____ | ___°

Phase | Season:

- ○ Breathe & drop in
- ○ Moonthly tracking
- ○ Gratitude practice
- ○ Celebrate yourself!

Physical State — Flow | Fluids

Emotional & Mental State

Self-Care — Sleep | Dreams

M • AUG 11

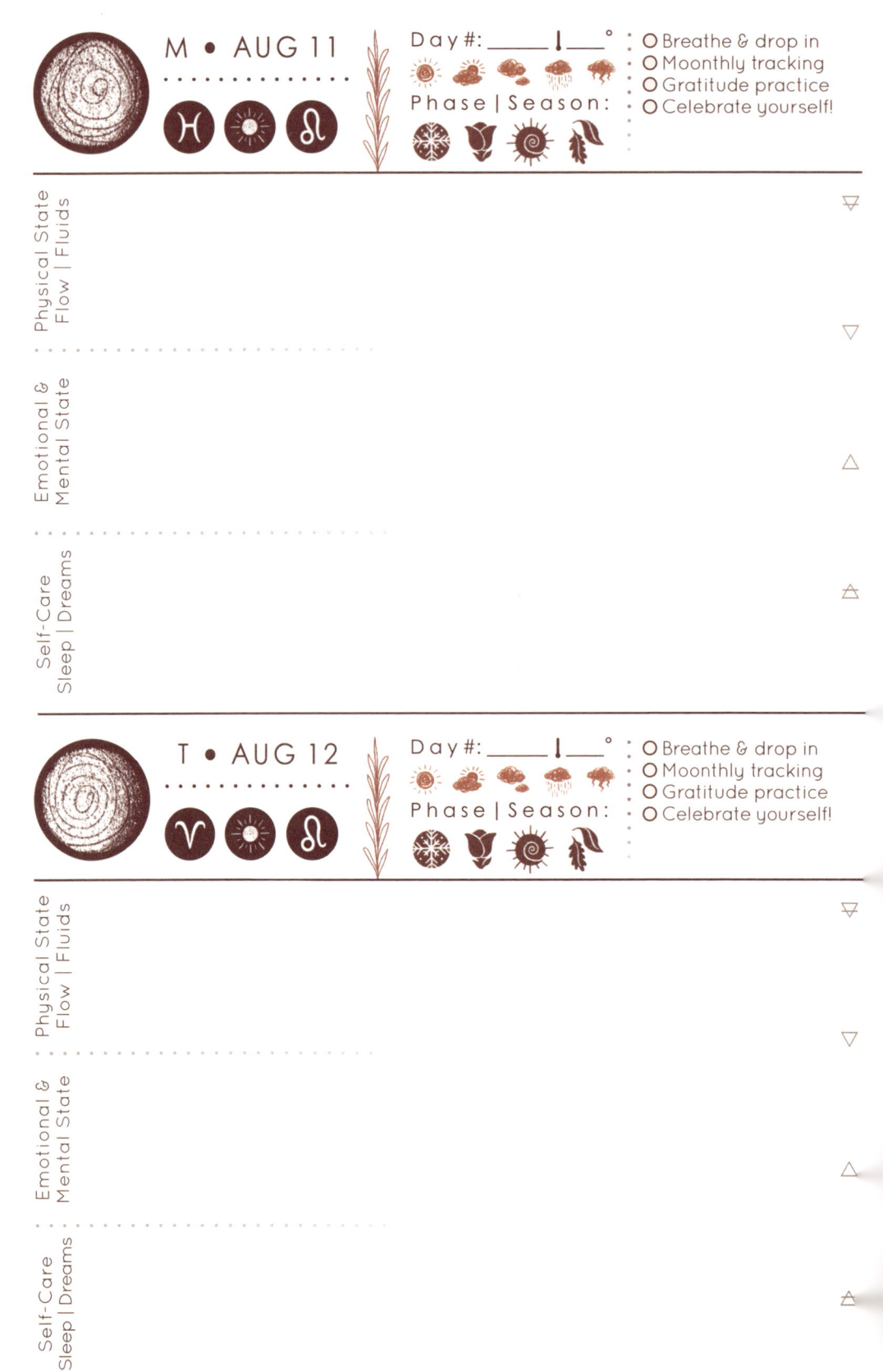

Day #: _____ | _____°

Phase | Season:

- Breathe & drop in
- Moonthly tracking
- Gratitude practice
- Celebrate yourself!

Physical State — Flow | Fluids

Emotional & Mental State

Self-Care — Sleep | Dreams

T • AUG 12

Day #: _____ | _____°

Phase | Season:

- Breathe & drop in
- Moonthly tracking
- Gratitude practice
- Celebrate yourself!

Physical State — Flow | Fluids

Emotional & Mental State

Self-Care — Sleep | Dreams

W • AUG 13

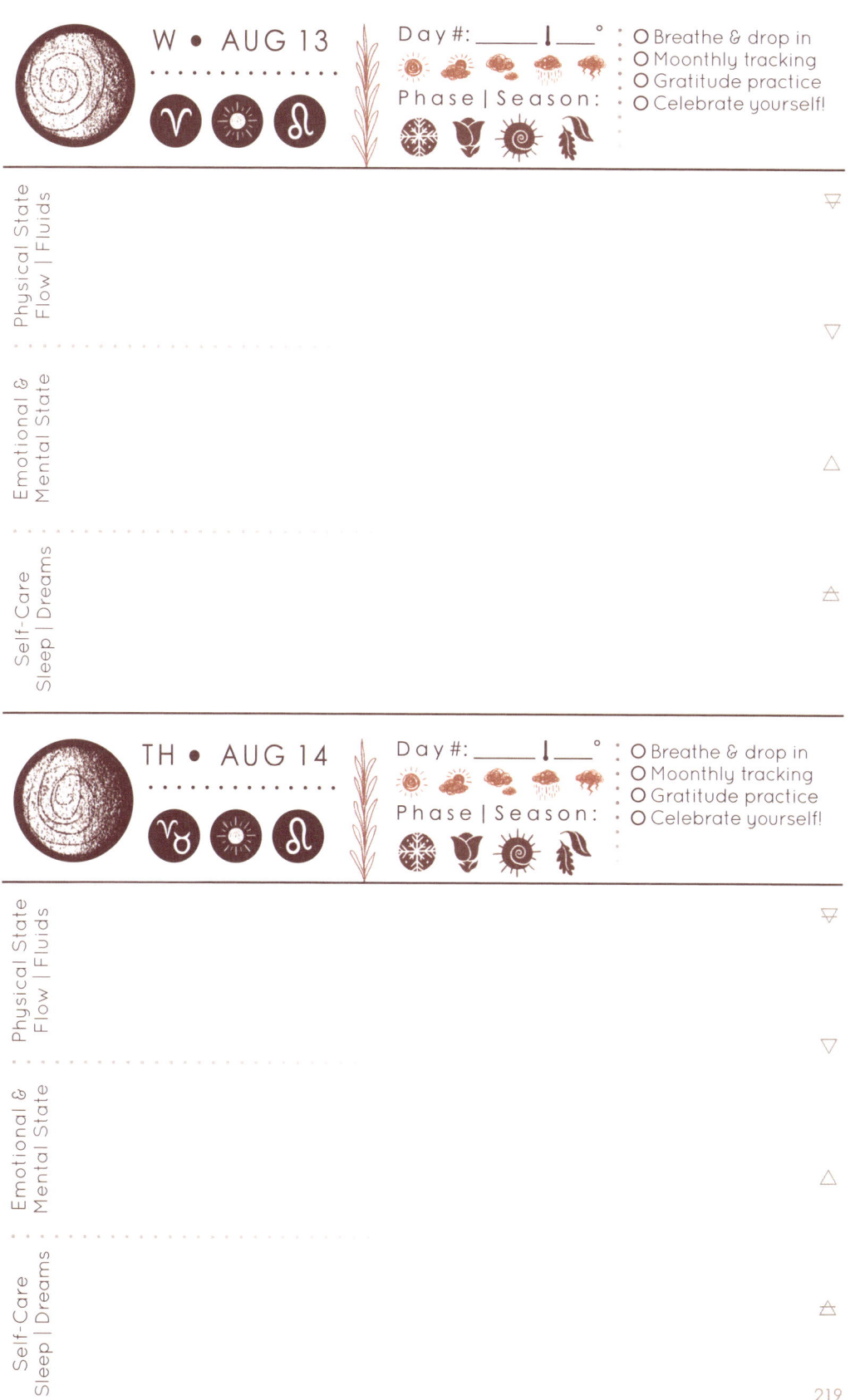

♈ ☉ ♌

Day #: _____ | _____°

Phase | Season:

- Breathe & drop in
- Moonthly tracking
- Gratitude practice
- Celebrate yourself!

Physical State
Flow | Fluids

Emotional &
Mental State

Self-Care
Sleep | Dreams

TH • AUG 14

♑ ☉ ♌

Day #: _____ | _____°

Phase | Season:

- Breathe & drop in
- Moonthly tracking
- Gratitude practice
- Celebrate yourself!

Physical State
Flow | Fluids

Emotional &
Mental State

Self-Care
Sleep | Dreams

F • AUG 15

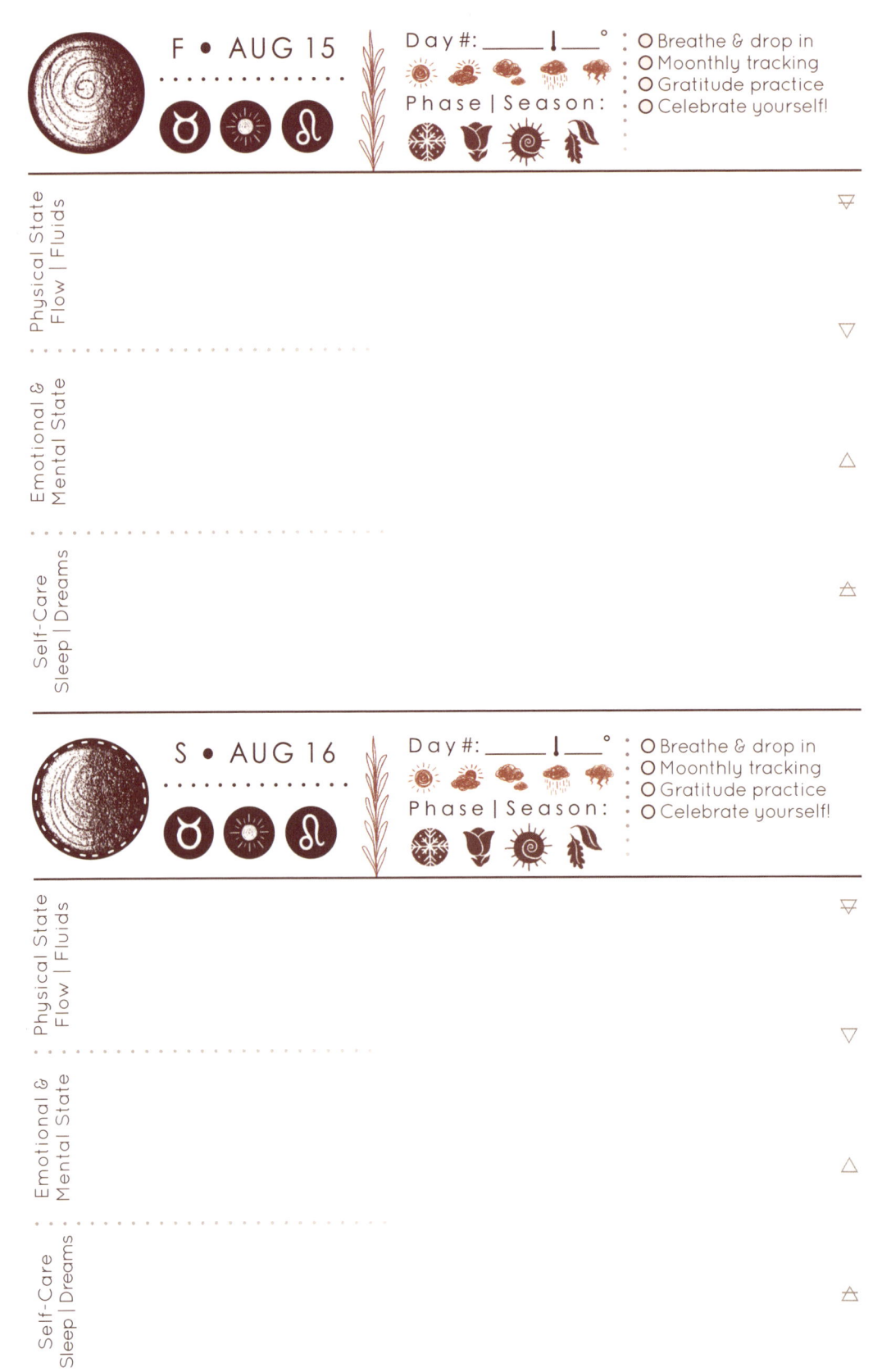

♉ ☀ ♌

Day #: _____ | _____°

Phase | Season:

○ Breathe & drop in
○ Moonthly tracking
○ Gratitude practice
○ Celebrate yourself!

Physical State
Flow | Fluids

Emotional &
Mental State

Self-Care
Sleep | Dreams

S • AUG 16

♉ ☀ ♌

Day #: _____ | _____°

Phase | Season:

○ Breathe & drop in
○ Moonthly tracking
○ Gratitude practice
○ Celebrate yourself!

Physical State
Flow | Fluids

Emotional &
Mental State

Self-Care
Sleep | Dreams

LAST QUARTER IN TAURUS

A deep surrender in allowing traditions to shift & evolve with respect

What am I leaving behind this lunar cycle?

Where can I make more space for reflection &/or integration?

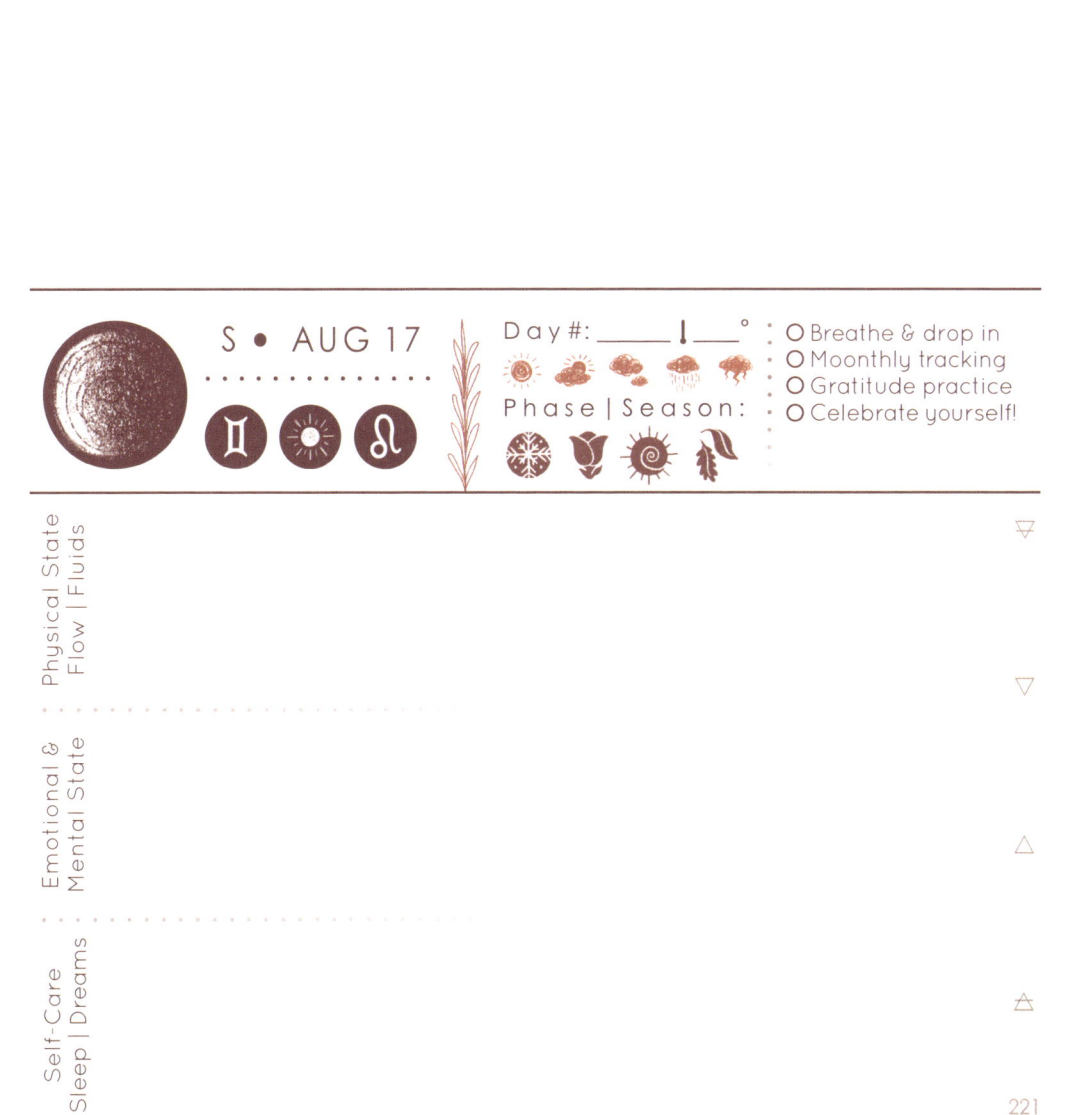

S • AUG 17

Day #: _____ | _____°

Phase | Season:

- ○ Breathe & drop in
- ○ Moonthly tracking
- ○ Gratitude practice
- ○ Celebrate yourself!

Physical State
Flow | Fluids

Emotional &
Mental State

Self-Care
Sleep | Dreams

M • AUG 18

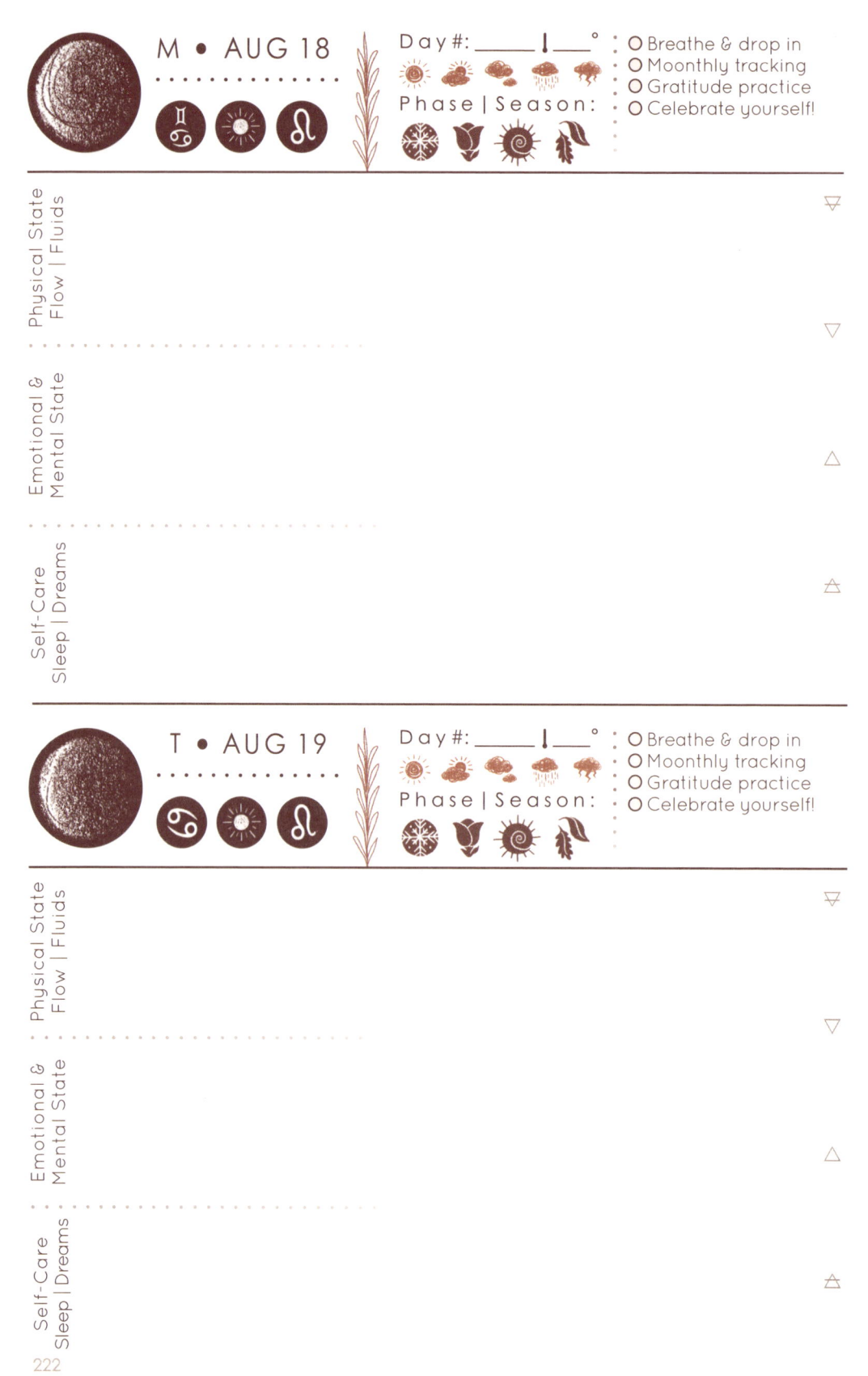

Day #: _____ | _____°
Phase | Season:

○ Breathe & drop in
○ Moonthly tracking
○ Gratitude practice
○ Celebrate yourself!

Physical State
Flow | Fluids

Emotional &
Mental State

Self-Care
Sleep | Dreams

T • AUG 19

Day #: _____ | _____°
Phase | Season:

○ Breathe & drop in
○ Moonthly tracking
○ Gratitude practice
○ Celebrate yourself!

Physical State
Flow | Fluids

Emotional &
Mental State

Self-Care
Sleep | Dreams

222

W • AUG 20

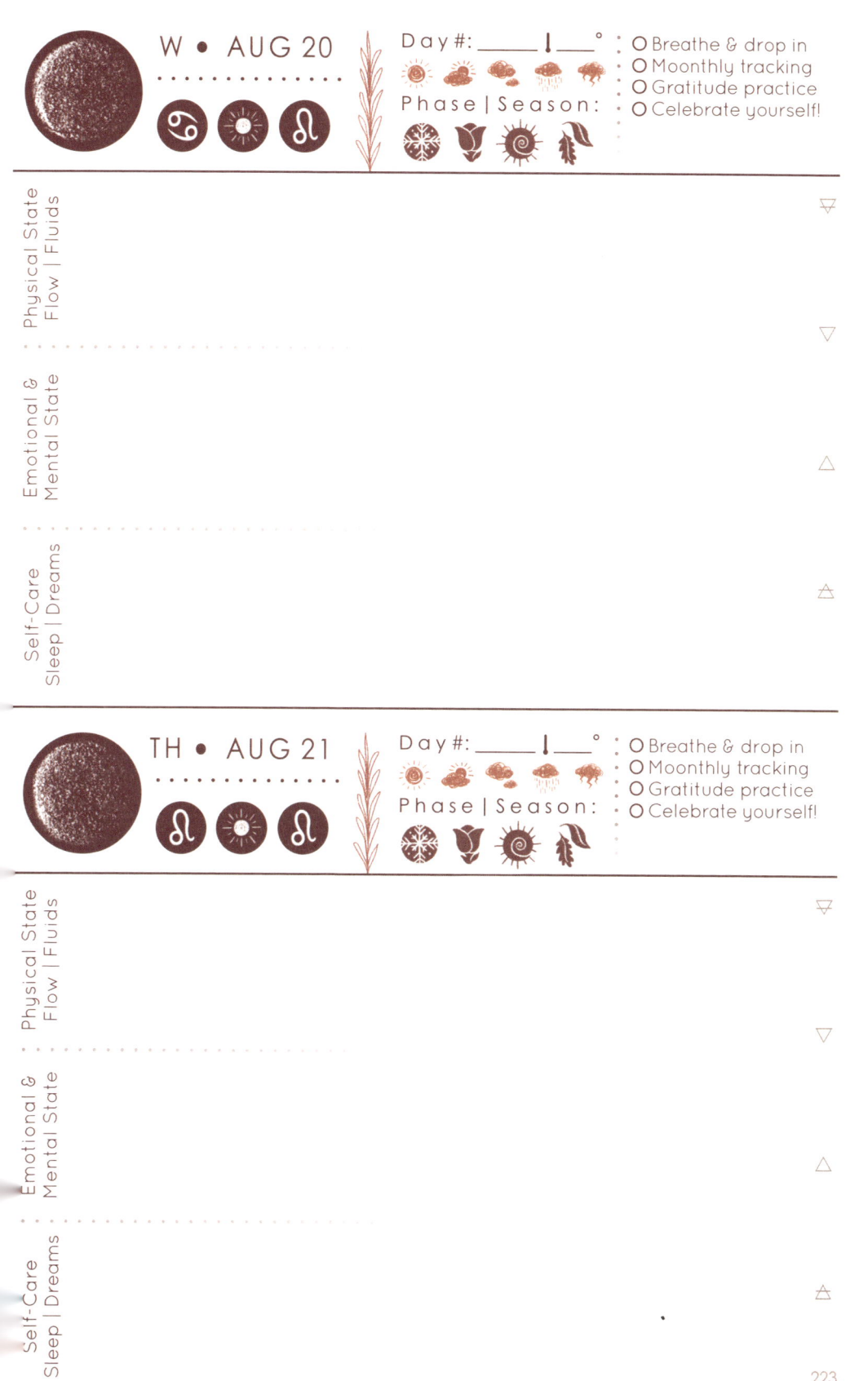

Day #: _____ | _____°

Phase | Season:

○ Breathe & drop in
○ Moonthly tracking
○ Gratitude practice
○ Celebrate yourself!

Physical State / Flow | Fluids

Emotional & Mental State

Self-Care / Sleep | Dreams

TH • AUG 21

Day #: _____ | _____°

Phase | Season:

○ Breathe & drop in
○ Moonthly tracking
○ Gratitude practice
○ Celebrate yourself!

Physical State / Flow | Fluids

Emotional & Mental State

Self-Care / Sleep | Dreams

☾ 7th
07 | 24
08 | 22

CHECK IN & REFLECT

Last Cycle Day 1: _____

Last Cycle Length: _____

Circle the phase you bled near:

○ ☾ ☾ ☾ ☾ ● ● ● ☽ ☽ ☽ ○

Caution Days: (days I needed space)

Bliss Days: (days I felt great)

Use this space to reflect on your experiences & findings from this ending lunar cycle or your last menstrual cycle. Use cycle day #s if you bleed, or moon phases if you don't.

DAYS TO NOTE — Which cycle days stood out?

OBSERVATIONS — Notice any changes or patterns?

SELF-CARE — What was helpful & nourishing?

PLAN & PREPARE

Next Predicted Cycle:
🩸 ☾ _____

CHECKLIST

Add the following to any other planners or calendars for your next cycle, then check it off.

- ☐ Predicted "days to note" _____
- ☐ Days to slow down (pre-bleed) _____
- ☐ Rest day(s) (next bleed) _____
- ☐ Date with yourself _____
- ☐ _____

- ☐ Self chest/breast exam
- ☐ Meal plan with cycle
- ☐ _____
- ☐ _____
- ☐ _____

OPEN SPACE

Use this space how you wish, or print out one of our free templates to paste here for BBT charting, dream tracking, or something else:

Moon Sign Medicine: Astrological Tarot Spread

by Iris Rivera (they/them) • Astrologer, Witch, Psychic & Reiki Practitioner • @iristhebrujx • iristhebrujx.com •

Many of us are on lifelong journeys of learning how to love ourselves more skillfully. Our astrological Moon sign can help identify how to nurture ourselves compassionately and how to listen to our inner wisdom. The Moon represents our physical/emotional body, our caregiver or mother and intuition.

You can think of this spread as an interview, you are asking your Moon sign questions about what it needs and how you can tenderly care for it. Use what you know or can research about your Moon sign to complement how you interpret the tarot card.

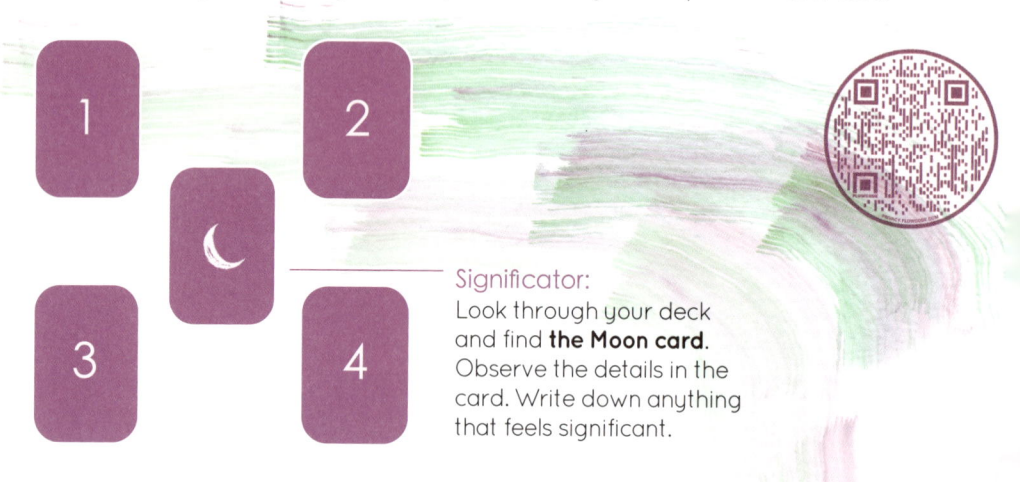

Significator: Look through your deck and find **the Moon card**. Observe the details in the card. Write down anything that feels significant.

Card 1: **How does my Moon sign need to be nurtured?**

For example, if you are an Air Moon and you draw The Empress, there is a need to physically ground in your body instead of spending so much time in your head overthinking.

Card 2: **How does my Moon sign offer a sense of belonging with others?**

For example, if you are an Earth Moon and you draw The Star, you are so materially driven and invested in progress that can be seen. You need a community that inspires idealism and makes space for your hopes and dreams to take flight.

Card 3: **What does my Moon sign struggle with most?**

For example, if you are a Fire Moon and you draw the Ace of Cups, you struggle with the intensity of your feelings. You can be overwhelmed by your own passion.

Card 4: **What medicine does my Moon sign offer me?**

For example, if you are a Water Moon and you draw the Queen of Pentacles, your Moon sign offers the medicine of intuitive nurturing. You are naturally gifted at translating your love into demonstrative acts of care for yourself and others.

Phasic Overview & In-Betweens

Use this space to focus on the phases of the moonth and the in-betweens of the peak lunations.

One way of using this space is to designate one column for your goal-planning, intention-setting or focus per phase/week. Use the other column for reflections, dream themes, nutrition tracking, cards pulls, etc!

F • AUG 22

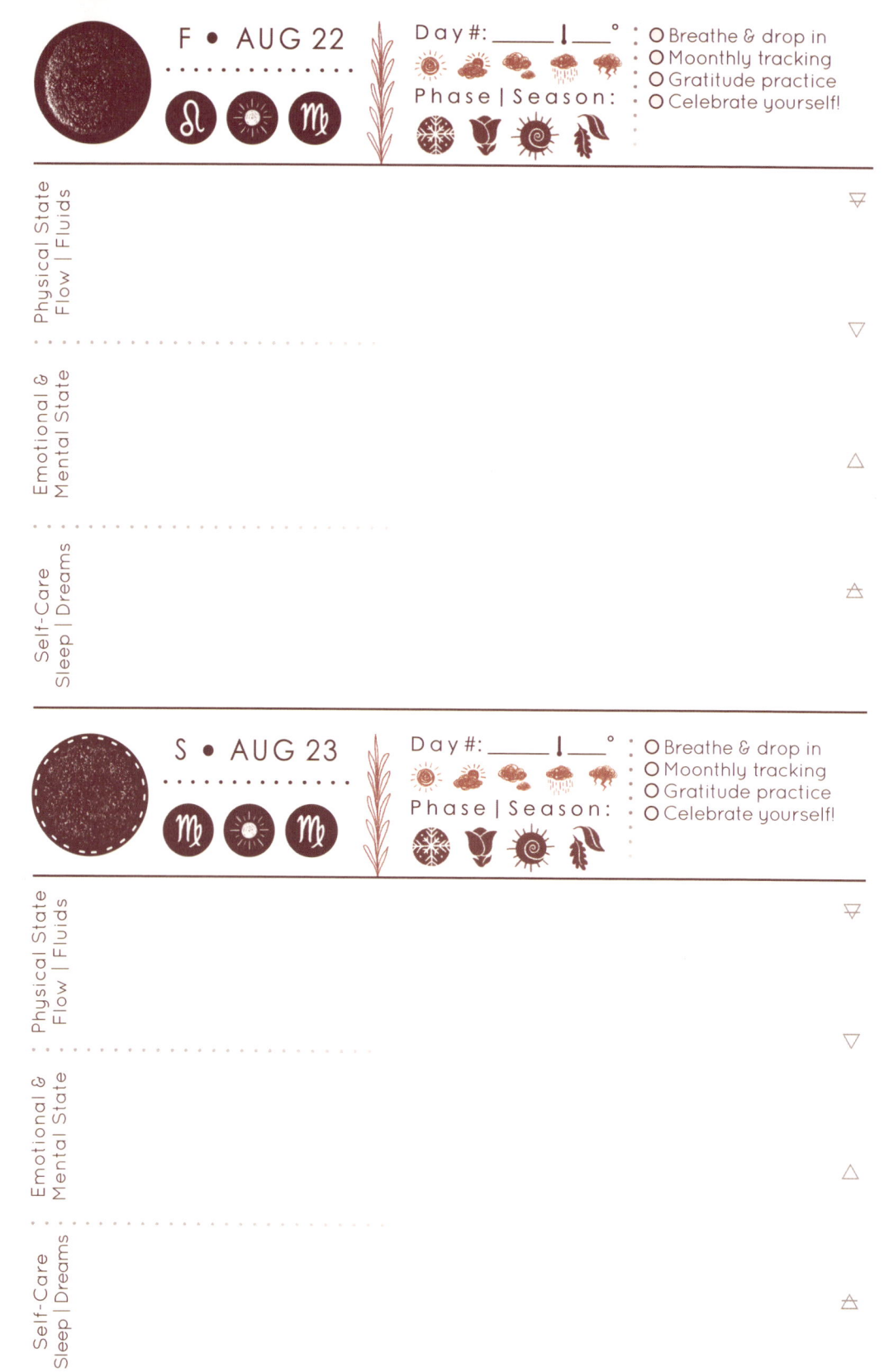

Day #: _____ | _____°

Phase | Season:

- ○ Breathe & drop in
- ○ Moonthly tracking
- ○ Gratitude practice
- ○ Celebrate yourself!

Physical State / Flow | Fluids

Emotional & Mental State

Self-Care / Sleep | Dreams

S • AUG 23

Day #: _____ | _____°

Phase | Season:

- ○ Breathe & drop in
- ○ Moonthly tracking
- ○ Gratitude practice
- ○ Celebrate yourself!

Physical State / Flow | Fluids

Emotional & Mental State

Self-Care / Sleep | Dreams

NEW MOON IN VIRGO

Opening up to alternate routines that honor earthly vessels

What do I want to grow & focus on during this lunar cycle?

How will I hold space for this?

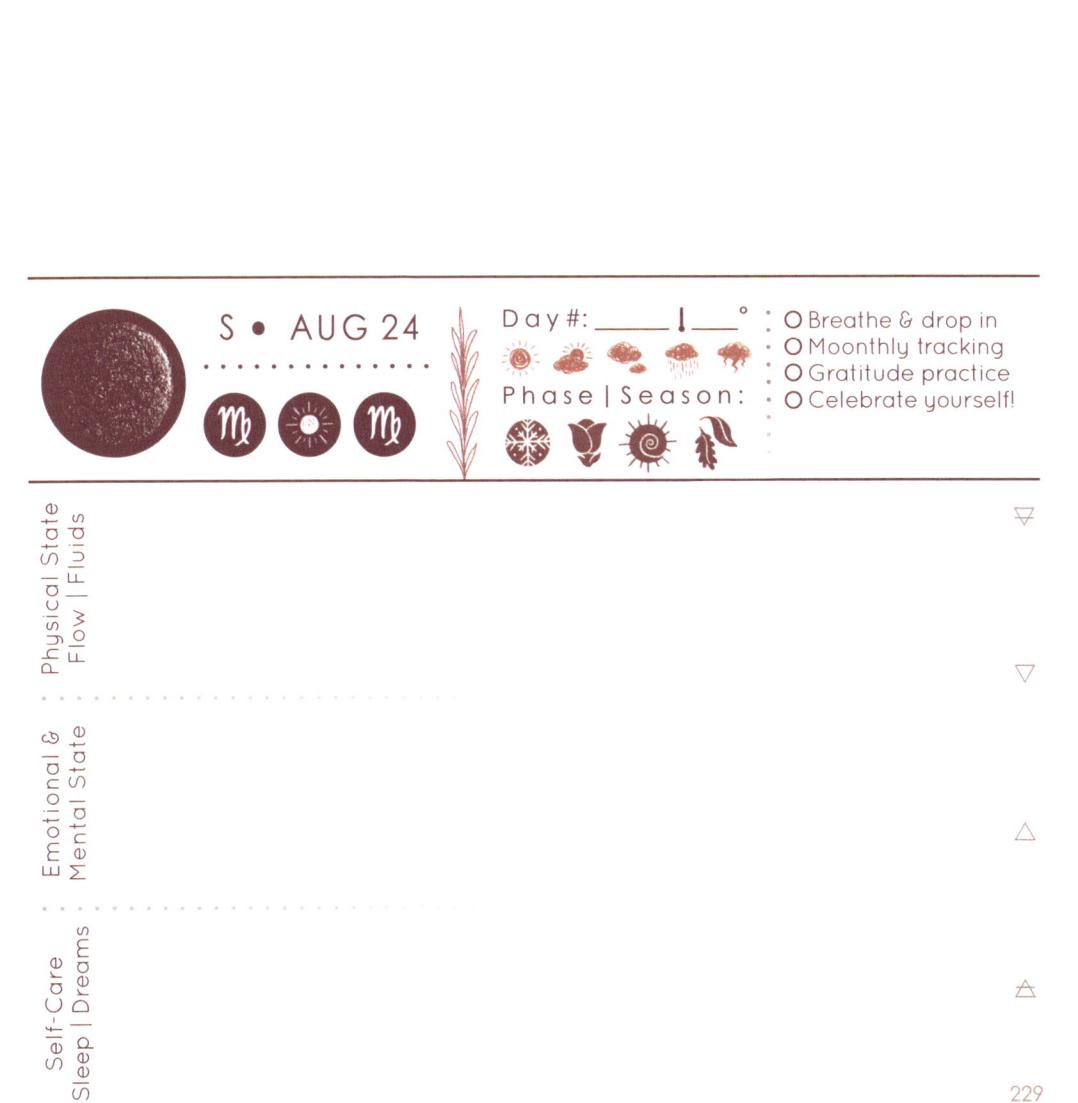

S • AUG 24

Day #: _____ | _____°

Phase | Season:

- ○ Breathe & drop in
- ○ Moonthly tracking
- ○ Gratitude practice
- ○ Celebrate yourself!

Physical State
Flow | Fluids

Emotional &
Mental State

Self-Care
Sleep | Dreams

M • AUG 25

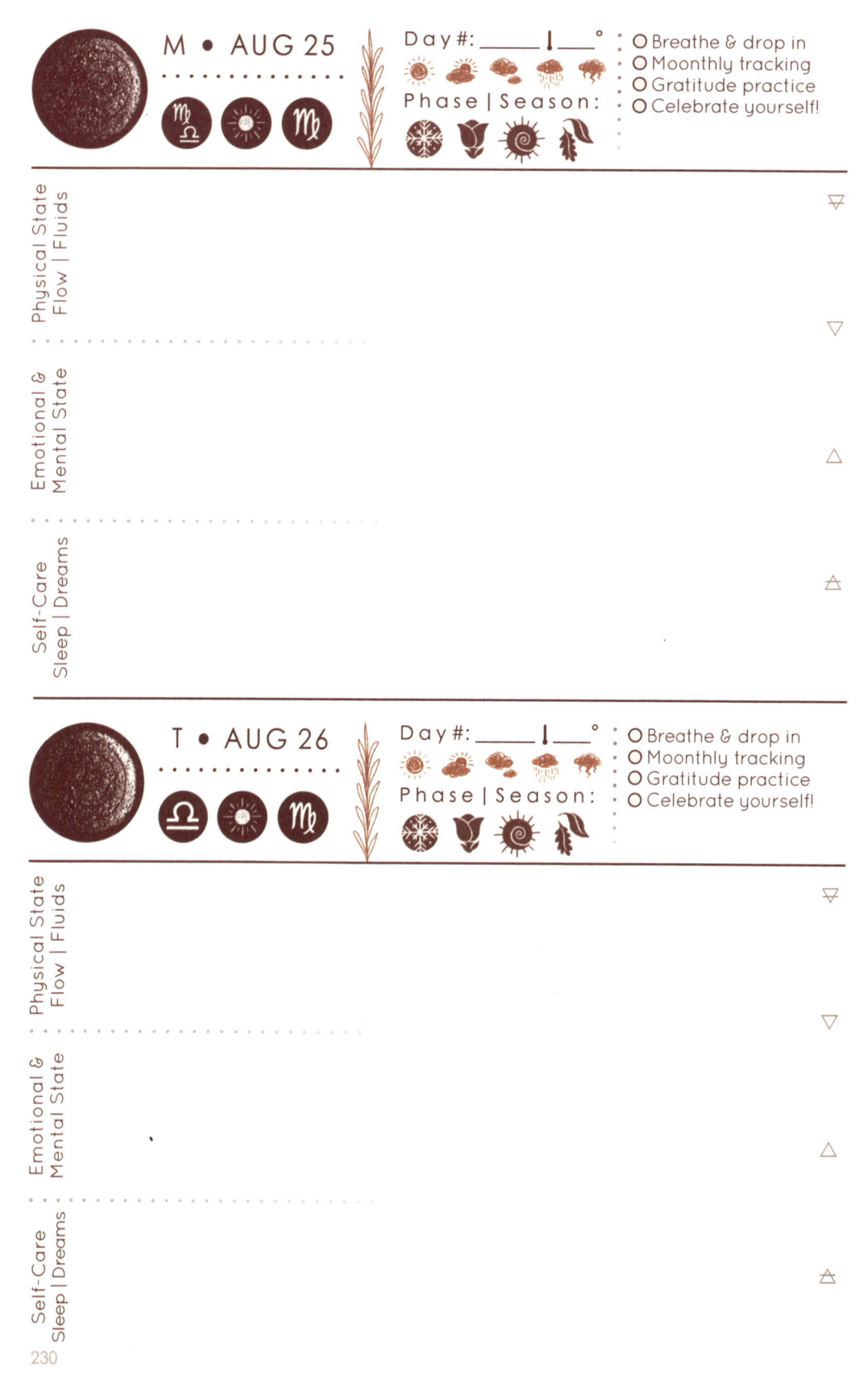

Day #: _____ | _____°

Phase | Season:

- ○ Breathe & drop in
- ○ Moonthly tracking
- ○ Gratitude practice
- ○ Celebrate yourself!

Physical State / Flow | Fluids

Emotional & Mental State

Self-Care / Sleep | Dreams

T • AUG 26

Day #: _____ | _____°

Phase | Season:

- ○ Breathe & drop in
- ○ Moonthly tracking
- ○ Gratitude practice
- ○ Celebrate yourself!

Physical State / Flow | Fluids

Emotional & Mental State

Self-Care / Sleep | Dreams

W • AUG 27

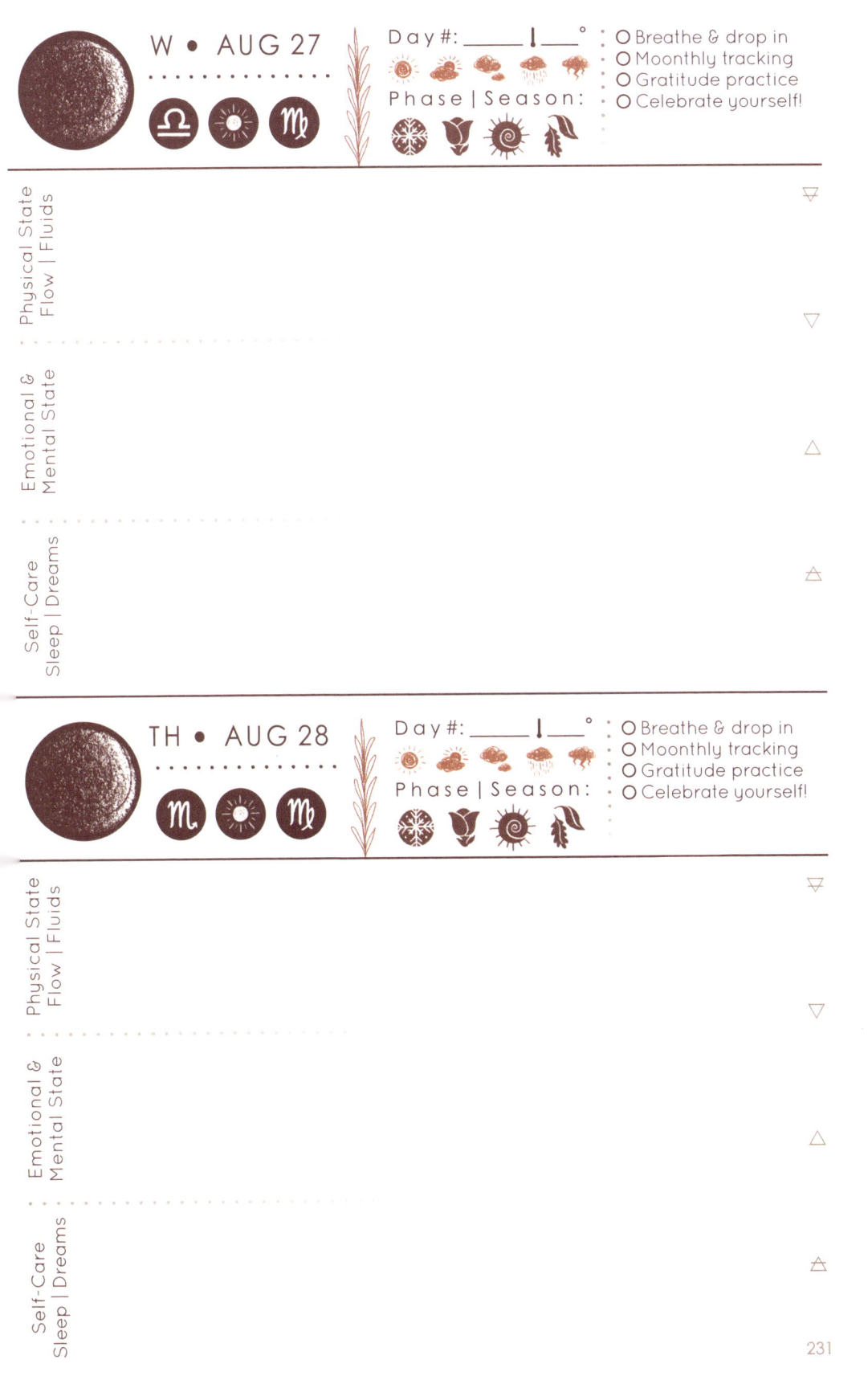

Day #: _____ | _____°

Phase | Season:

- Breathe & drop in
- Moonthly tracking
- Gratitude practice
- Celebrate yourself!

Physical State
Flow | Fluids

Emotional &
Mental State

Self-Care
Sleep | Dreams

TH • AUG 28

Day #: _____ | _____°

Phase | Season:

- Breathe & drop in
- Moonthly tracking
- Gratitude practice
- Celebrate yourself!

Physical State
Flow | Fluids

Emotional &
Mental State

Self-Care
Sleep | Dreams

F • AUG 29

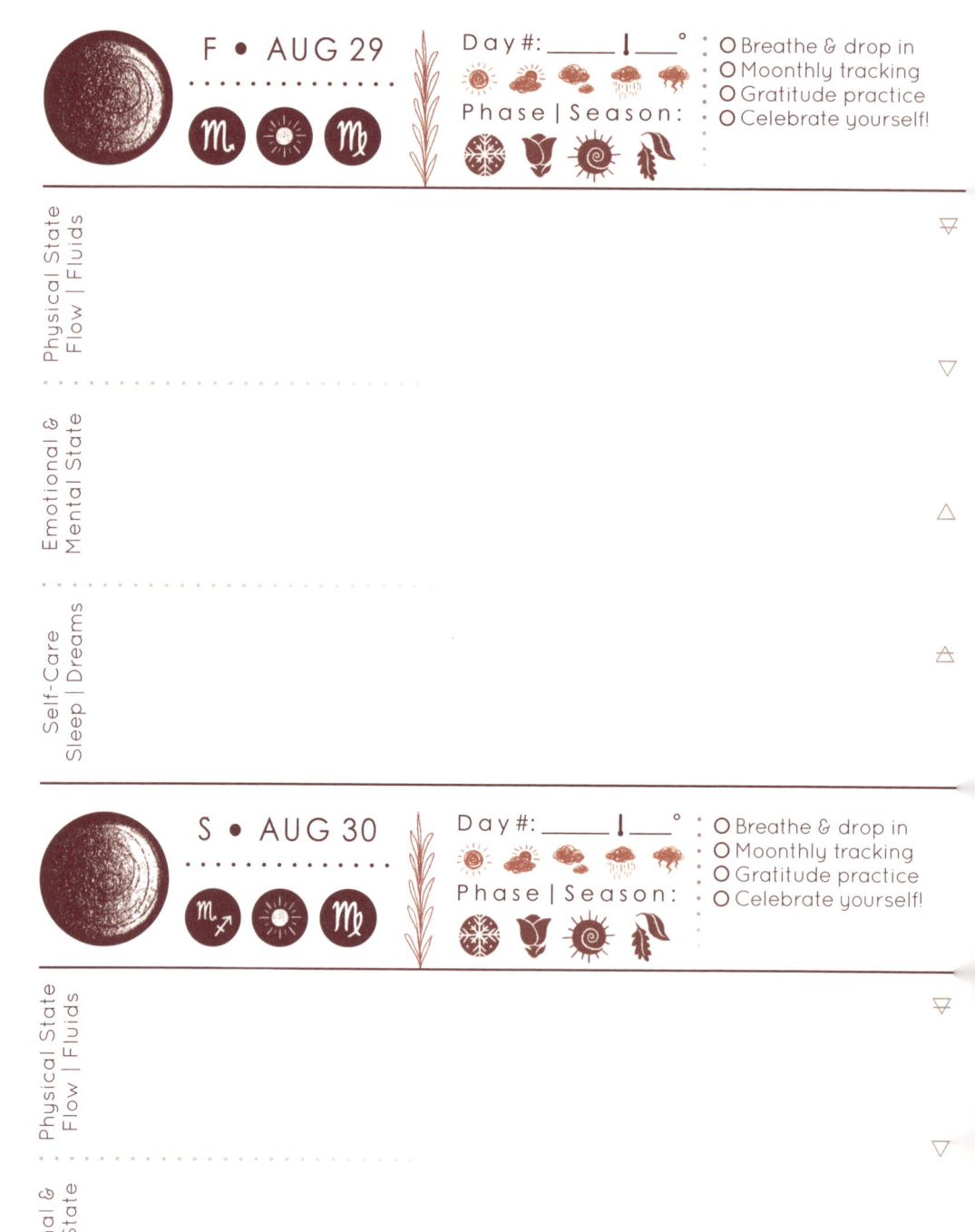

Day #: _____ | _____°

Phase | Season:

- ○ Breathe & drop in
- ○ Moonthly tracking
- ○ Gratitude practice
- ○ Celebrate yourself!

Physical State / Flow | Fluids

Emotional & Mental State

Self-Care / Sleep | Dreams

S • AUG 30

Day #: _____ | _____°

Phase | Season:

- ○ Breathe & drop in
- ○ Moonthly tracking
- ○ Gratitude practice
- ○ Celebrate yourself!

Physical State / Flow | Fluids

Emotional & Mental State

Self-Care / Sleep | Dreams

S • AUG 31

Day #: _____ | _____°

Phase | Season:

- O Breathe & drop in
- O Moonthly tracking
- O Gratitude practice
- O Celebrate yourself!

Physical State / Flow | Fluids

Emotional & Mental State

Self-Care / Sleep | Dreams

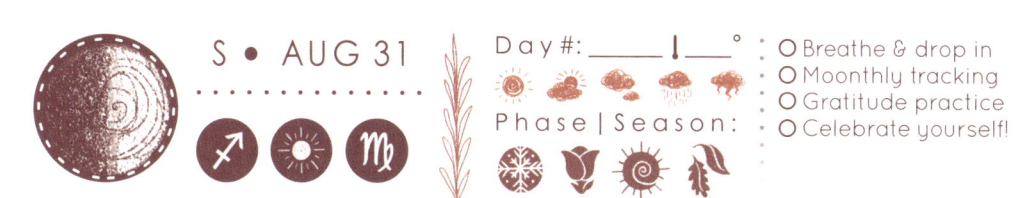

FIRST QUARTER IN SAGITTARIUS

Exploring layers of meaning in unfurling teachings

What is sprouting & coming into awareness?

What can I release to make space for further growth & grounding?

M • SEPT 1

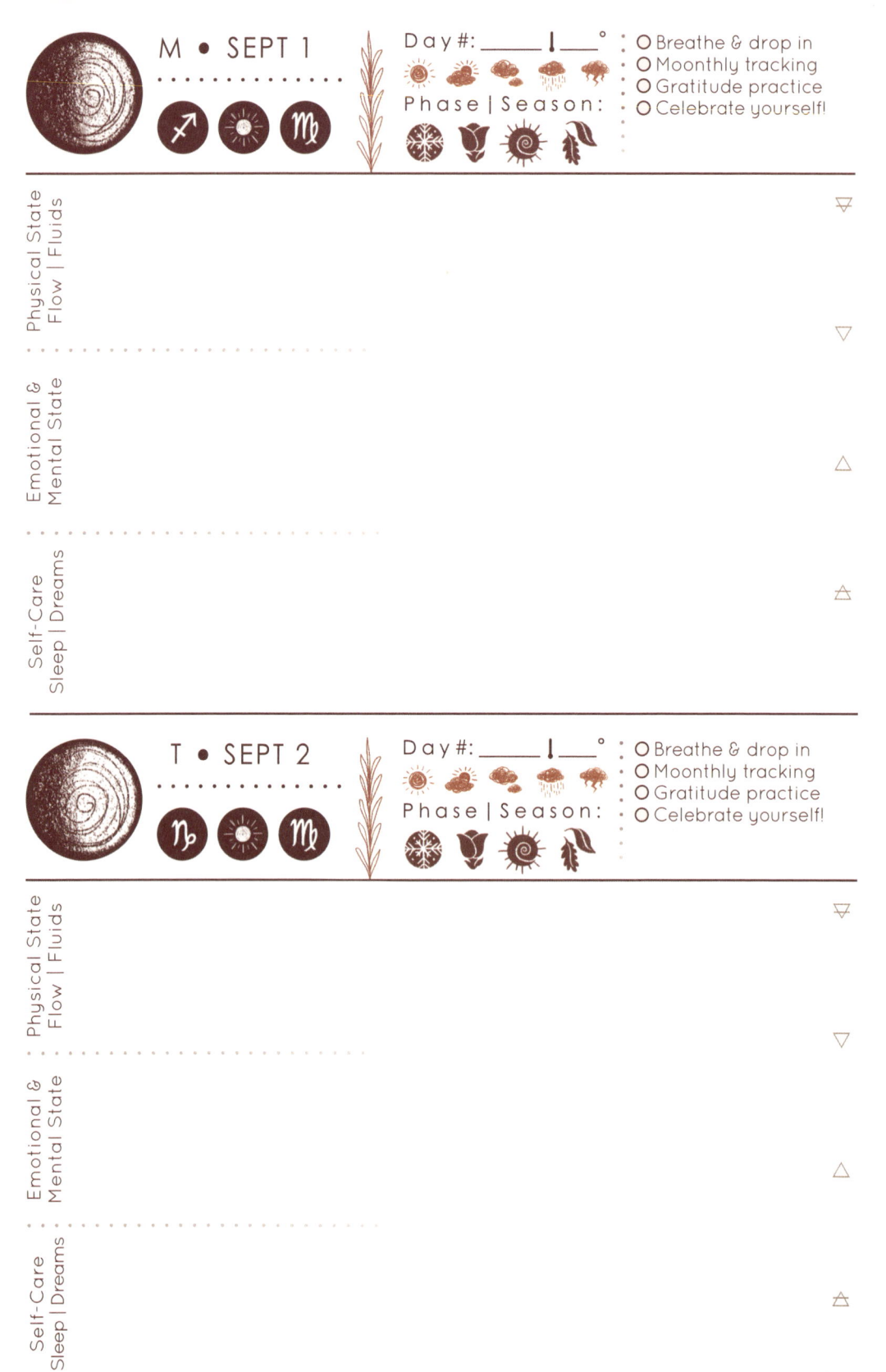

Day #: _____ | _____°

Phase | Season:

- ○ Breathe & drop in
- ○ Moonthly tracking
- ○ Gratitude practice
- ○ Celebrate yourself!

Physical State / Flow | Fluids

Emotional & Mental State

Self-Care / Sleep | Dreams

T • SEPT 2

Day #: _____ | _____°

Phase | Season:

- ○ Breathe & drop in
- ○ Moonthly tracking
- ○ Gratitude practice
- ○ Celebrate yourself!

Physical State / Flow | Fluids

Emotional & Mental State

Self-Care / Sleep | Dreams

W • SEPT 3

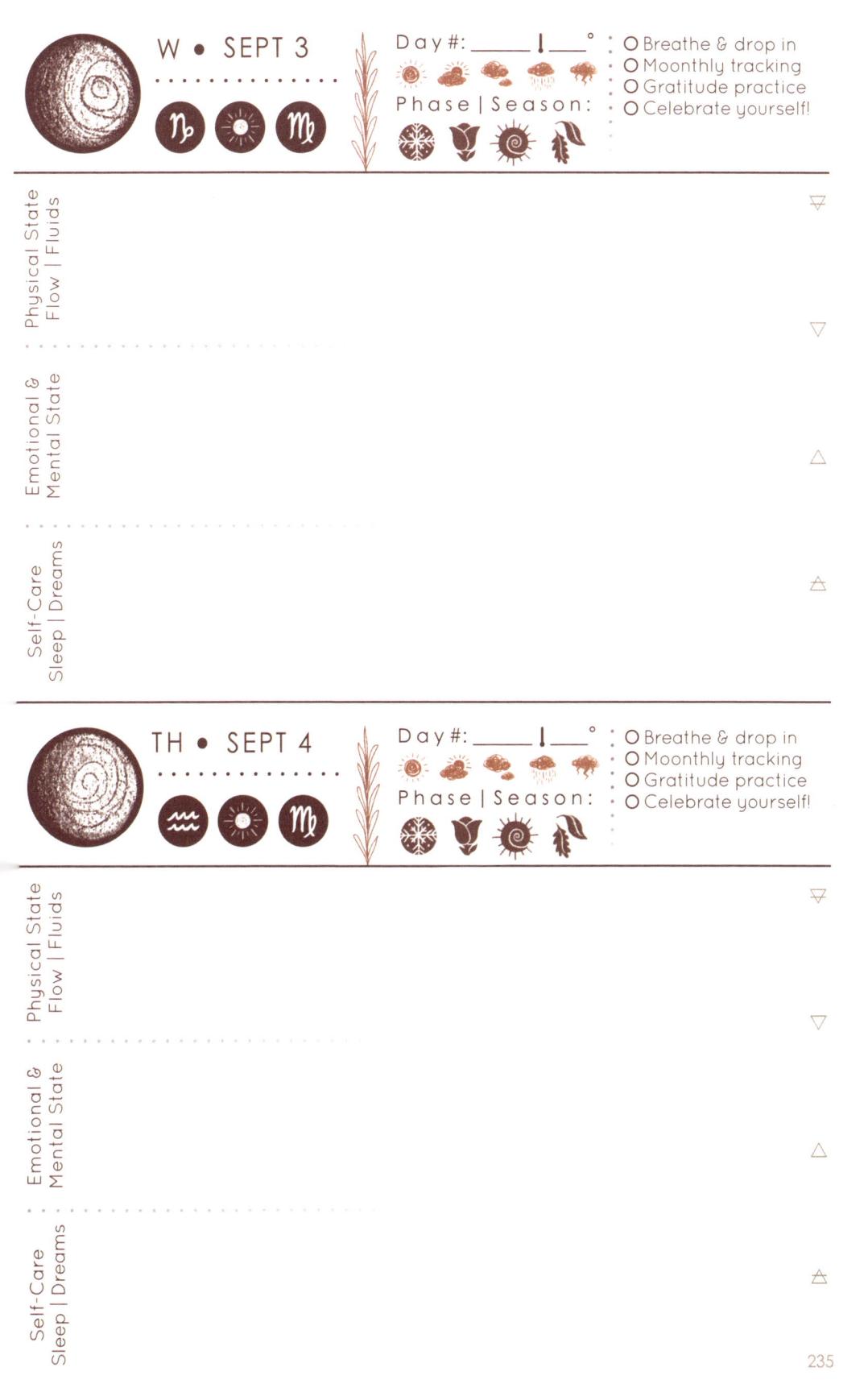

♑ ☉ ♍

Day #: _____ | _____°

Phase | Season:

- Breathe & drop in
- Moonthly tracking
- Gratitude practice
- Celebrate yourself!

Physical State / Flow | Fluids

Emotional & Mental State

Self-Care / Sleep | Dreams

TH • SEPT 4

♒ ☉ ♍

Day #: _____ | _____°

Phase | Season:

- Breathe & drop in
- Moonthly tracking
- Gratitude practice
- Celebrate yourself!

Physical State / Flow | Fluids

Emotional & Mental State

Self-Care / Sleep | Dreams

F • SEPT 5

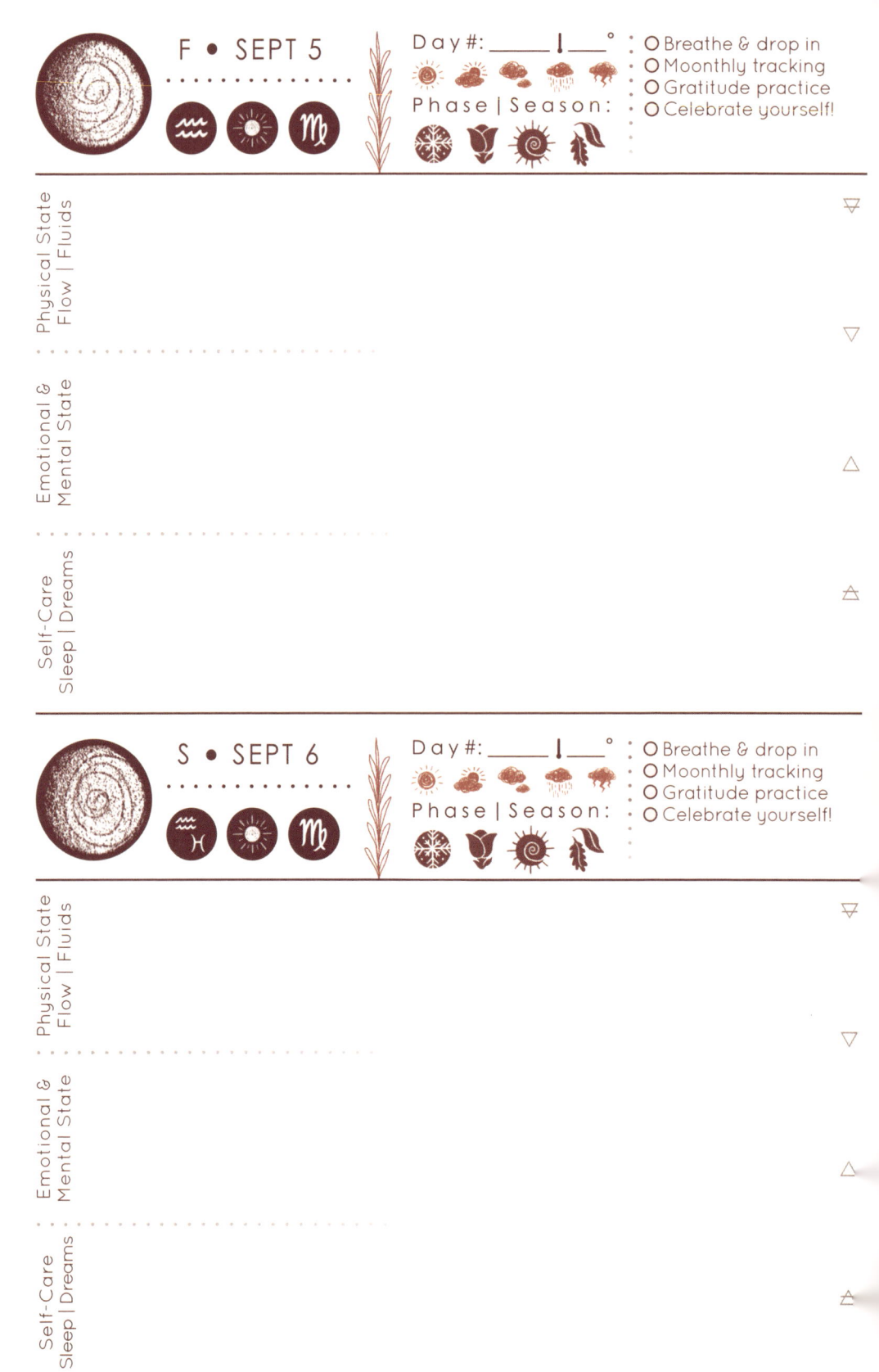

Day #: _____ | _____°

Phase | Season:

- ○ Breathe & drop in
- ○ Moonthly tracking
- ○ Gratitude practice
- ○ Celebrate yourself!

Physical State
Flow | Fluids

Emotional &
Mental State

Self-Care
Sleep | Dreams

S • SEPT 6

Day #: _____ | _____°

Phase | Season:

- ○ Breathe & drop in
- ○ Moonthly tracking
- ○ Gratitude practice
- ○ Celebrate yourself!

Physical State
Flow | Fluids

Emotional &
Mental State

Self-Care
Sleep | Dreams

S • SEPT 7

Day #: _____ | ___°

Phase | Season:

- ○ Breathe & drop in
- ○ Moonthly tracking
- ○ Gratitude practice
- ○ Celebrate yourself!

Physical State / Flow | Fluids

Emotional & Mental State

Self-Care / Sleep | Dreams

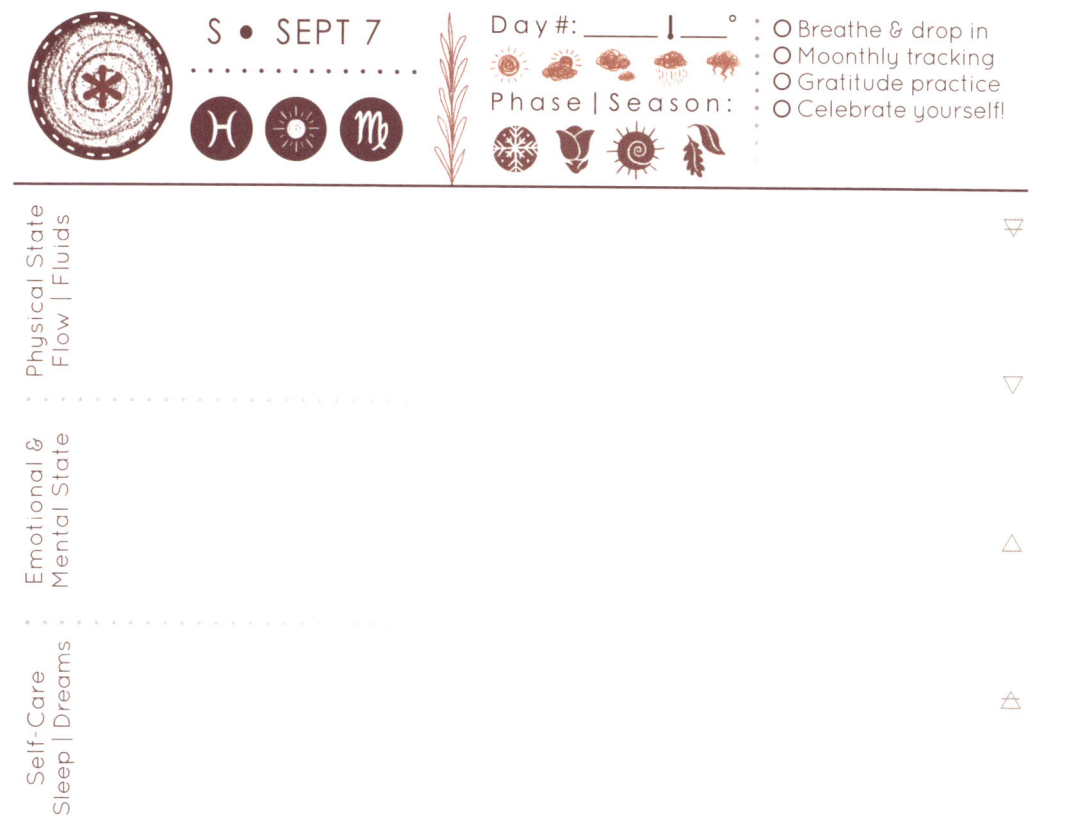

FULL MOON LUNAR ECLIPSE IN PISCES

Diving deep into the universal abundance within, guided from beyond

What is being illuminated?

give gratitude for what is & what is becoming:

M • SEPT 8

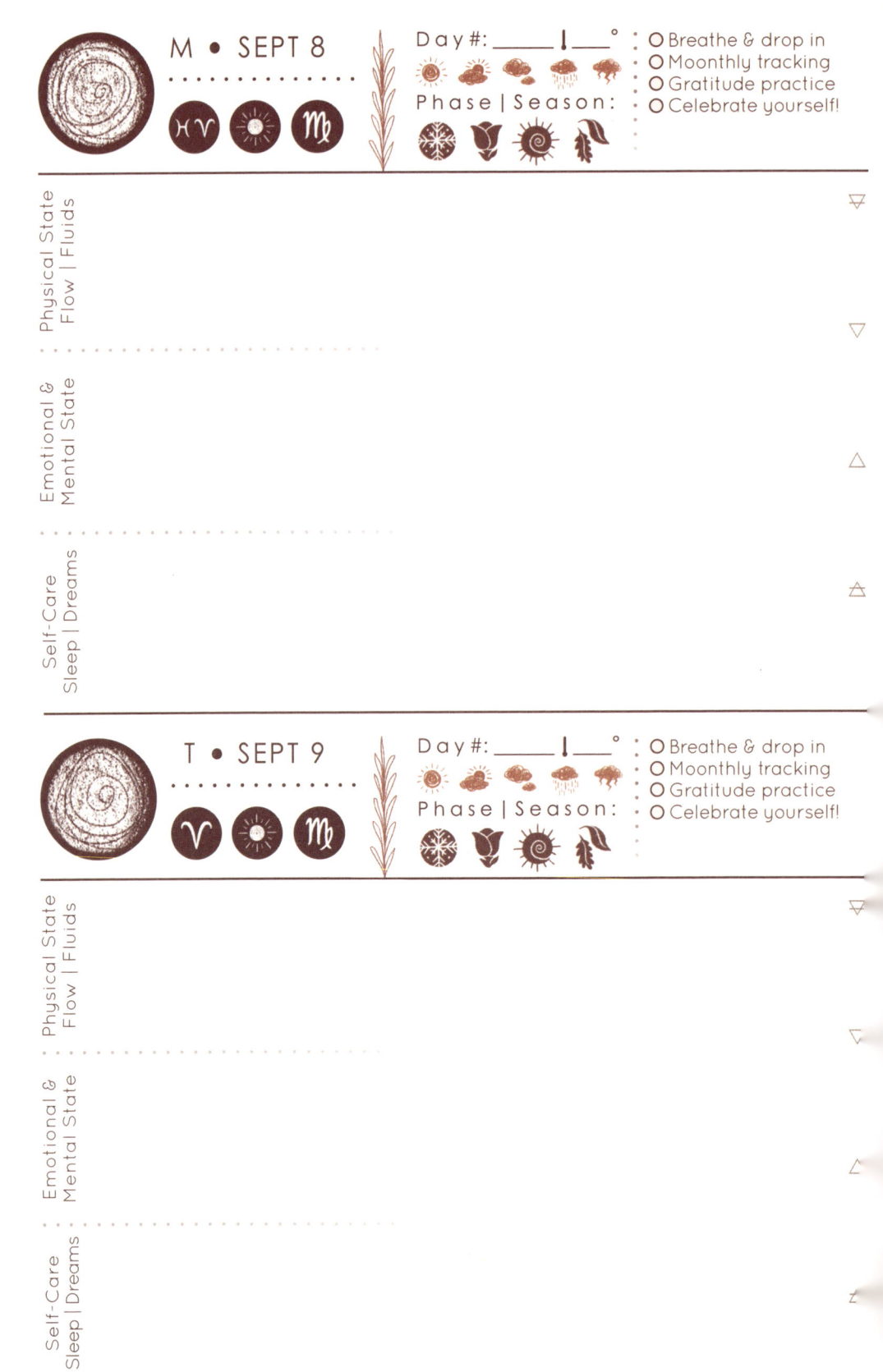

Day #: _____ | ___°

Phase | Season:

- Breathe & drop in
- Moonthly tracking
- Gratitude practice
- Celebrate yourself!

Physical State / Flow | Fluids

Emotional & Mental State

Self-Care / Sleep | Dreams

T • SEPT 9

Day #: _____ | ___°

Phase | Season:

- Breathe & drop in
- Moonthly tracking
- Gratitude practice
- Celebrate yourself!

Physical State / Flow | Fluids

Emotional & Mental State

Self-Care / Sleep | Dreams

W • SEPT 10

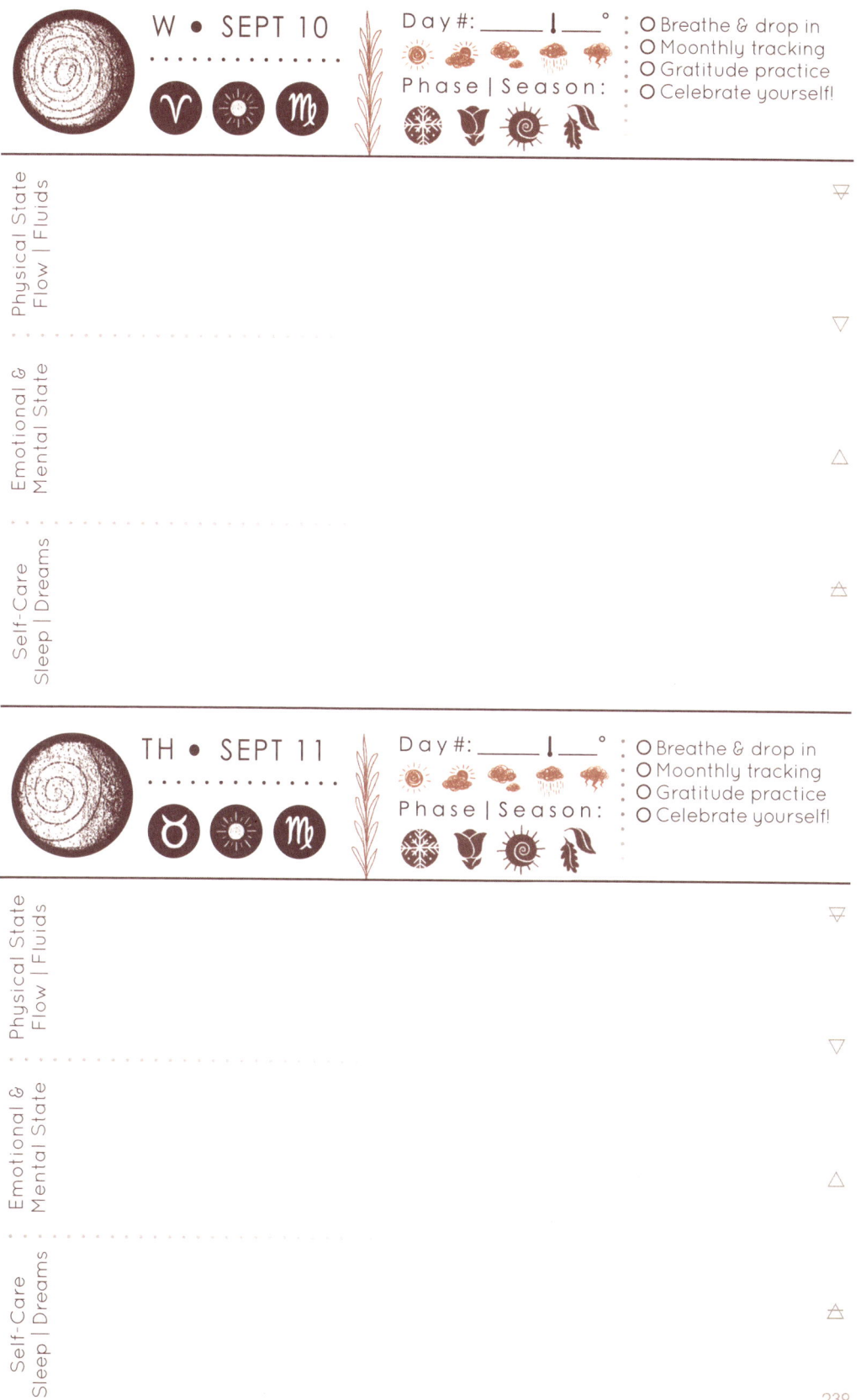

♈ ☀ ♍

Day #: _____ | ___°

Phase | Season:

- Breathe & drop in
- Moonthly tracking
- Gratitude practice
- Celebrate yourself!

Physical State / Flow | Fluids

Emotional & Mental State

Self-Care / Sleep | Dreams

TH • SEPT 11

♉ ☀ ♍

Day #: _____ | ___°

Phase | Season:

- Breathe & drop in
- Moonthly tracking
- Gratitude practice
- Celebrate yourself!

Physical State / Flow | Fluids

Emotional & Mental State

Self-Care / Sleep | Dreams

F • SEPT 12

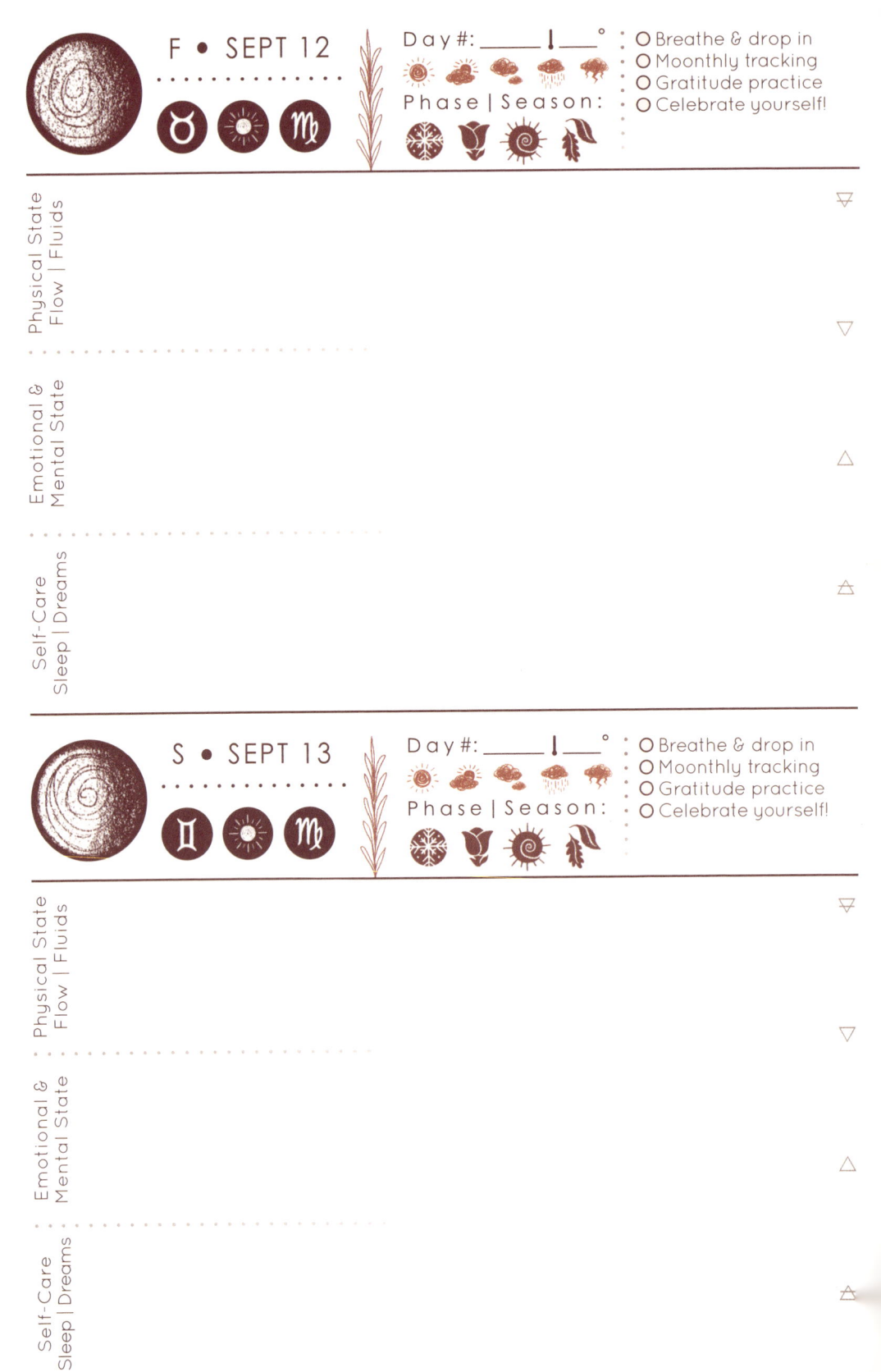

Day #: _____ | _____°

Phase | Season:

- ○ Breathe & drop in
- ○ Moonthly tracking
- ○ Gratitude practice
- ○ Celebrate yourself!

Physical State / Flow | Fluids

Emotional & Mental State

Self-Care / Sleep | Dreams

S • SEPT 13

Day #: _____ | _____°

Phase | Season:

- ○ Breathe & drop in
- ○ Moonthly tracking
- ○ Gratitude practice
- ○ Celebrate yourself!

Physical State / Flow | Fluids

Emotional & Mental State

Self-Care / Sleep | Dreams

S • SEPT 14

Day #: _____ | _____°

Phase | Season:

- ○ Breathe & drop in
- ○ Moonthly tracking
- ○ Gratitude practice
- ○ Celebrate yourself!

Physical State
Flow | Fluids

Emotional &
Mental State

Self-Care
Sleep | Dreams

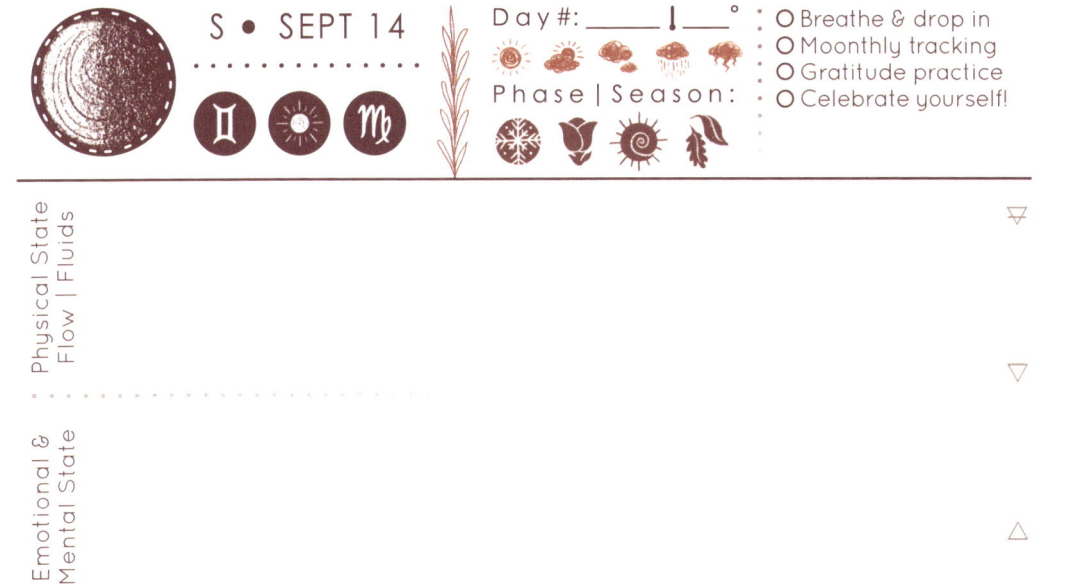

LAST QUARTER IN GEMINI

Finding space between breaths & allowing pauses before processing

What am I leaving behind this lunar cycle?

Where can I make more space for reflection &/or integration?

M • SEPT 15

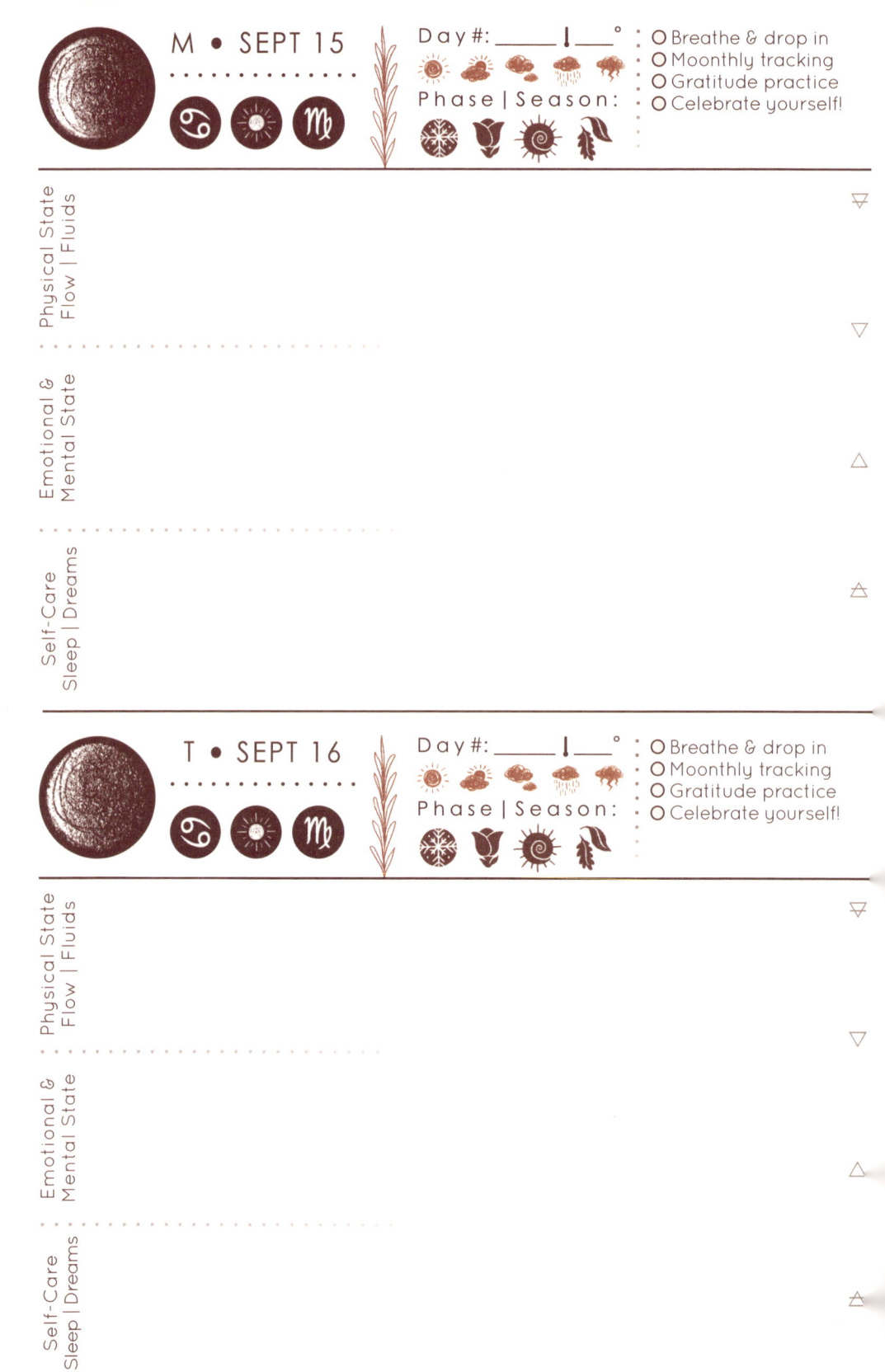

Day #: _____ | _____°

Phase | Season:

- ◯ Breathe & drop in
- ◯ Moonthly tracking
- ◯ Gratitude practice
- ◯ Celebrate yourself!

Physical State
Flow | Fluids

Emotional & Mental State

Self-Care
Sleep | Dreams

T • SEPT 16

Day #: _____ | _____°

Phase | Season:

- ◯ Breathe & drop in
- ◯ Moonthly tracking
- ◯ Gratitude practice
- ◯ Celebrate yourself!

Physical State
Flow | Fluids

Emotional & Mental State

Self-Care
Sleep | Dreams

W • SEPT 17

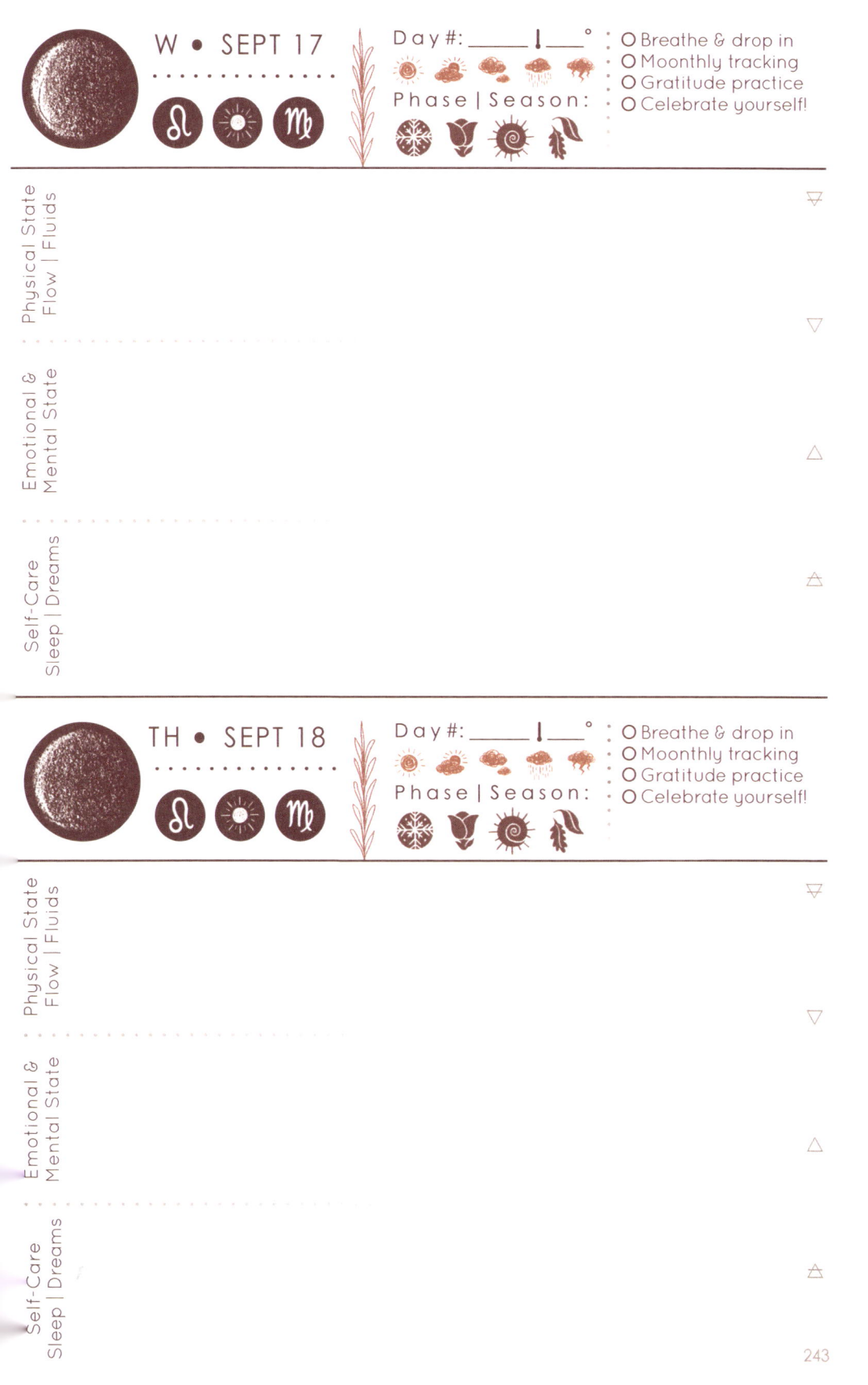

Day #: _____ | _____°

Phase | Season:

- Breathe & drop in
- Moonthly tracking
- Gratitude practice
- Celebrate yourself!

Physical State / Flow | Fluids

Emotional & Mental State

Self-Care / Sleep | Dreams

TH • SEPT 18

Day #: _____ | _____°

Phase | Season:

- Breathe & drop in
- Moonthly tracking
- Gratitude practice
- Celebrate yourself!

Physical State / Flow | Fluids

Emotional & Mental State

Self-Care / Sleep | Dreams

☾ 8th
08 | 23
09 | 20

CHECK IN & REFLECT

Last Cycle Day 1: _____

Last Cycle Length: _____

Circle the phase you bled near:

○ ☾ ☾ ☾ ☾ ● ● ● ☽ ☽ ☽ ○

Use this space to reflect on your experiences & findings from this ending lunar cycle or your last menstrual cycle. Use cycle day #s if you bleed, or moon phases if you don't.

Caution Days: (days I needed space)

Bliss Days: (days I felt great)

DAYS TO NOTE — Which cycle days stood out?

OBSERVATIONS — Notice any changes or patterns?

SELF-CARE — What was helpful & nourishing?

PLAN & PREPARE

Next Predicted Cycle:
🩸 ☾ _____

CHECKLIST

Add the following to any other planners or calendars for your next cycle, then check it off.

- ☐ Predicted "days to note" _____
- ☐ Days to slow down (pre-bleed) _____
- ☐ Rest day(s) (next bleed) _____
- ☐ Date with yourself _____
- ☐ _____

- ☐ Self chest/breast exam
- ☐ Meal plan with cycle
- ☐ _____
- ☐ _____
- ☐ _____

OPEN SPACE

Use this space how you wish, or print out one of our free templates to paste here for BBT charting, dream tracking, or something else:

How to Make Pelvic Exams More Comfortable

by Melissa Haley (they/them) of Wyld Garden Chicago Doula • Full Spectrum Doula & Placenta Encapsulator • @wyld_garden • wyld-garden.com •

The cervix is shaped like a mini powdered donut. It's delicate but firm and the center for many nerve endings. It is the gateway between your insides and your outsides. It can metabolize itself during birth to open a gateway for life.

Getting cervical exams can be overwhelming for many reasons: it's vulnerable, the experience doesn't center the patient, and for some it brings up body dysphoria. The first time I intentionally touched mine, I got lightheaded. Cervixes hold a lot of emotion and sometimes trauma.

Your cervix deserves to be treated with care!

Every provider should tell you each step and WAIT for your consent before beginning.

Shop around and find someone you are comfortable with. Online forums and midwives are both good places to start. Here are some ways to make an exam more comfortable:

- With a trusted provider, talk with clothes on beforehand

- Request to not use the stirrups, instead prop your feet on the table and tilt your knees open

- Request a pillow or cushion for under your bottom, to tilt your pelvis and make your cervix more easily visible

- Ensure that the speculum is warmed and lubricated

- Speculums come in 3 sizes; ask for the correct size for your body

- Request to insert the speculum yourself

- Ask to see your cervix; my midwife even took a picture for me!

- Wear a dress, skirt, or long t-shirt that you can keep on during the exam

- Explore your cervix at home: touch it with clean hands in the shower or buy a speculum online and use a mirror to see your cervix.

Phasic Overview & In-Betweens

Use this space to focus on the phases of the moonth and the in-betweens of the peak lunations.

One way of using this space is to designate one column for your goal-planning, intention-setting or focus per phase/week. Use the other column for reflections, dream themes, nutrition tracking, cards pulls, etc!

F • SEPT 19

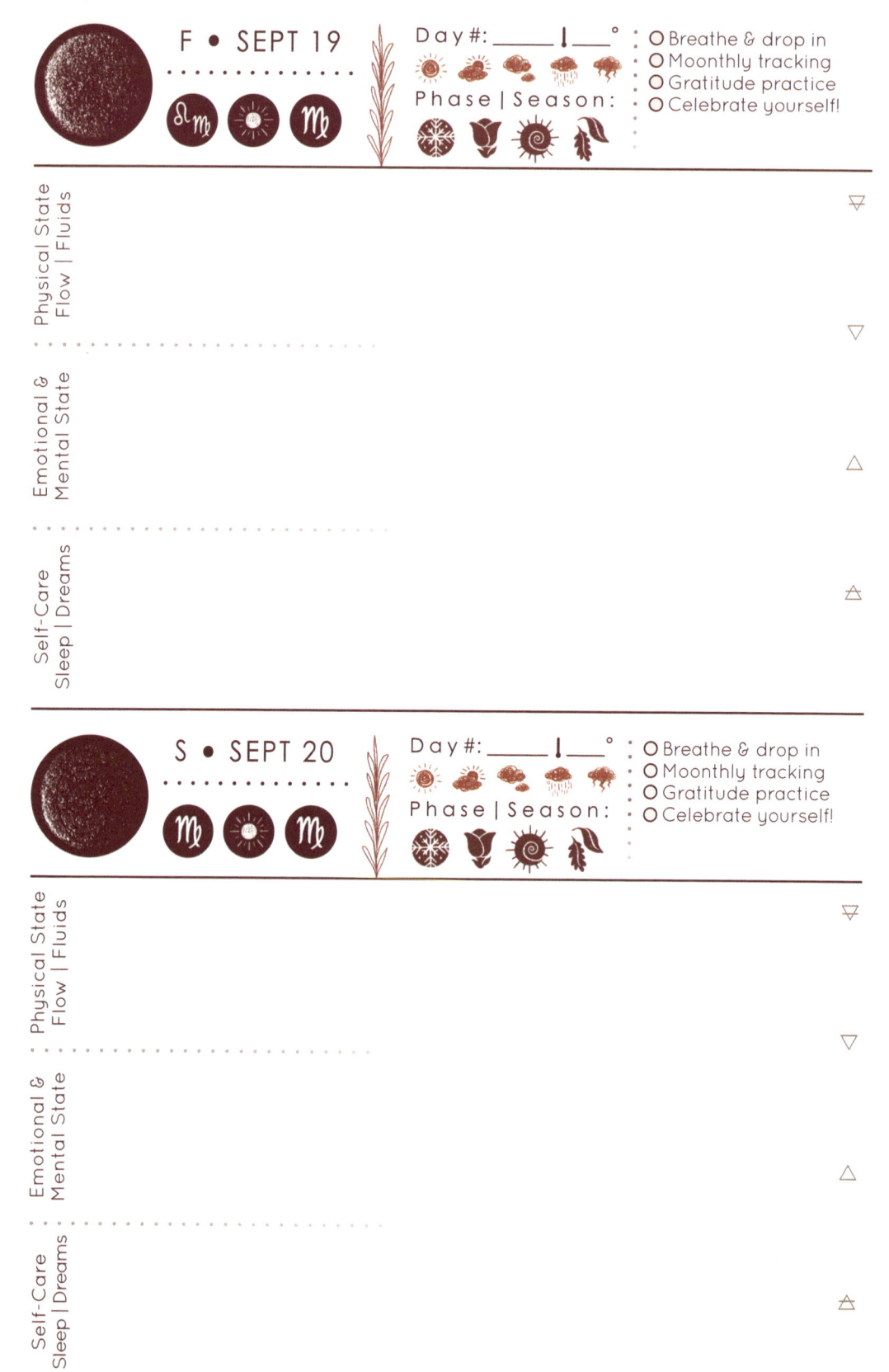

Day #: _____ | _____°

Phase | Season:

- ○ Breathe & drop in
- ○ Moonthly tracking
- ○ Gratitude practice
- ○ Celebrate yourself!

Physical State
Flow | Fluids

Emotional & Mental State

Self-Care
Sleep | Dreams

S • SEPT 20

Day #: _____ | _____°

Phase | Season:

- ○ Breathe & drop in
- ○ Moonthly tracking
- ○ Gratitude practice
- ○ Celebrate yourself!

Physical State
Flow | Fluids

Emotional & Mental State

Self-Care
Sleep | Dreams

S • SEPT 21

Day #: _____ | _____°

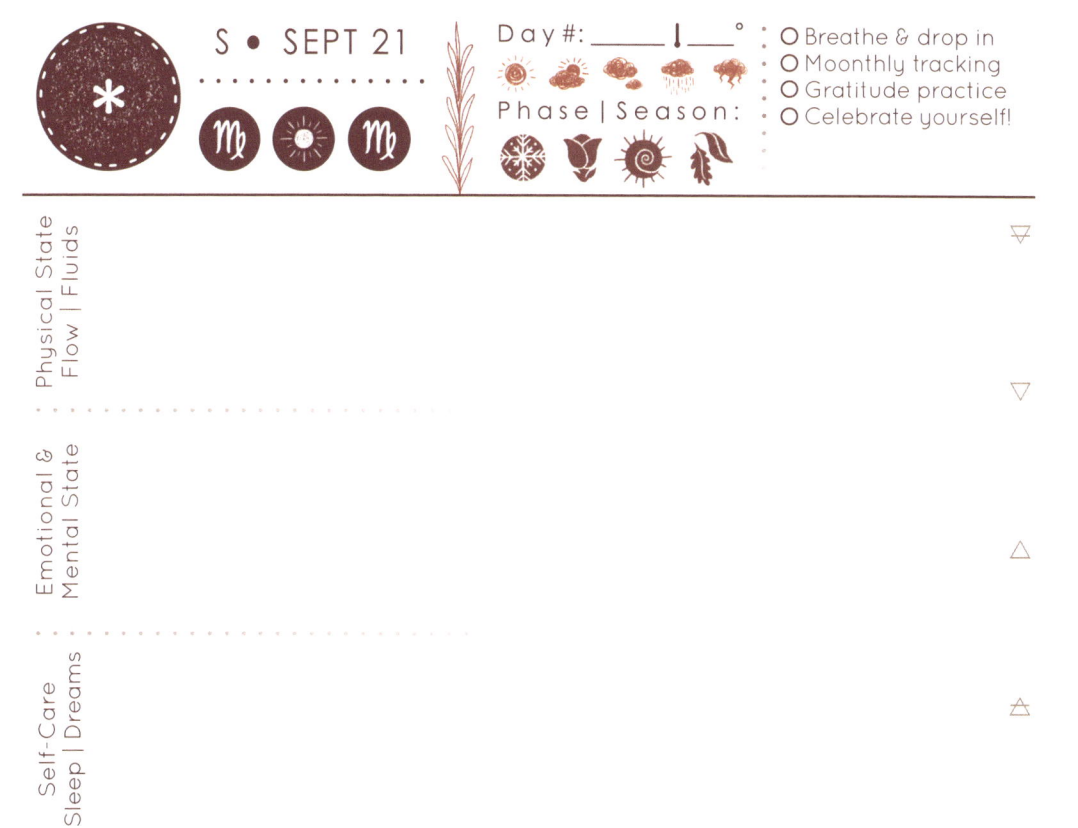

Phase | Season:

- ○ Breathe & drop in
- ○ Moonthly tracking
- ○ Gratitude practice
- ○ Celebrate yourself!

Physical State
Flow | Fluids

Emotional & Mental State

Self-Care
Sleep | Dreams

NEW MOON SOLAR ECLIPSE IN VIRGO

A signal for simplification and efficiency for the sake of true sustainability

What do I want to grow & focus on during this lunar cycle?

How will I hold space for this?

M • SEPT 22
·· EQUINOX ··

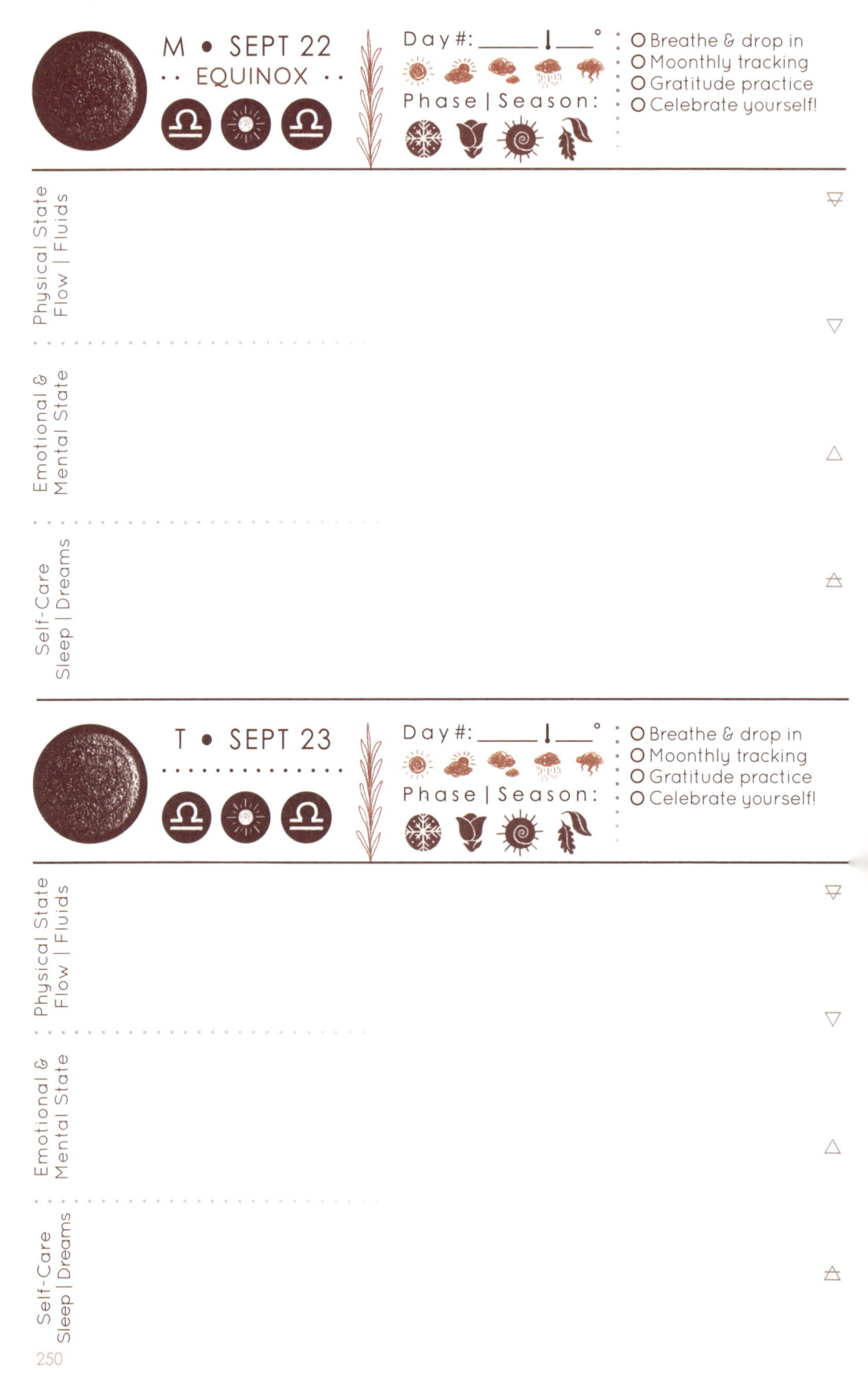

♎ ☀ ♎

Day #: _____ | _____°

Phase | Season:

O Breathe & drop in
O Moonthly tracking
O Gratitude practice
O Celebrate yourself!

Physical State / Flow | Fluids

Emotional & Mental State

Self-Care / Sleep | Dreams

T • SEPT 23

♎ ☀ ♎

Day #: _____ | _____°

Phase | Season:

O Breathe & drop in
O Moonthly tracking
O Gratitude practice
O Celebrate yourself!

Physical State / Flow | Fluids

Emotional & Mental State

Self-Care / Sleep | Dreams

W • SEPT 24

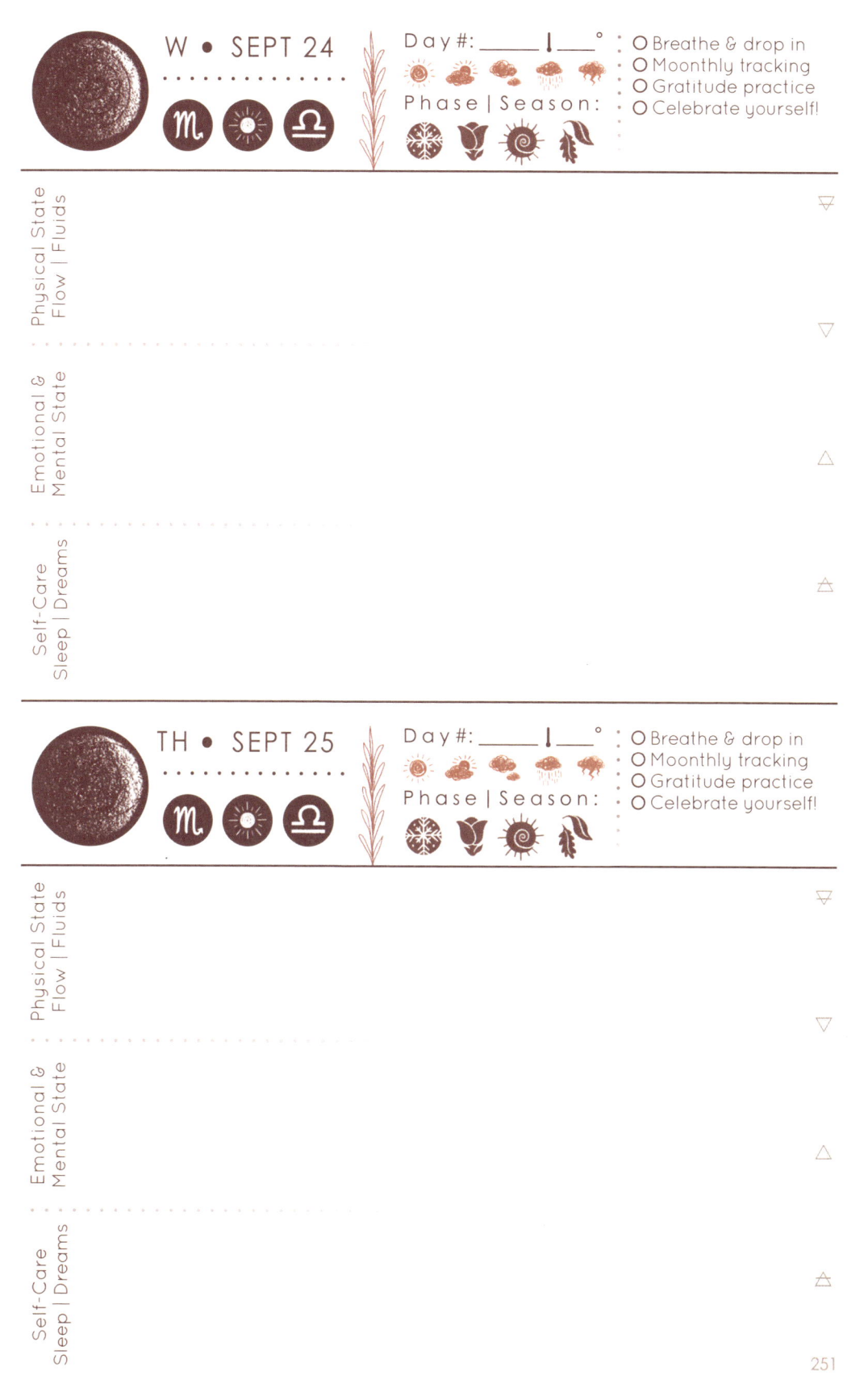

♏ ☀ ♎

Day #: _____ | _____°

Phase | Season:

- ○ Breathe & drop in
- ○ Moonthly tracking
- ○ Gratitude practice
- ○ Celebrate yourself!

Physical State
Flow | Fluids

Emotional & Mental State

Self-Care
Sleep | Dreams

TH • SEPT 25

♏ ☀ ♎

Day #: _____ | _____°

Phase | Season:

- ○ Breathe & drop in
- ○ Moonthly tracking
- ○ Gratitude practice
- ○ Celebrate yourself!

Physical State
Flow | Fluids

Emotional & Mental State

Self-Care
Sleep | Dreams

F • SEPT 26

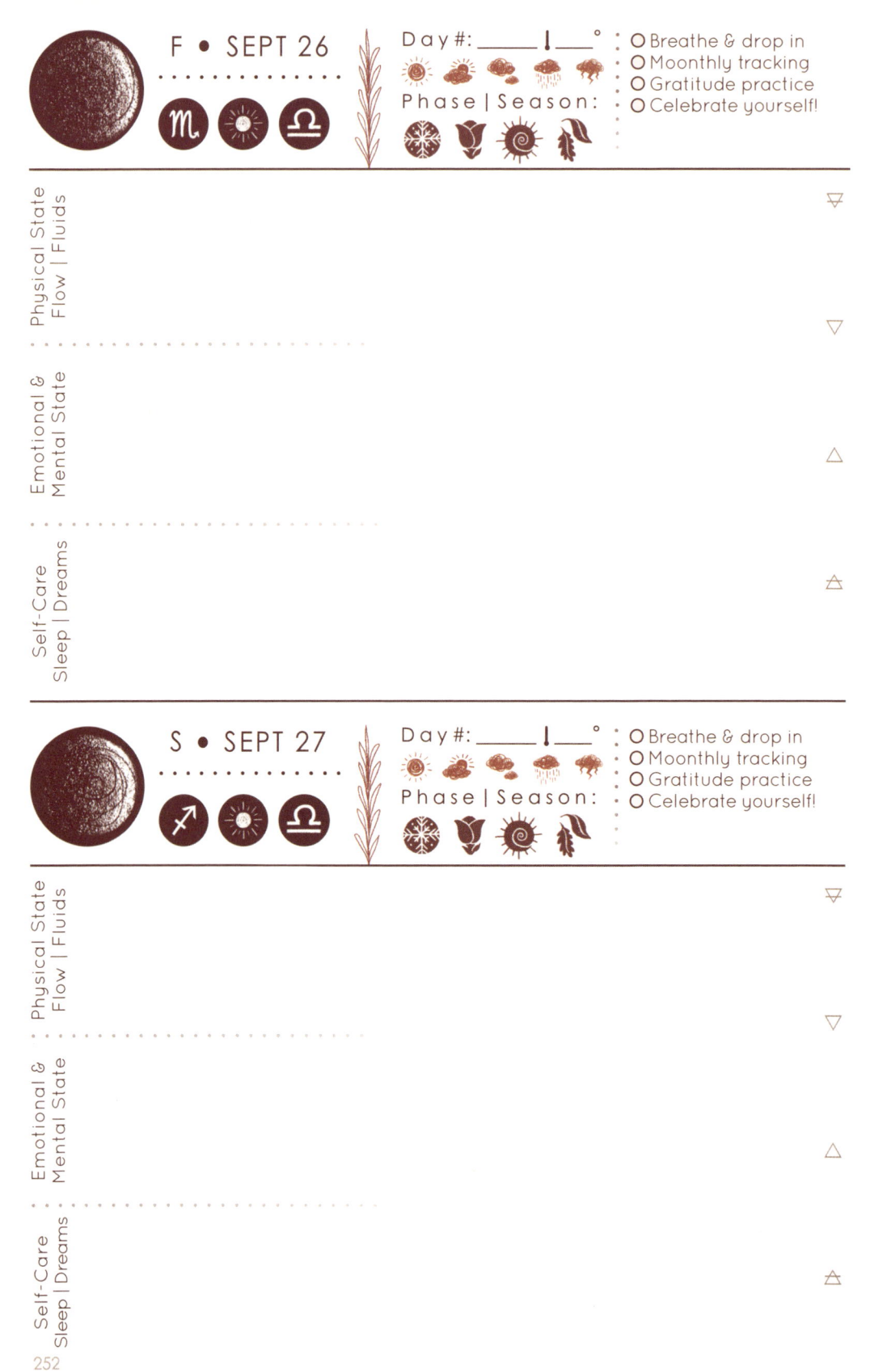

Day #: _____ | _____°

Phase | Season:

- ○ Breathe & drop in
- ○ Moonthly tracking
- ○ Gratitude practice
- ○ Celebrate yourself!

Physical State
Flow | Fluids

Emotional &
Mental State

Self-Care
Sleep | Dreams

S • SEPT 27

Day #: _____ | _____°

Phase | Season:

- ○ Breathe & drop in
- ○ Moonthly tracking
- ○ Gratitude practice
- ○ Celebrate yourself!

Physical State
Flow | Fluids

Emotional &
Mental State

Self-Care
Sleep | Dreams

S • SEPT 28

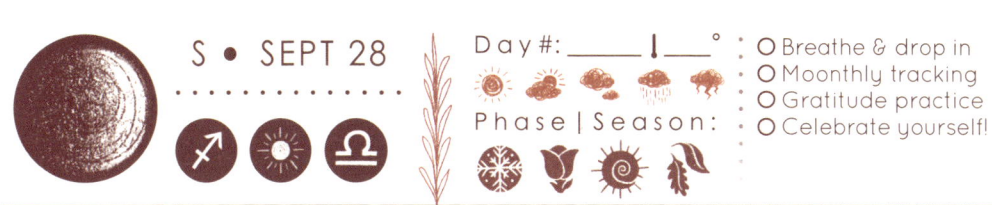

Day #: _____ | _____°

Phase | Season:

- ○ Breathe & drop in
- ○ Moonthly tracking
- ○ Gratitude practice
- ○ Celebrate yourself!

Physical State | Flow | Fluids

Emotional & Mental State

Self-Care | Sleep | Dreams

M • SEPT 29

Day #: ____ | ____°

Phase | Season:

- ○ Breathe & drop in
- ○ Moonthly tracking
- ○ Gratitude practice
- ○ Celebrate yourself!

Physical State / Flow | Fluids

Emotional & Mental State

Self-Care / Sleep | Dreams

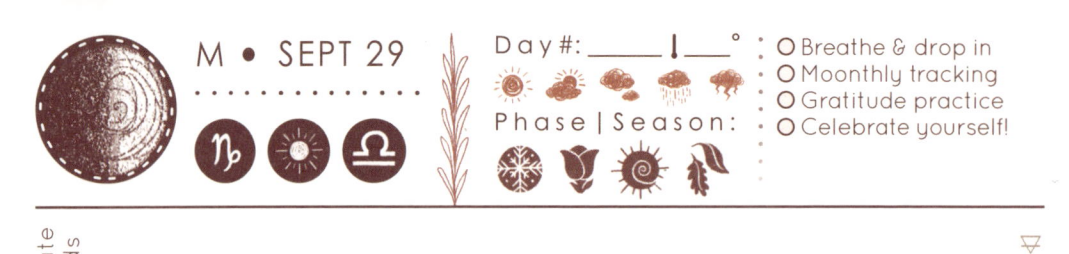

FIRST QUARTER IN CAPRICORN

Growing awareness around the form and flow of currency

What is sprouting & coming into awareness?

What can I release to make space for further growth & grounding?

T • SEPT 30

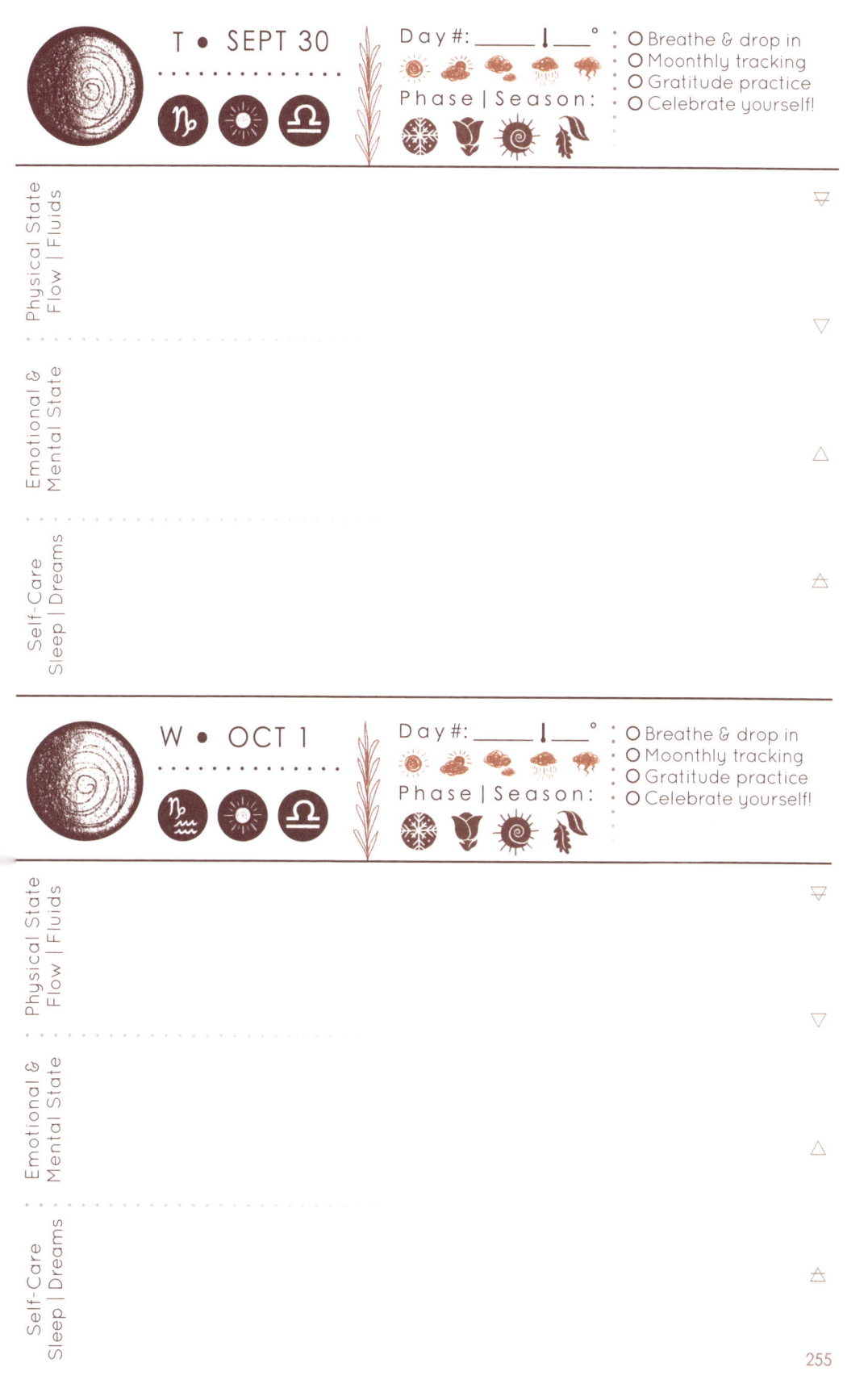

Day #: _____ | _____°

Phase | Season:

- Breathe & drop in
- Moonthly tracking
- Gratitude practice
- Celebrate yourself!

Physical State
Flow | Fluids

Emotional & Mental State

Self-Care
Sleep | Dreams

W • OCT 1

Day #: _____ | _____°

Phase | Season:

- Breathe & drop in
- Moonthly tracking
- Gratitude practice
- Celebrate yourself!

Physical State
Flow | Fluids

Emotional & Mental State

Self-Care
Sleep | Dreams

TH • OCT 2

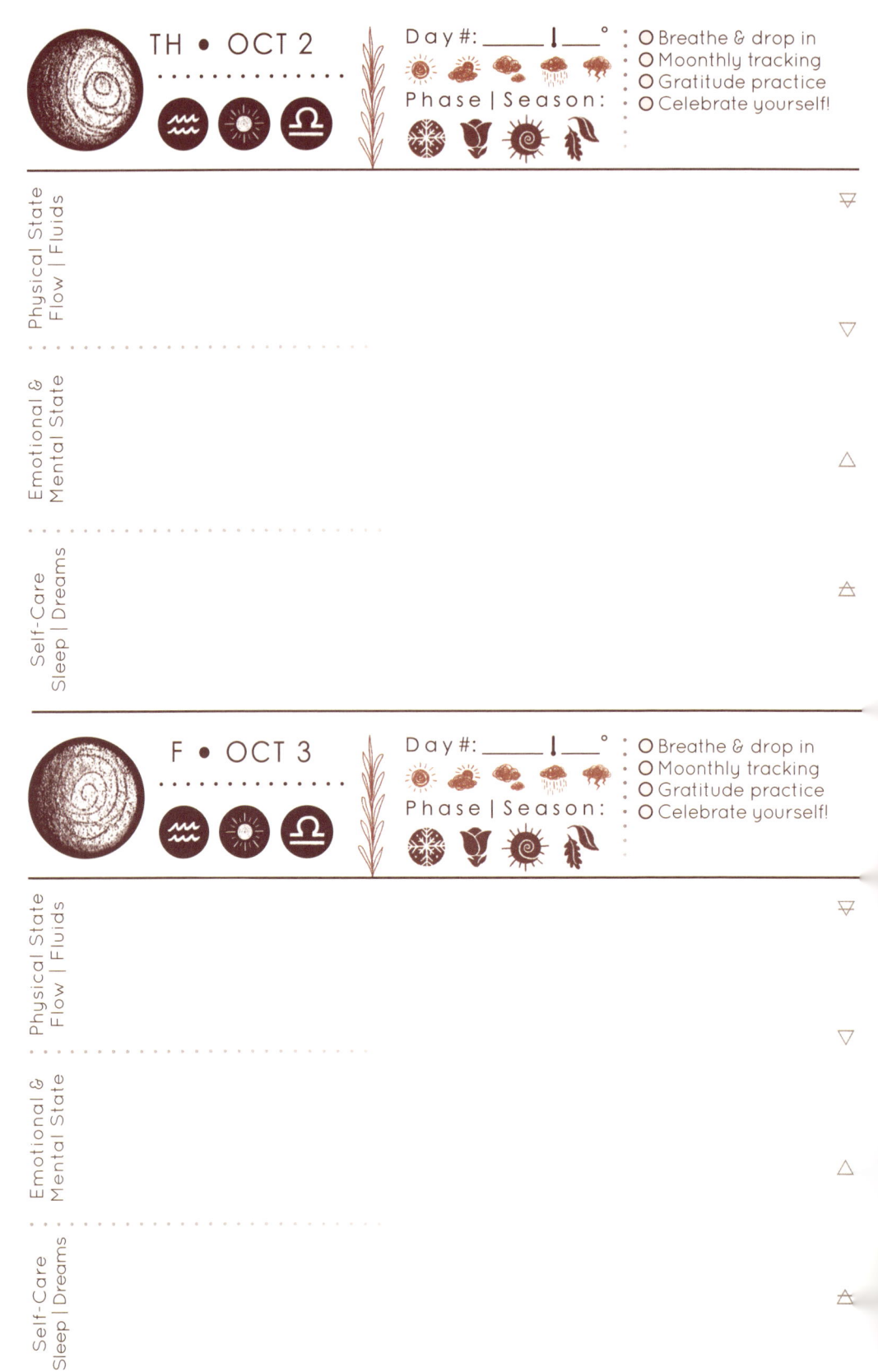

Day #: _____ | _____°

Phase | Season:

- O Breathe & drop in
- O Moonthly tracking
- O Gratitude practice
- O Celebrate yourself!

Physical State
Flow | Fluids

Emotional & Mental State

Self-Care
Sleep | Dreams

F • OCT 3

Day #: _____ | _____°

Phase | Season:

- O Breathe & drop in
- O Moonthly tracking
- O Gratitude practice
- O Celebrate yourself!

Physical State
Flow | Fluids

Emotional & Mental State

Self-Care
Sleep | Dreams

T • OCT 7

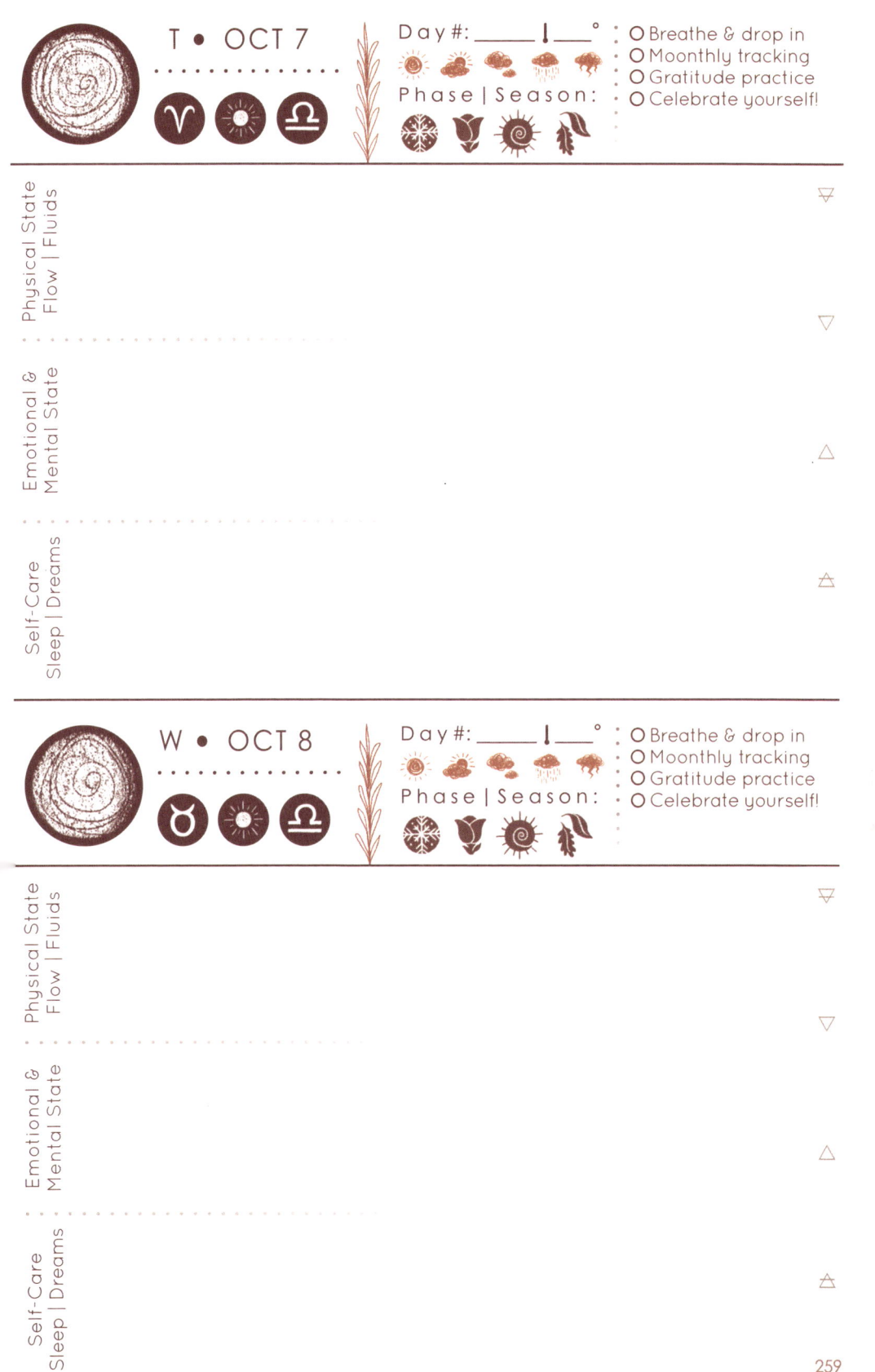

Day #: _____ | _____°

Phase | Season:

- ◯ Breathe & drop in
- ◯ Moonthly tracking
- ◯ Gratitude practice
- ◯ Celebrate yourself!

Physical State / Flow | Fluids

Emotional & Mental State

Self-Care / Sleep | Dreams

W • OCT 8

Day #: _____ | _____°

Phase | Season:

- ◯ Breathe & drop in
- ◯ Moonthly tracking
- ◯ Gratitude practice
- ◯ Celebrate yourself!

Physical State / Flow | Fluids

Emotional & Mental State

Self-Care / Sleep | Dreams

TH • OCT 9

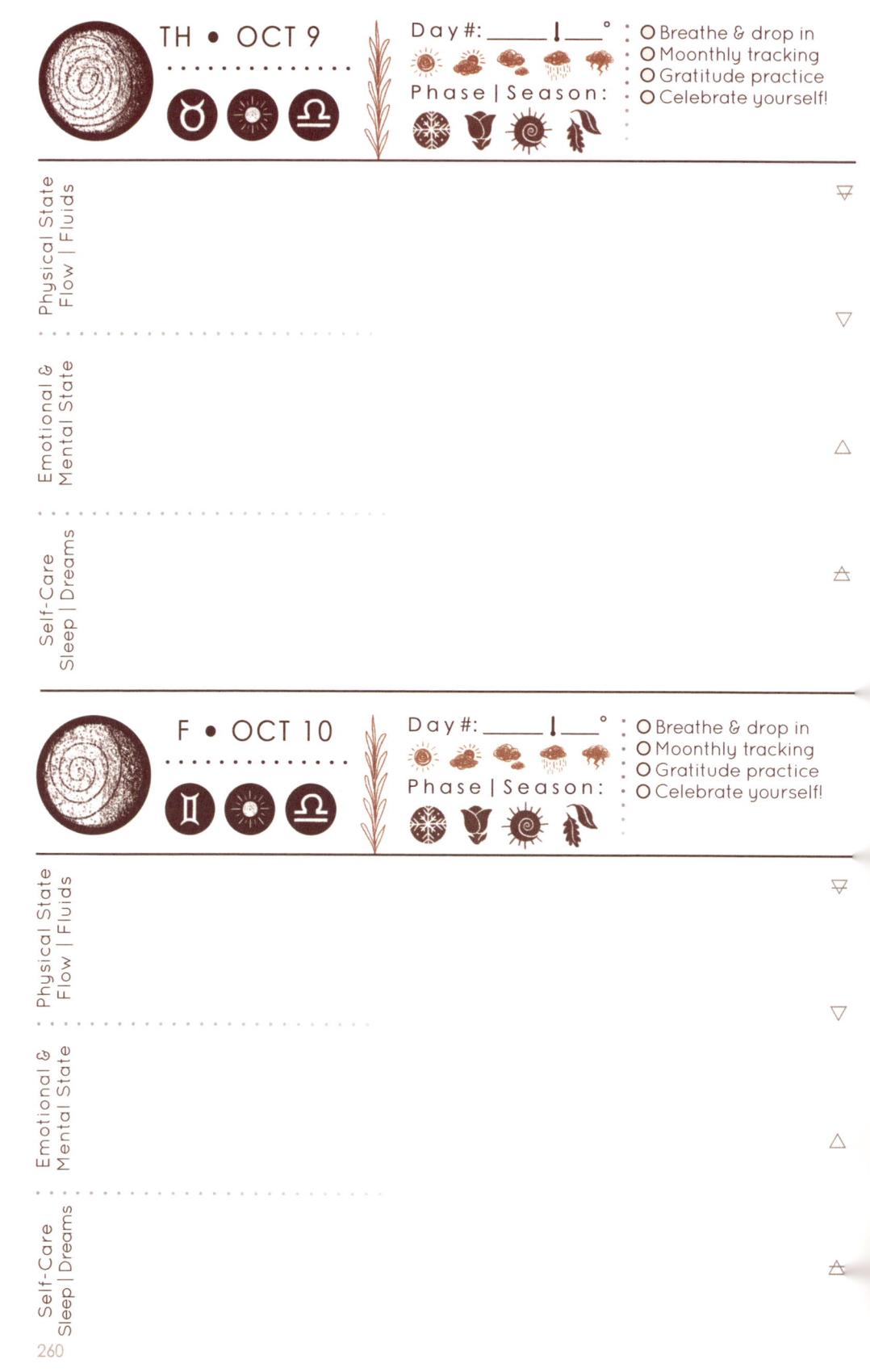

Day #: _____ | _____°

Phase | Season:

- Breathe & drop in
- Moonthly tracking
- Gratitude practice
- Celebrate yourself!

Physical State
Flow | Fluids

Emotional & Mental State

Self-Care
Sleep | Dreams

F • OCT 10

Day #: _____ | _____°

Phase | Season:

- Breathe & drop in
- Moonthly tracking
- Gratitude practice
- Celebrate yourself!

Physical State
Flow | Fluids

Emotional & Mental State

Self-Care
Sleep | Dreams

S • OCT 11

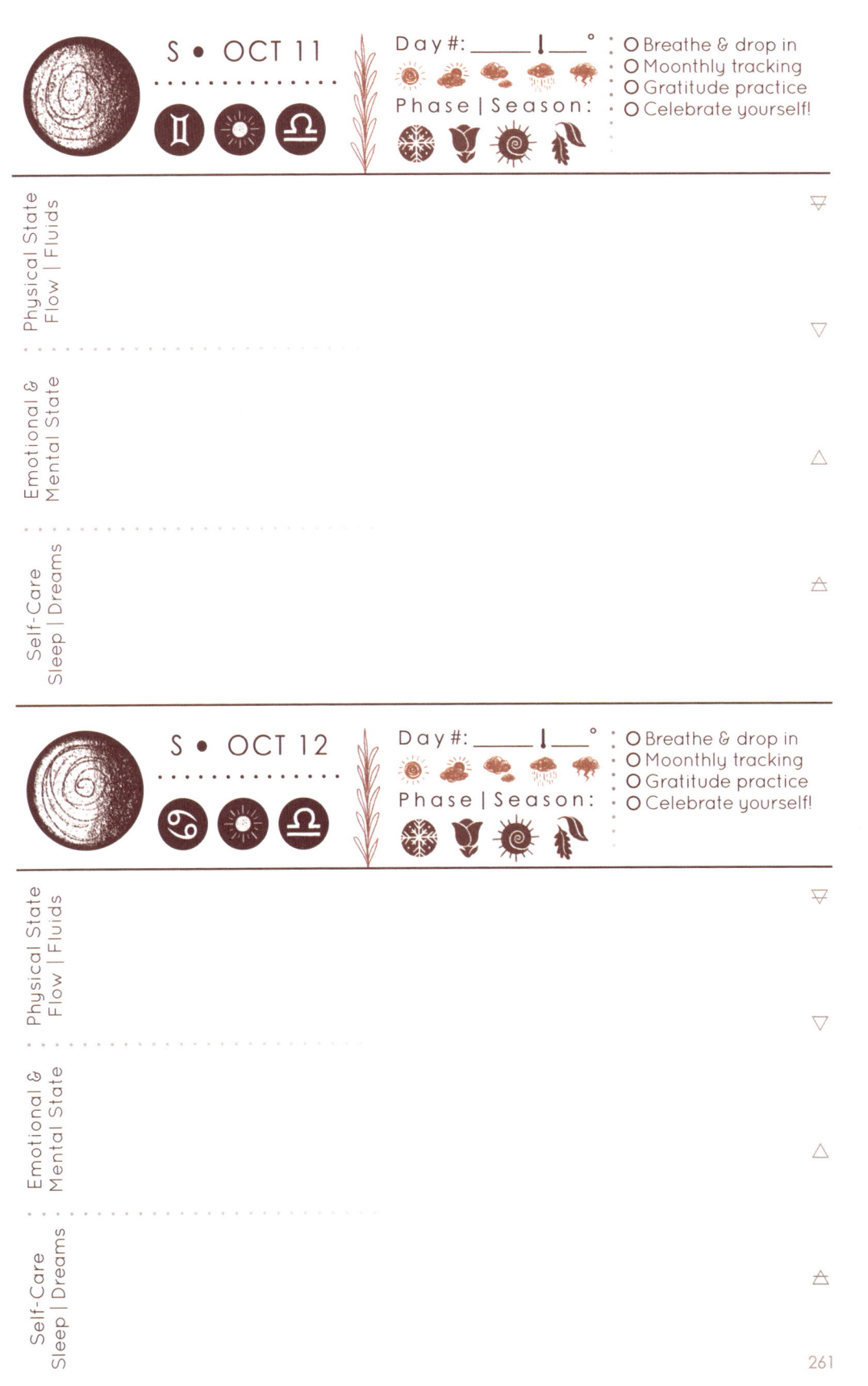

♊ ☉ ♎

Day #: _____ | ___°

Phase | Season:

- O Breathe & drop in
- O Moonthly tracking
- O Gratitude practice
- O Celebrate yourself!

Physical State
Flow | Fluids

Emotional &
Mental State

Self-Care
Sleep | Dreams

S • OCT 12

♋ ☉ ♎

Day #: _____ | ___°

Phase | Season:

- O Breathe & drop in
- O Moonthly tracking
- O Gratitude practice
- O Celebrate yourself!

Physical State
Flow | Fluids

Emotional &
Mental State

Self-Care
Sleep | Dreams

M • OCT 13

Day #: _____ | _____°

Phase | Season:

- ○ Breathe & drop in
- ○ Moonthly tracking
- ○ Gratitude practice
- ○ Celebrate yourself!

Physical State / Flow | Fluids

Emotional & Mental State

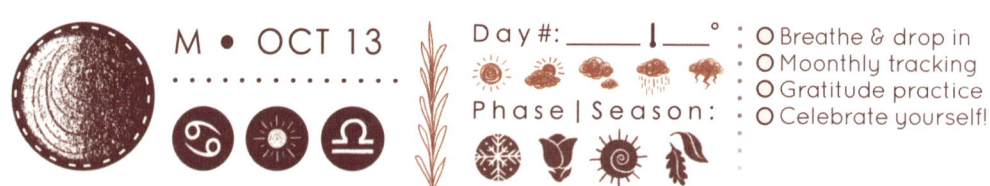

Self-Care / Sleep | Dreams

LAST QUARTER IN CANCER

Moving stuck emotions & feelings blocking connection

What am I leaving behind this lunar cycle?

Where can I make more space for reflection &/or integration?

T • OCT 14

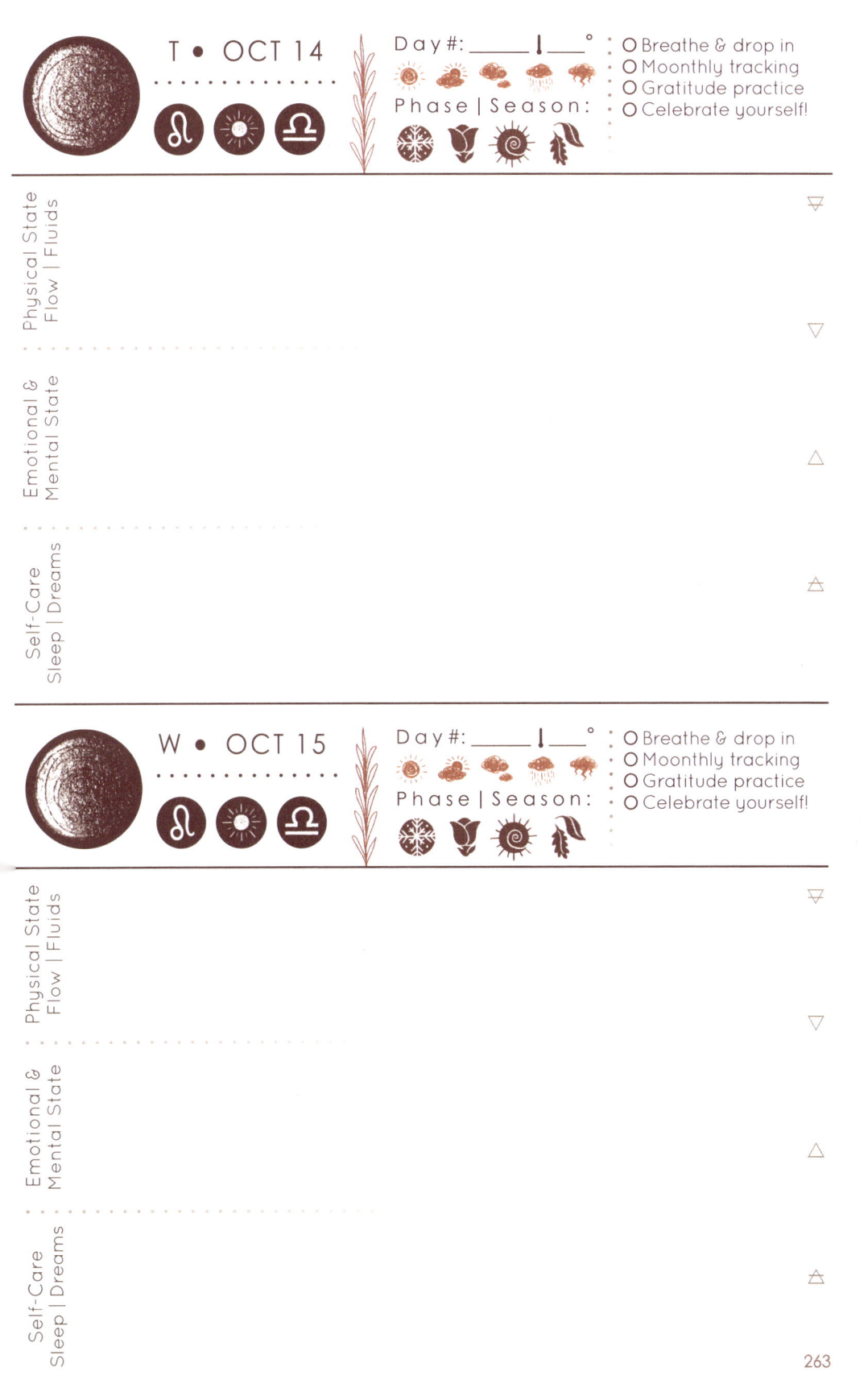

♌ ☉ ♎

Day #: _____ | _____°
Phase | Season:

- ○ Breathe & drop in
- ○ Moonthly tracking
- ○ Gratitude practice
- ○ Celebrate yourself!

Physical State / Flow | Fluids

Emotional & Mental State

Self-Care / Sleep | Dreams

W • OCT 15

♌ ☉ ♎

Day #: _____ | _____°
Phase | Season:

- ○ Breathe & drop in
- ○ Moonthly tracking
- ○ Gratitude practice
- ○ Celebrate yourself!

Physical State / Flow | Fluids

Emotional & Mental State

Self-Care / Sleep | Dreams

TH • OCT 16

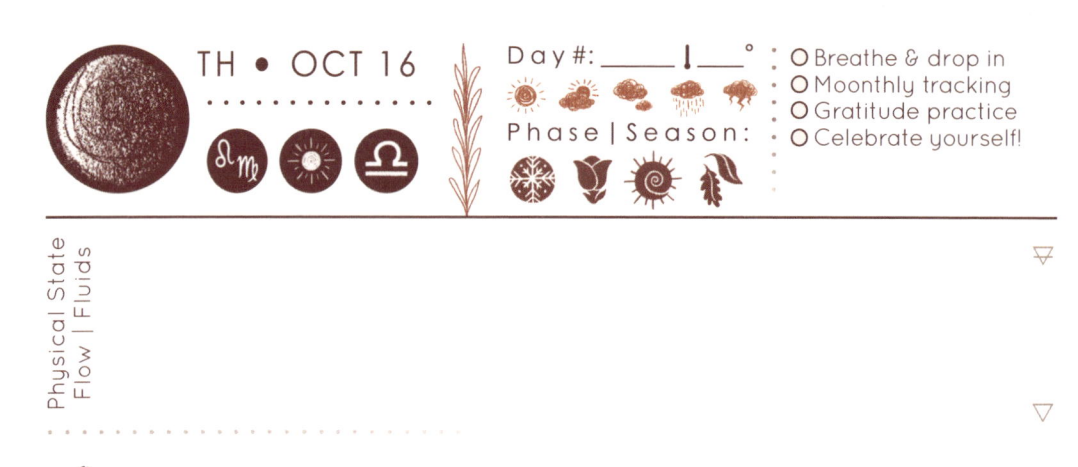

♌♍ ☉ ♎

Day #: _____ | _____°

Phase | Season:

- O Breathe & drop in
- O Moonthly tracking
- O Gratitude practice
- O Celebrate yourself!

Physical State
Flow | Fluids

Emotional & Mental State

Self-Care
Sleep | Dreams

F • OCT 17

♍ ☉ ♎

Day #: _____ | _____°

Phase | Season:

- O Breathe & drop in
- O Moonthly tracking
- O Gratitude practice
- O Celebrate yourself!

Physical State
Flow | Fluids

Emotional & Mental State

Self-Care
Sleep | Dreams

S • OCT 18

Day #: _____ | _____°

Phase | Season:

- Breathe & drop in
- Moonthly tracking
- Gratitude practice
- Celebrate yourself!

Physical State / Flow | Fluids

Emotional & Mental State

Self-Care / Sleep | Dreams

S • OCT 19

Day #: _____ | _____°

Phase | Season:

- Breathe & drop in
- Moonthly tracking
- Gratitude practice
- Celebrate yourself!

Physical State / Flow | Fluids

Emotional & Mental State

Self-Care / Sleep | Dreams

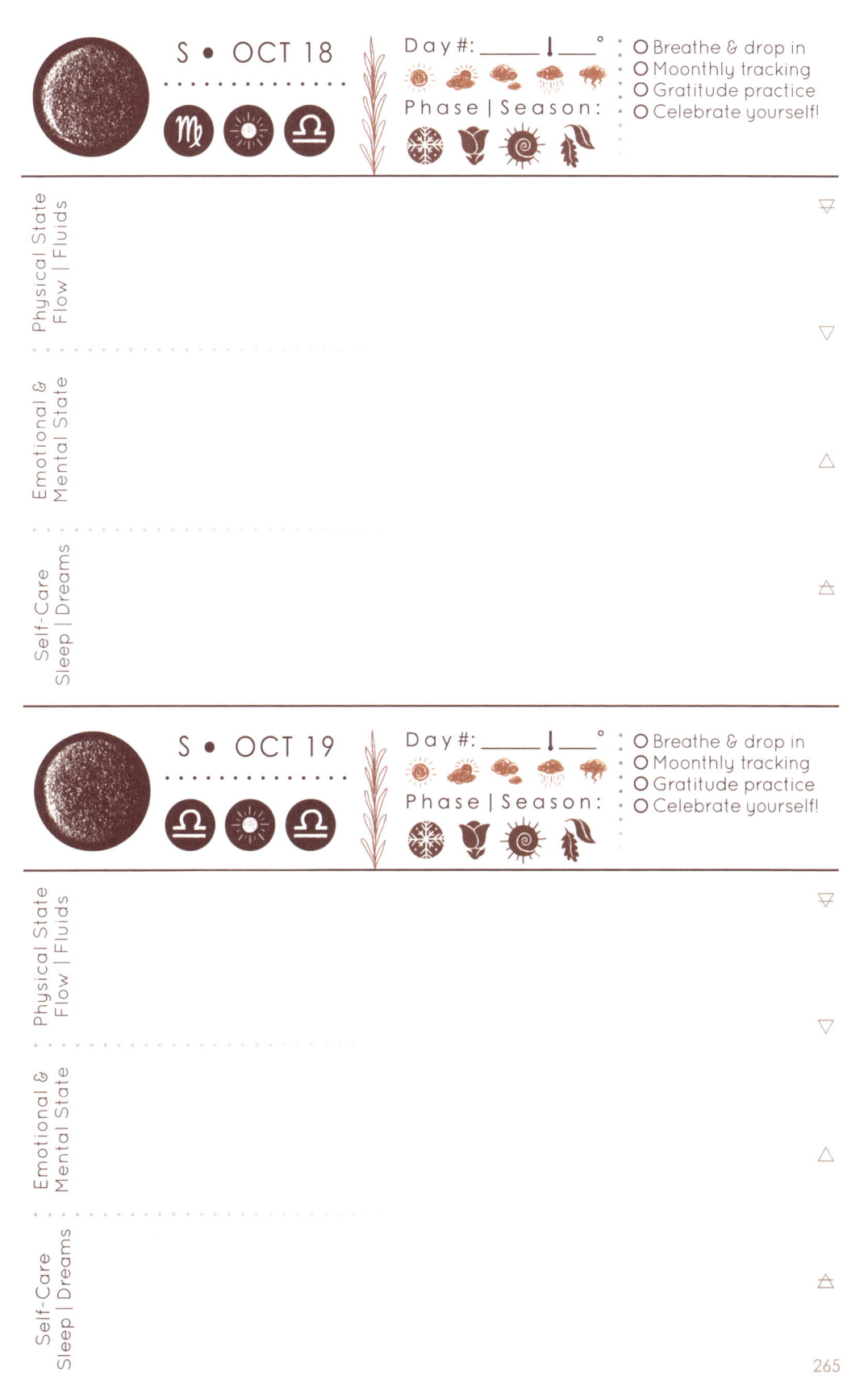

☾ 9th
09 | 21
10 | 20

CHECK IN & REFLECT

Use this space to reflect on your experiences & findings from this ending lunar cycle or your last menstrual cycle. Use cycle day #s if you bleed, or moon phases if you don't.

Last Cycle Day 1: _____

Last Cycle Length: _____

Circle the phase you bled near:

○ ☾ ☾ ☾ ● ● ● ● ● ☽ ☽ ☽ ○

Caution Days: (days I needed space)

Bliss Days: (days I felt great)

DAYS TO NOTE — Which cycle days stood out?

OBSERVATIONS — Notice any changes or patterns?

SELF-CARE — What was helpful & nourishing?

PLAN & PREPARE

Next Predicted Cycle:

🩸 ☾ _____

CHECKLIST

Add the following to any other planners or calendars for your next cycle, then check it off.

- ☐ Predicted "days to note" _____
- ☐ Days to slow down (pre-bleed) _____
- ☐ Rest day(s) (next bleed) _____
- ☐ Date with yourself _____
- ☐ _____

- ☐ Self chest/breast exam
- ☐ Meal plan with cycle
- ☐ _____
- ☐ _____
- ☐ _____

OPEN SPACE

Use this space how you wish, or print out one of our free templates to paste here for BBT charting, dream tracking, or something else:

Color Wheel Of Emotions

by Lauren Schwind-Lipson (she/her) aka Subnormal Child • Artist, Art Teacher, Art Ritual Facilitator • @subnormalchild • subnormalchild.com •

Disclaimer: This is an art ritual!
Part of art as ritual is about these three principals:

Use these three principles in this creative process or any creative magic you dive into! Less judgment and more flow is what it's all about!

Our emotions are ever-changing, and one effective way to track these shifts and explore them is to envision our emotions as colors.

This approach allows us to connect with these colors in various contexts, aiding our efforts to understand and make peace with these diverse emotions.

So you can dress or paint with these emotional colors to call in more of or make peace with.

Draw a large circle on a piece of paper and break it into as many slices as you feel called. Start with six slices to get started, and you can always make another if you want to explore even more emotional ranges.

Each slice of the proverbial pie will act as a space holder for an emotion. So fill in each slice with the name of an emotion, think simply, and fit other emotions to start. Examples include Sad, Angry, Happy, Calm, Anxious, Excited, etc.

Sit with your little wheel of emotions and meditate for a moment with all your color-making materials around you.

When you're ready, begin to fill each slice with one color.

Decorate as you wish and place on your altar as a reminder of your emotional rainbow!

Use these colors in your journal to help you track your feelings or anything else you would like!

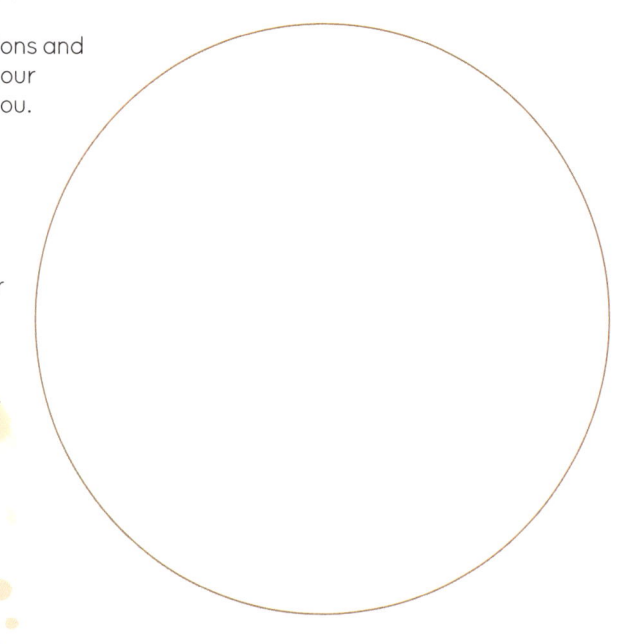

1. This is art about process not product. (Intuitive art)

2. Every mark is sacred. (even the "mistakes")

3. Everything that comes up is honored. (Especially emotions)

Phasic Overview & In-Betweens

Use this space to focus on the phases of the moonth and the in-betweens of the peak lunations.

One way of using this space is to designate one column for your goal-planning, intention-setting or focus per phase/week. Use the other column for reflections, dream themes, nutrition tracking, cards pulls, etc!

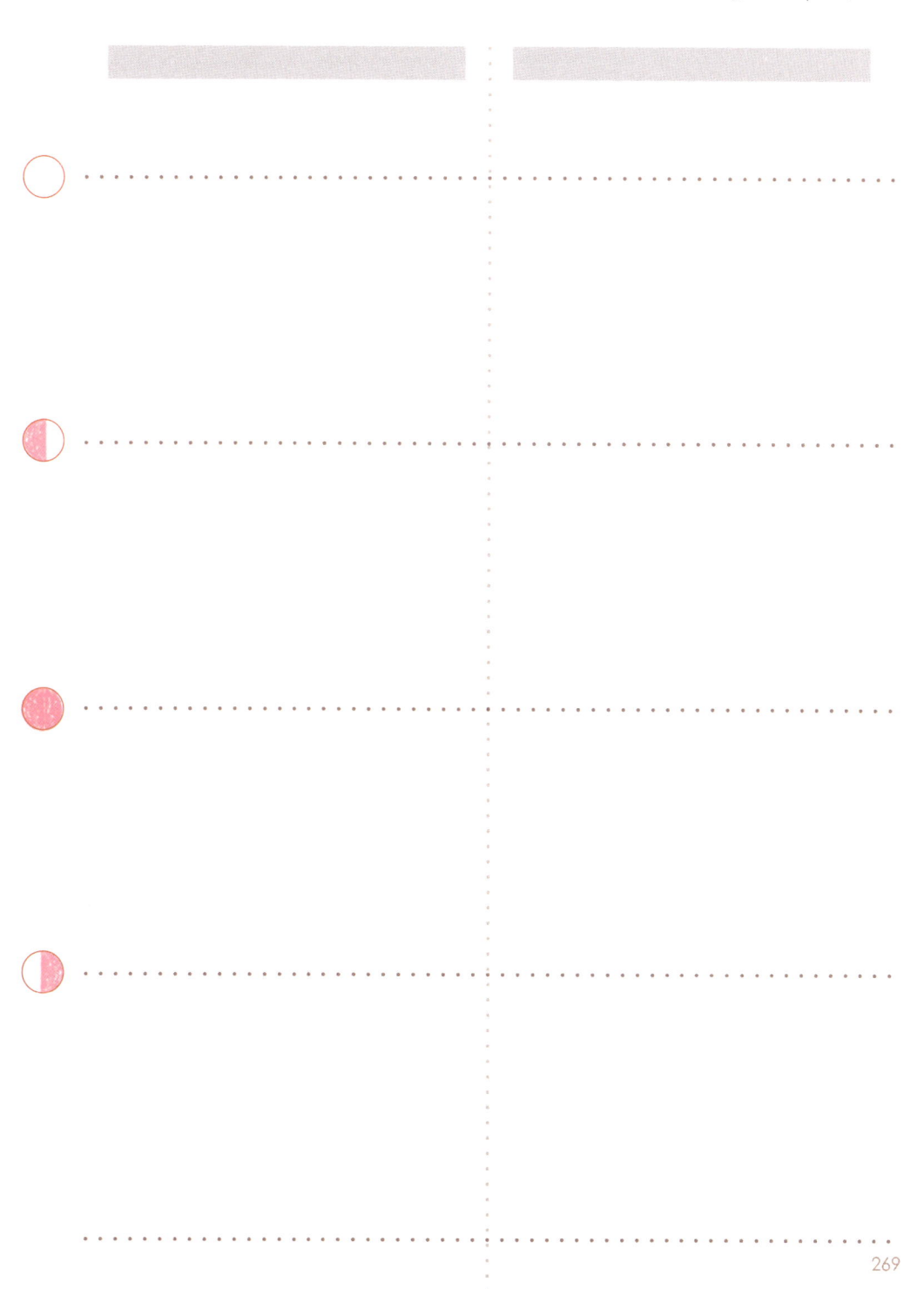

M • OCT 20

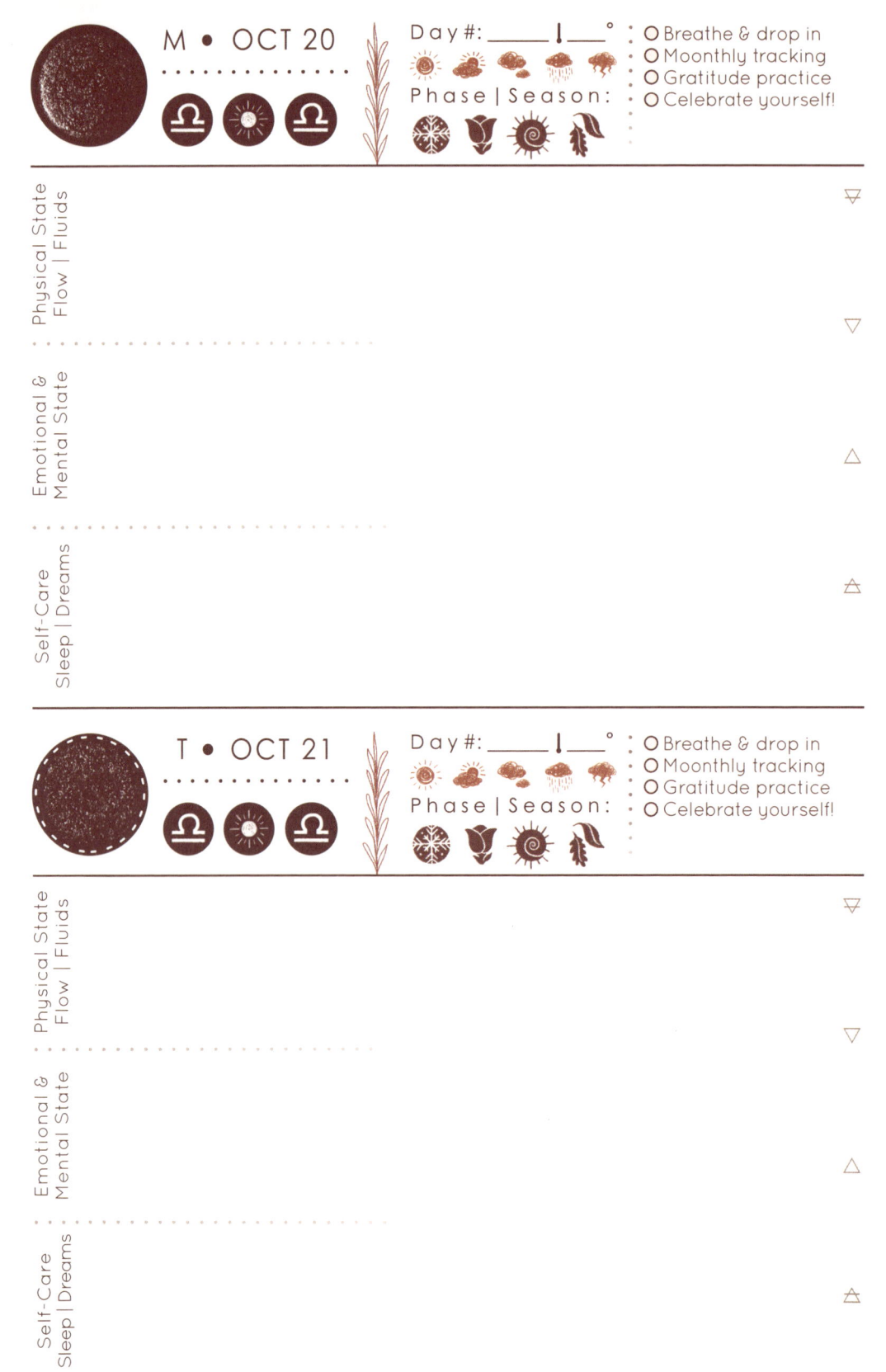

Day #: _____ | _____°

Phase | Season:

- ○ Breathe & drop in
- ○ Moonthly tracking
- ○ Gratitude practice
- ○ Celebrate yourself!

Physical State / Flow | Fluids

Emotional & Mental State

Self-Care / Sleep | Dreams

T • OCT 21

Day #: _____ | _____°

Phase | Season:

- ○ Breathe & drop in
- ○ Moonthly tracking
- ○ Gratitude practice
- ○ Celebrate yourself!

Physical State / Flow | Fluids

Emotional & Mental State

Self-Care / Sleep | Dreams

NEW MOON IN LIBRA

Viewing relational situations in a new perspective of presence

What do I want to grow & focus on during this lunar cycle?

How will I hold space for this?

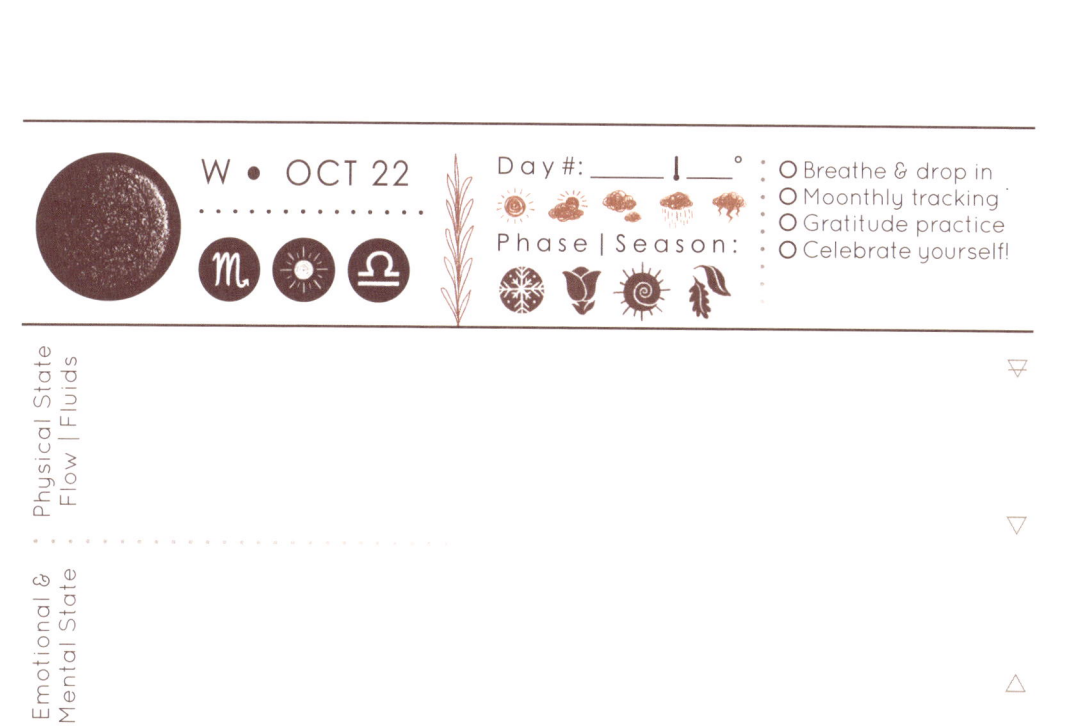

W • OCT 22

Day #: _____ | _____°

Phase | Season:

- ○ Breathe & drop in
- ○ Moonthly tracking
- ○ Gratitude practice
- ○ Celebrate yourself!

Physical State — Flow | Fluids

Emotional & Mental State

Self-Care — Sleep | Dreams

TH • OCT 23

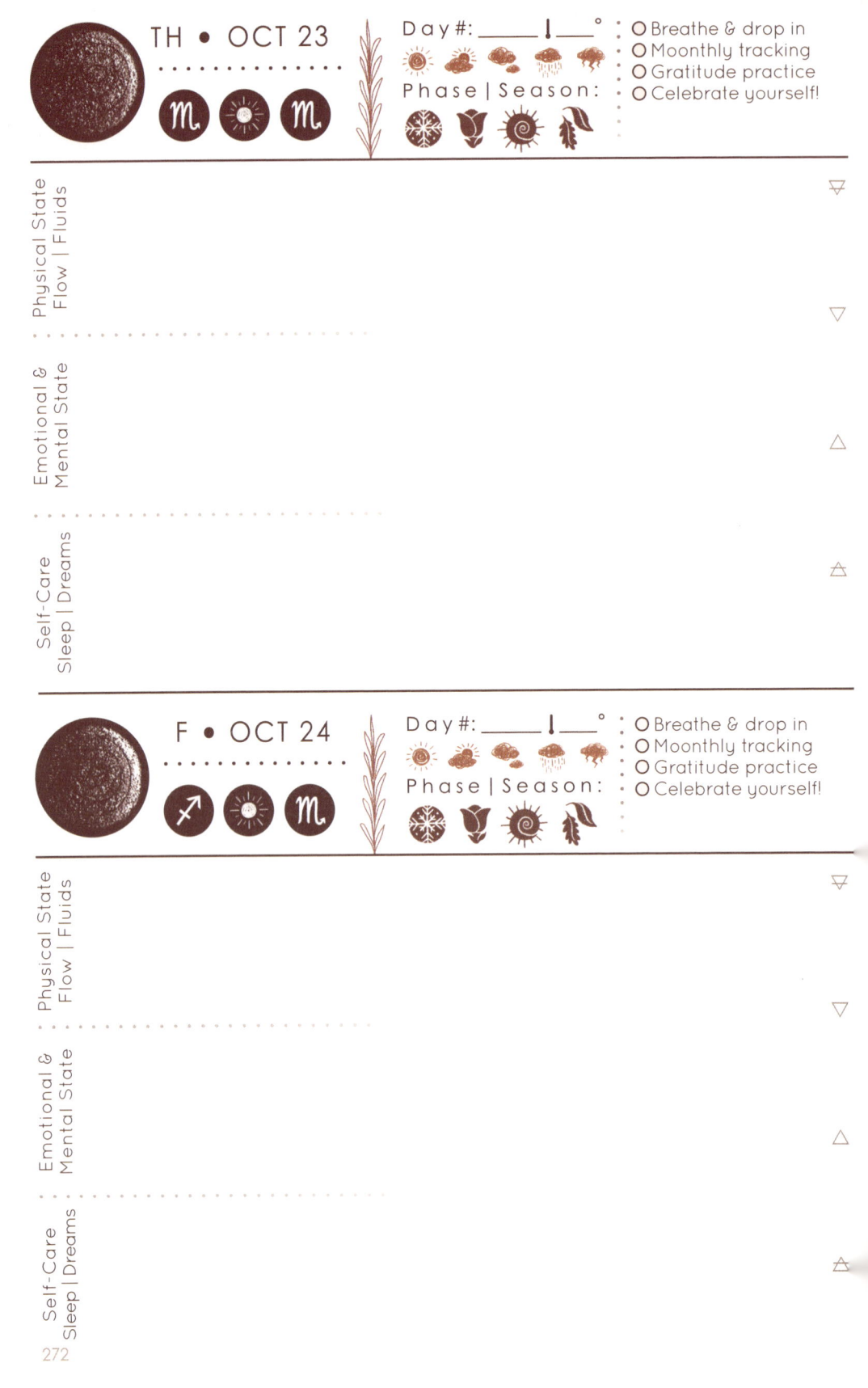

Day #: _____ | _____°

Phase | Season:

- ○ Breathe & drop in
- ○ Moonthly tracking
- ○ Gratitude practice
- ○ Celebrate yourself!

Physical State / Flow | Fluids

Emotional & Mental State

Self-Care / Sleep | Dreams

F • OCT 24

Day #: _____ | _____°

Phase | Season:

- ○ Breathe & drop in
- ○ Moonthly tracking
- ○ Gratitude practice
- ○ Celebrate yourself!

Physical State / Flow | Fluids

Emotional & Mental State

Self-Care / Sleep | Dreams

S • OCT 25

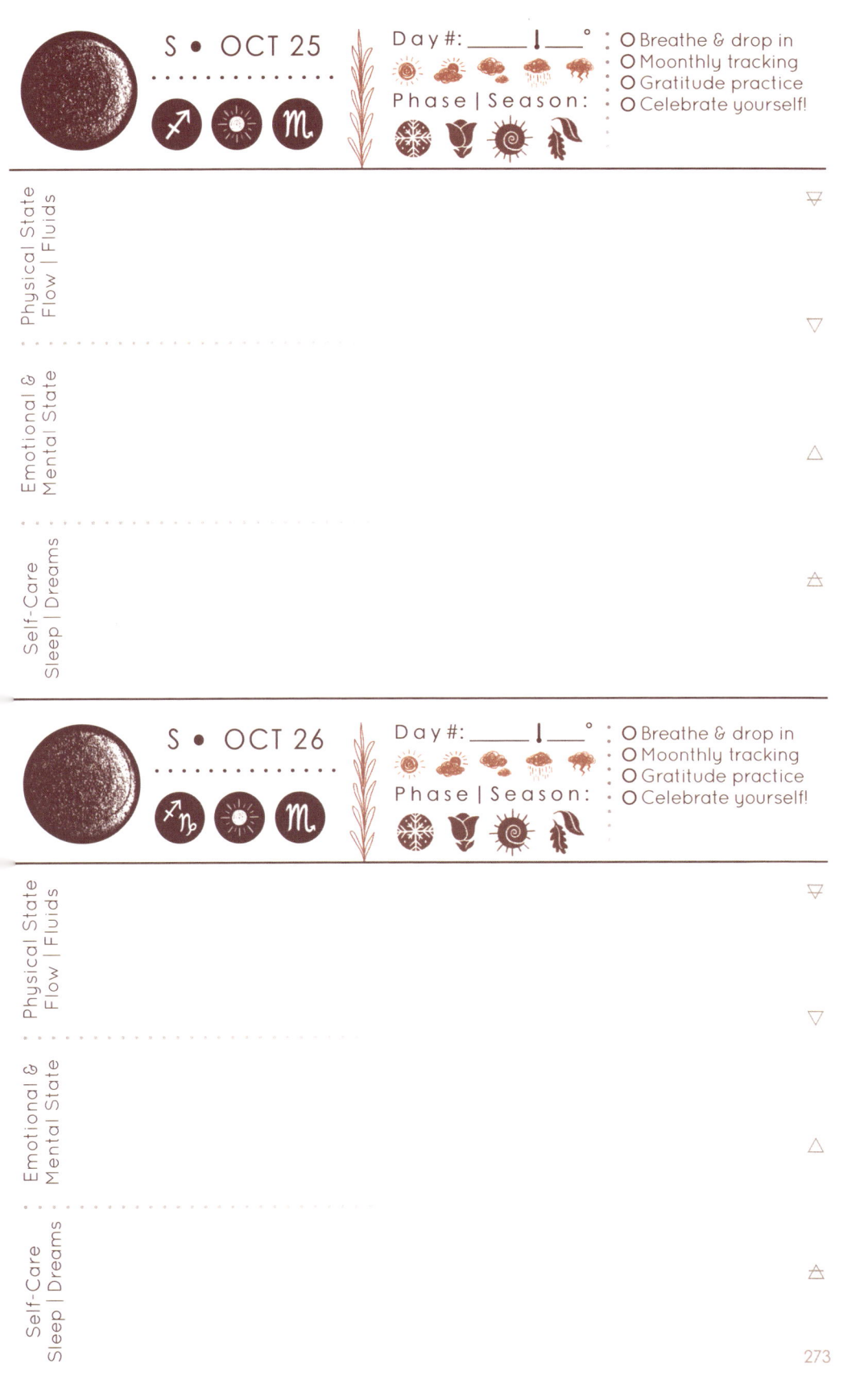

Day #: _____ | _____°

Phase | Season:

- Breathe & drop in
- Moonthly tracking
- Gratitude practice
- Celebrate yourself!

Physical State / Flow | Fluids

Emotional & Mental State

Self-Care / Sleep | Dreams

S • OCT 26

Day #: _____ | _____°

Phase | Season:

- Breathe & drop in
- Moonthly tracking
- Gratitude practice
- Celebrate yourself!

Physical State / Flow | Fluids

Emotional & Mental State

Self-Care / Sleep | Dreams

M • OCT 27

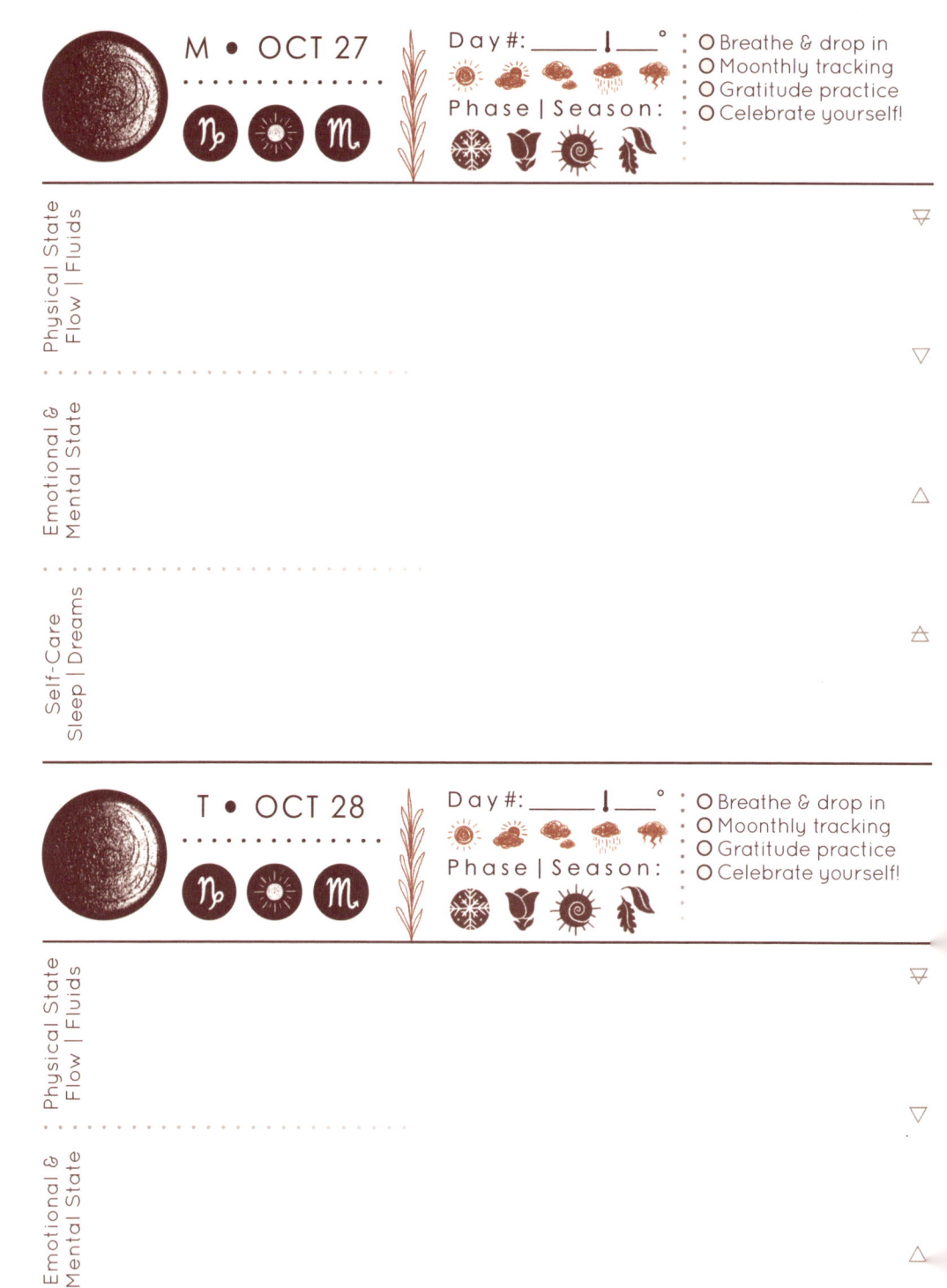

♑ ☉ ♏

Day #: _____ | _____°

Phase | Season:

- Breathe & drop in
- Moonthly tracking
- Gratitude practice
- Celebrate yourself!

Physical State
Flow | Fluids

Emotional &
Mental State

Self-Care
Sleep | Dreams

T • OCT 28

♑ ☉ ♏

Day #: _____ | _____°

Phase | Season:

- Breathe & drop in
- Moonthly tracking
- Gratitude practice
- Celebrate yourself!

Physical State
Flow | Fluids

Emotional &
Mental State

Self-Care
Sleep | Dreams

W • OCT 29

Day #: _____ | ____°

Phase | Season:

- ○ Breathe & drop in
- ○ Moonthly tracking
- ○ Gratitude practice
- ○ Celebrate yourself!

Physical State
Flow | Fluids

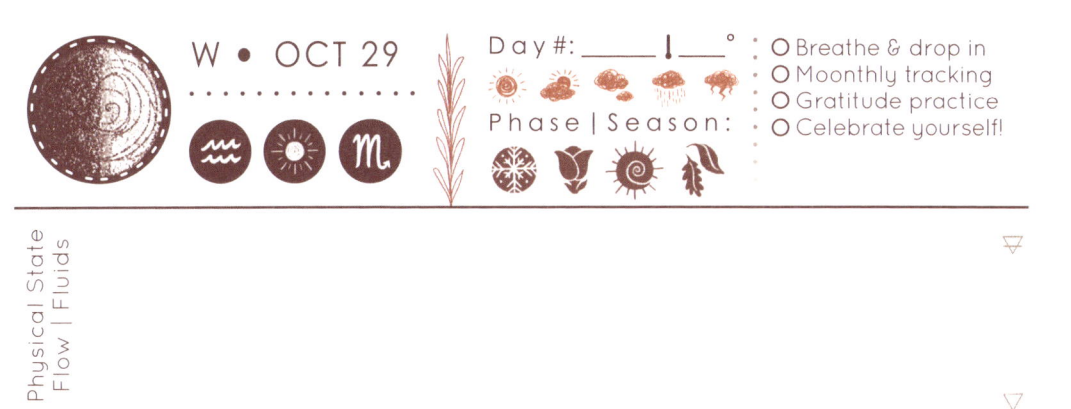

Emotional & Mental State

Self-Care
Sleep | Dreams

FIRST QUARTER IN AQUARIUS

Reflecting on the deep sense of interconnection that brings hope

What is sprouting & coming into awareness?

What can I release to make space for further growth & grounding?

TH • OCT 30

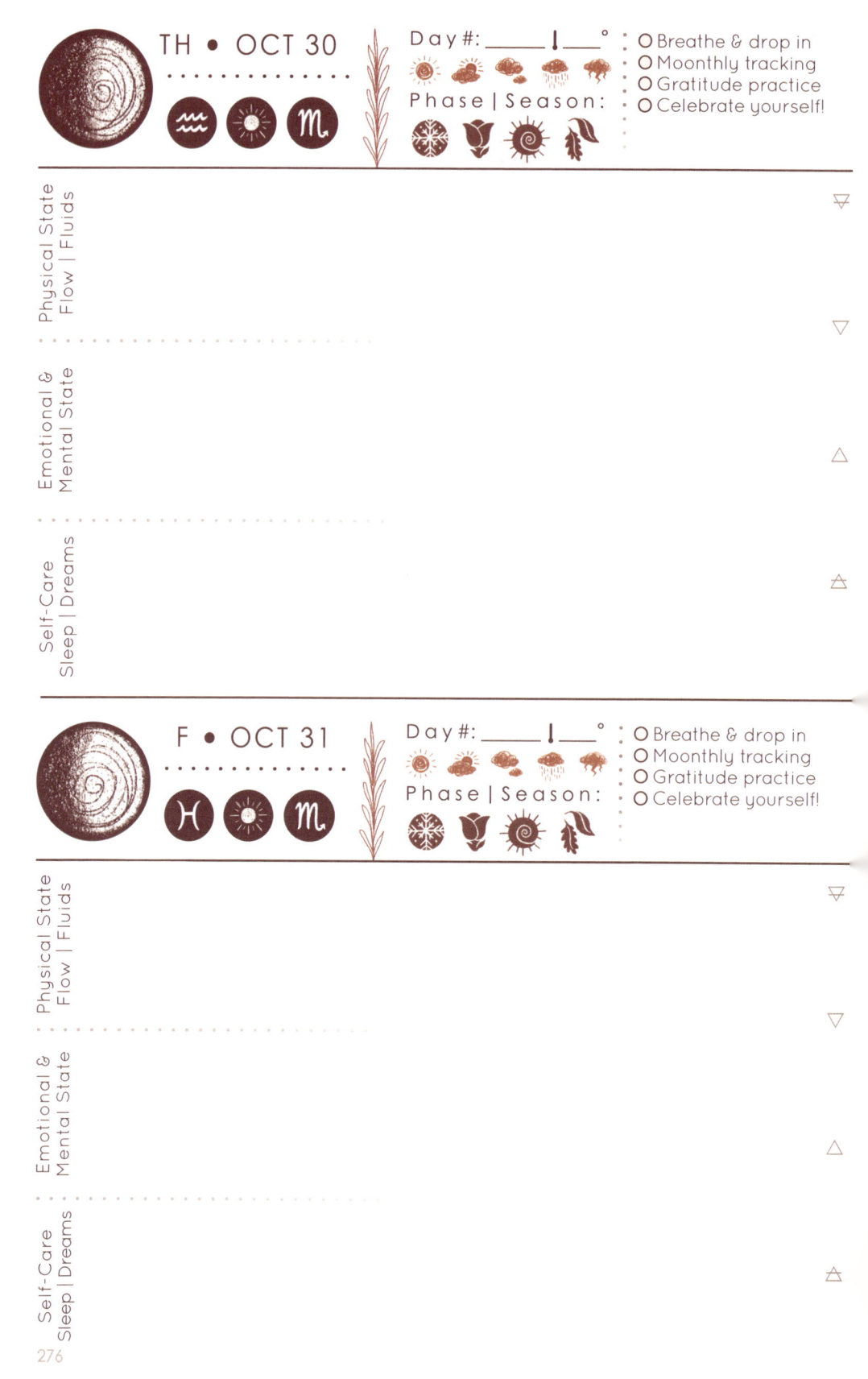

♒ ☀ ♏

Day #: _____ | _____°

Phase | Season:

- ○ Breathe & drop in
- ○ Moonthly tracking
- ○ Gratitude practice
- ○ Celebrate yourself!

Physical State
Flow | Fluids

Emotional & Mental State

Self-Care
Sleep | Dreams

F • OCT 31

♓ ☀ ♏

Day #: _____ | _____°

Phase | Season:

- ○ Breathe & drop in
- ○ Moonthly tracking
- ○ Gratitude practice
- ○ Celebrate yourself!

Physical State
Flow | Fluids

Emotional & Mental State

Self-Care
Sleep | Dreams

S • NOV 1

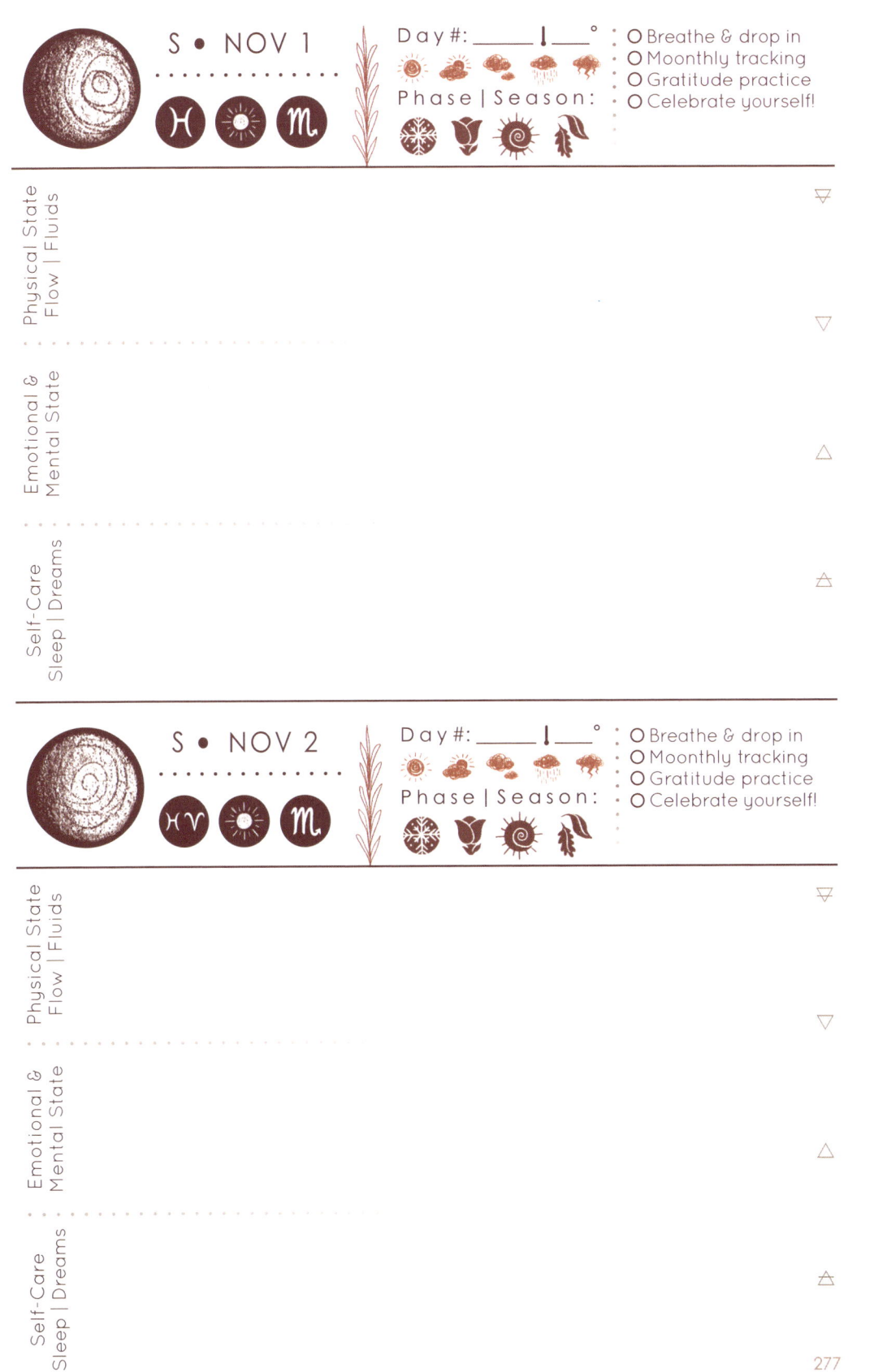

Day #: _____ | _____°

Phase | Season:

- ○ Breathe & drop in
- ○ Moonthly tracking
- ○ Gratitude practice
- ○ Celebrate yourself!

Physical State
Flow | Fluids

Emotional & Mental State

Self-Care
Sleep | Dreams

S • NOV 2

Day #: _____ | _____°

Phase | Season:

- ○ Breathe & drop in
- ○ Moonthly tracking
- ○ Gratitude practice
- ○ Celebrate yourself!

Physical State
Flow | Fluids

Emotional & Mental State

Self-Care
Sleep | Dreams

M • NOV 3

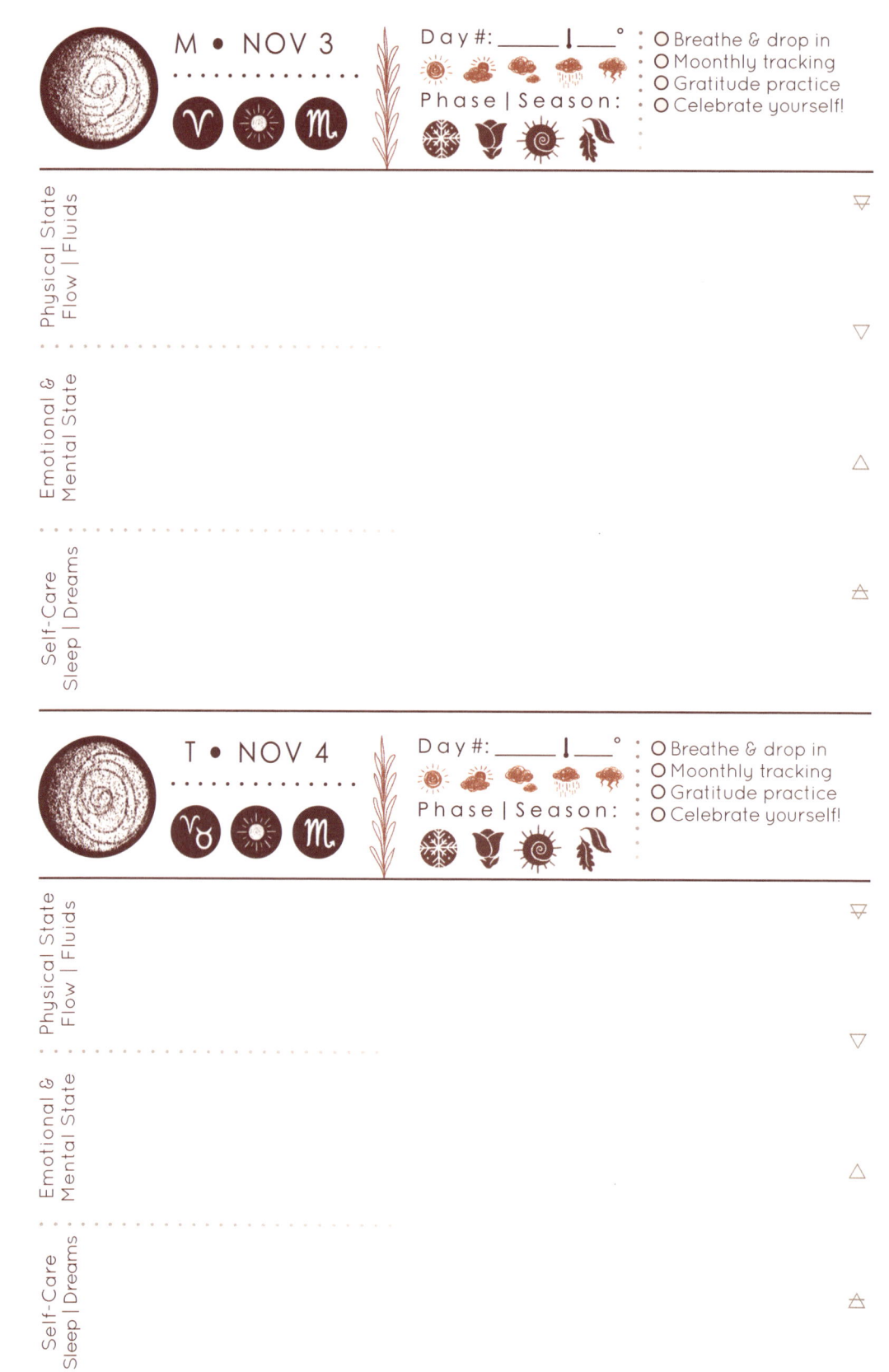

Day #: _____ | ____°

Phase | Season:

- ○ Breathe & drop in
- ○ Moonthly tracking
- ○ Gratitude practice
- ○ Celebrate yourself!

Physical State
Flow | Fluids

Emotional & Mental State

Self-Care
Sleep | Dreams

T • NOV 4

Day #: _____ | ____°

Phase | Season:

- ○ Breathe & drop in
- ○ Moonthly tracking
- ○ Gratitude practice
- ○ Celebrate yourself!

Physical State
Flow | Fluids

Emotional & Mental State

Self-Care
Sleep | Dreams

W • NOV 5

Day #: _____ | ____°

Phase | Season:

- ○ Breathe & drop in
- ○ Moonthly tracking
- ○ Gratitude practice
- ○ Celebrate yourself!

Physical State | Flow | Fluids

Emotional & Mental State

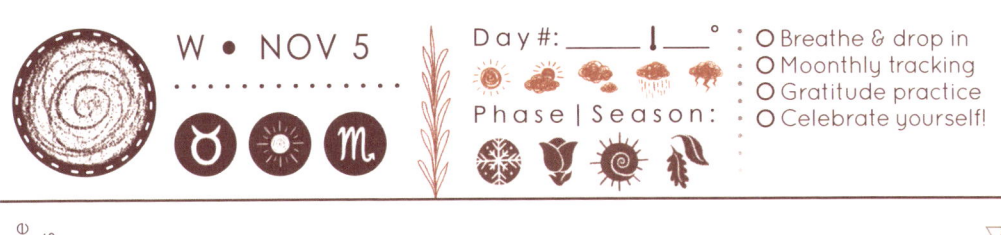

Self-Care | Sleep | Dreams

FULL MOON IN TAURUS

Affirming and forming compassionate boundaries

What is being illuminated?

I give gratitude for what is & what is becoming:

TH • NOV 6

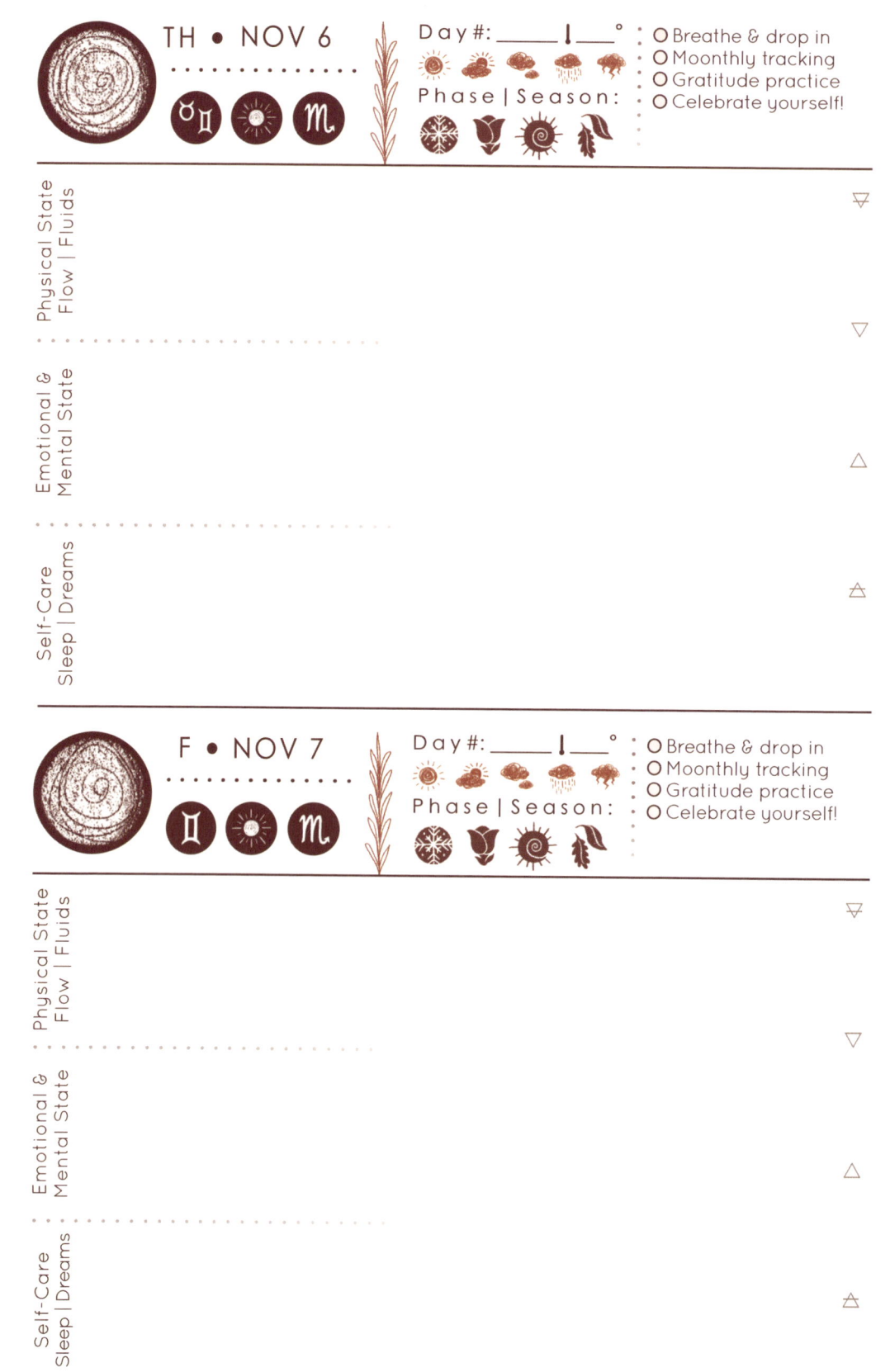

Day #: _____ | _____°

Phase | Season:

- ○ Breathe & drop in
- ○ Moonthly tracking
- ○ Gratitude practice
- ○ Celebrate yourself!

Physical State — Flow | Fluids

Emotional & Mental State

Self-Care — Sleep | Dreams

F • NOV 7

Day #: _____ | _____°

Phase | Season:

- ○ Breathe & drop in
- ○ Moonthly tracking
- ○ Gratitude practice
- ○ Celebrate yourself!

Physical State — Flow | Fluids

Emotional & Mental State

Self-Care — Sleep | Dreams

S • NOV 8

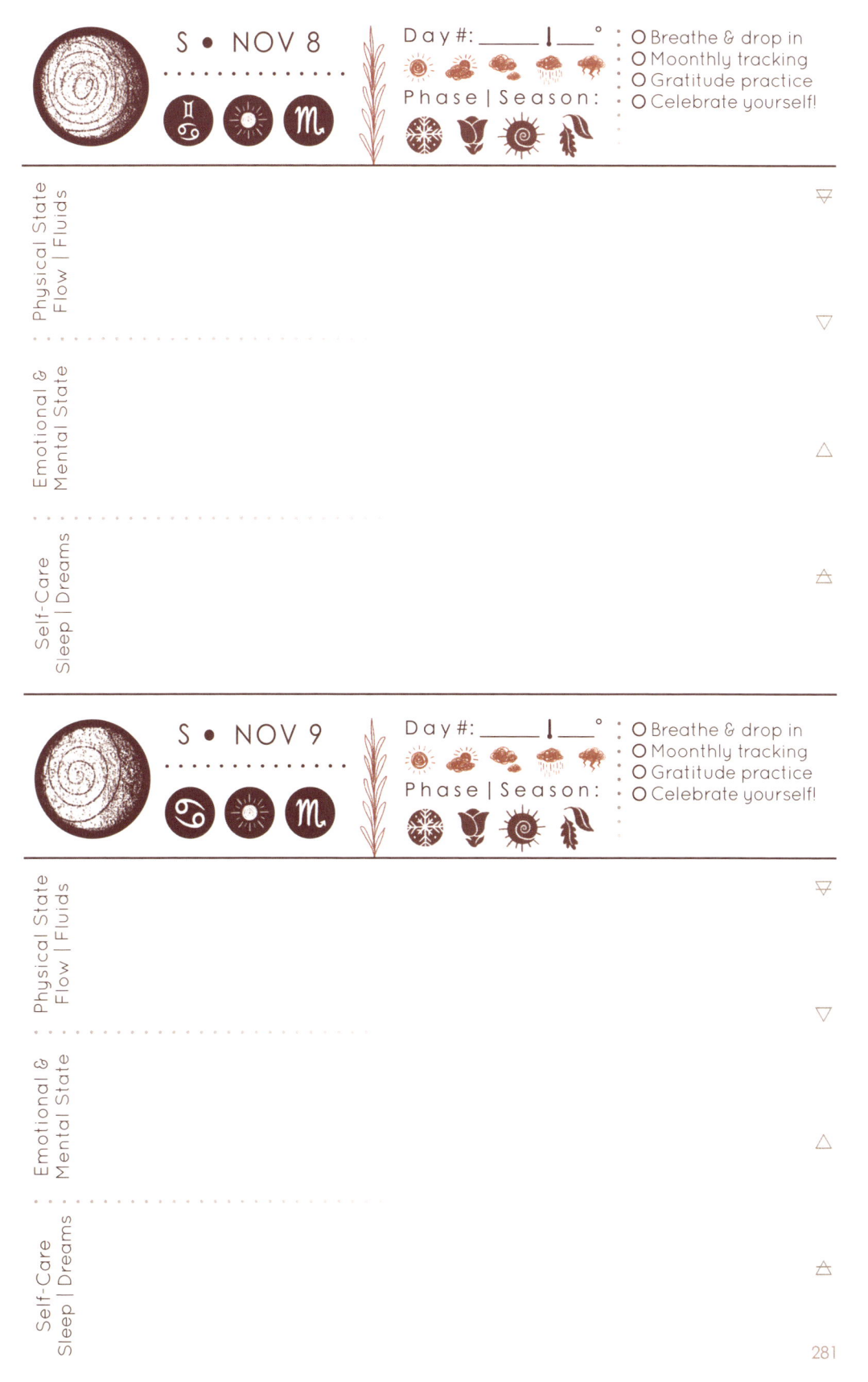

Day #: _____ | _____°

Phase | Season:

- ○ Breathe & drop in
- ○ Moonthly tracking
- ○ Gratitude practice
- ○ Celebrate yourself!

Physical State / Flow | Fluids

Emotional & Mental State

Self-Care / Sleep | Dreams

S • NOV 9

Day #: _____ | _____°

Phase | Season:

- ○ Breathe & drop in
- ○ Moonthly tracking
- ○ Gratitude practice
- ○ Celebrate yourself!

Physical State / Flow | Fluids

Emotional & Mental State

Self-Care / Sleep | Dreams

M • NOV 10

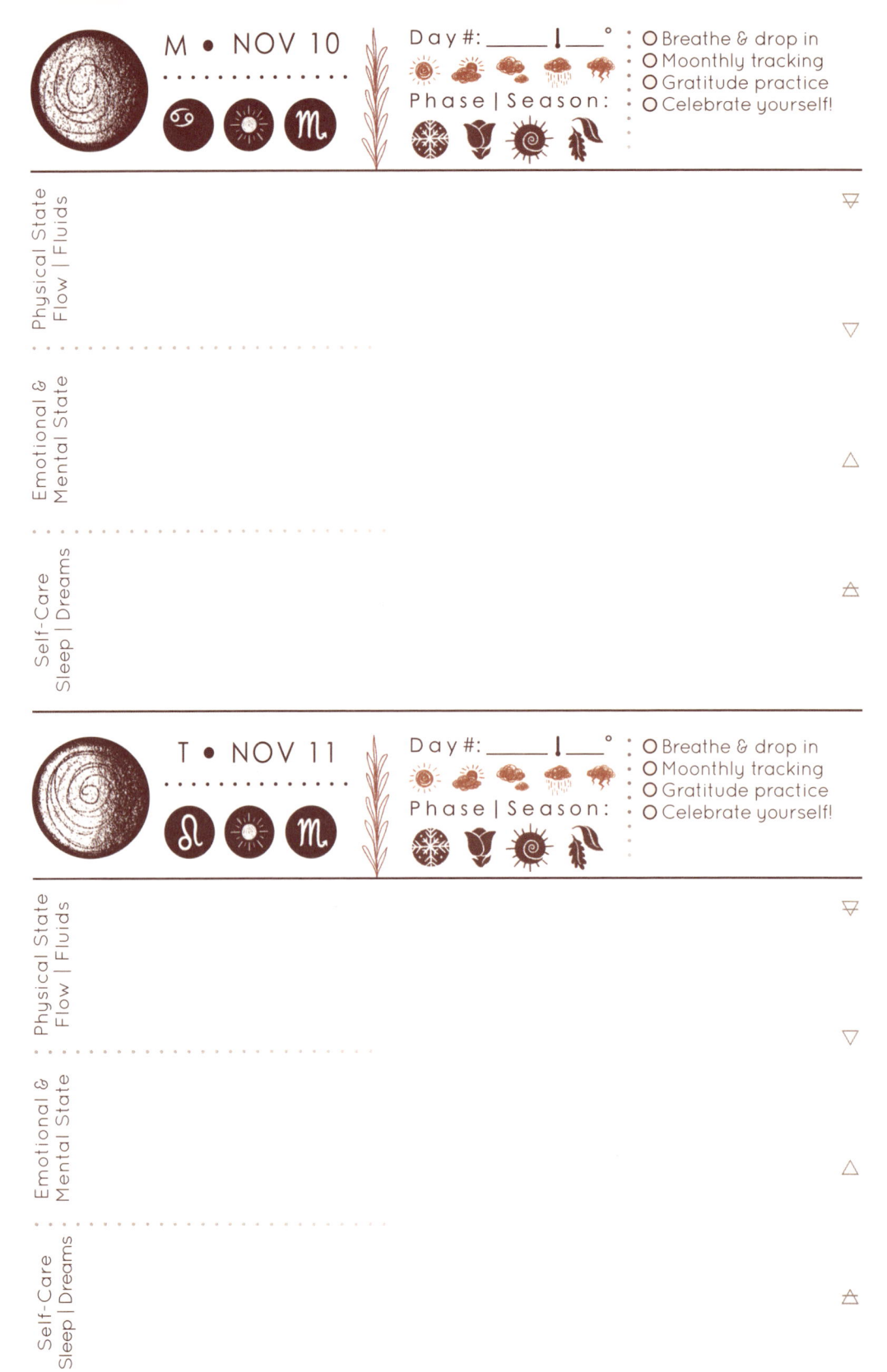

Day #: _____ | _____°

Phase | Season:

- Breathe & drop in
- Moonthly tracking
- Gratitude practice
- Celebrate yourself!

Physical State
Flow | Fluids

Emotional &
Mental State

Self-Care
Sleep | Dreams

T • NOV 11

Day #: _____ | _____°

Phase | Season:

- Breathe & drop in
- Moonthly tracking
- Gratitude practice
- Celebrate yourself!

Physical State
Flow | Fluids

Emotional &
Mental State

Self-Care
Sleep | Dreams

W • NOV 12

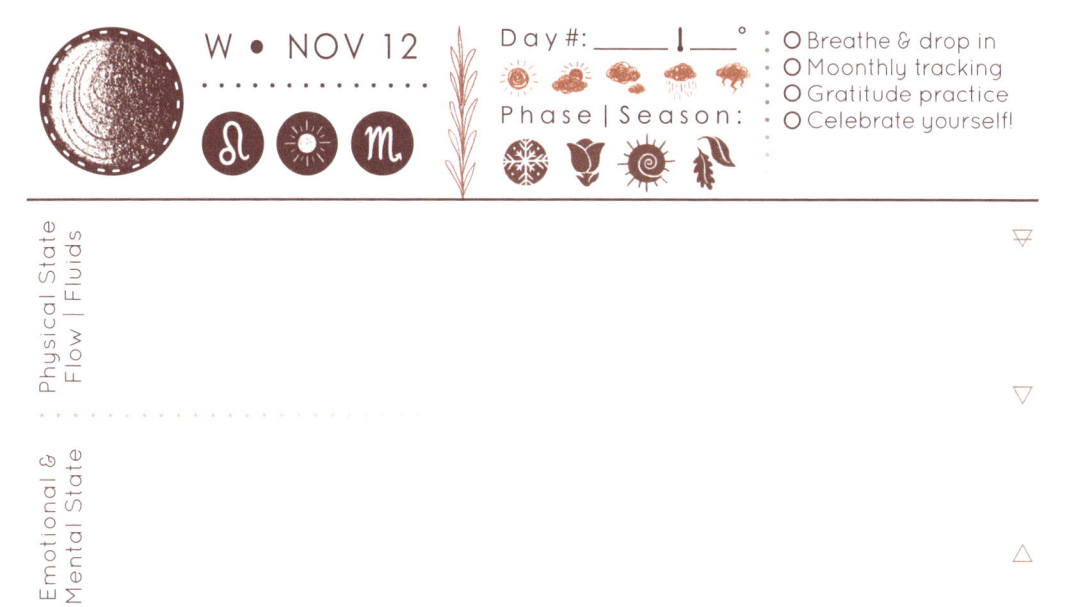

Day #: _____ | _____°

Phase | Season:

- ○ Breathe & drop in
- ○ Moonthly tracking
- ○ Gratitude practice
- ○ Celebrate yourself!

Physical State / Flow | Fluids

Emotional & Mental State

Self-Care / Sleep | Dreams

LAST QUARTER IN LEO

Releasing fear of how we are viewed or perceived

What am I leaving behind this lunar cycle?

Where can I make more space for reflection &/or integration?

TH • NOV 13

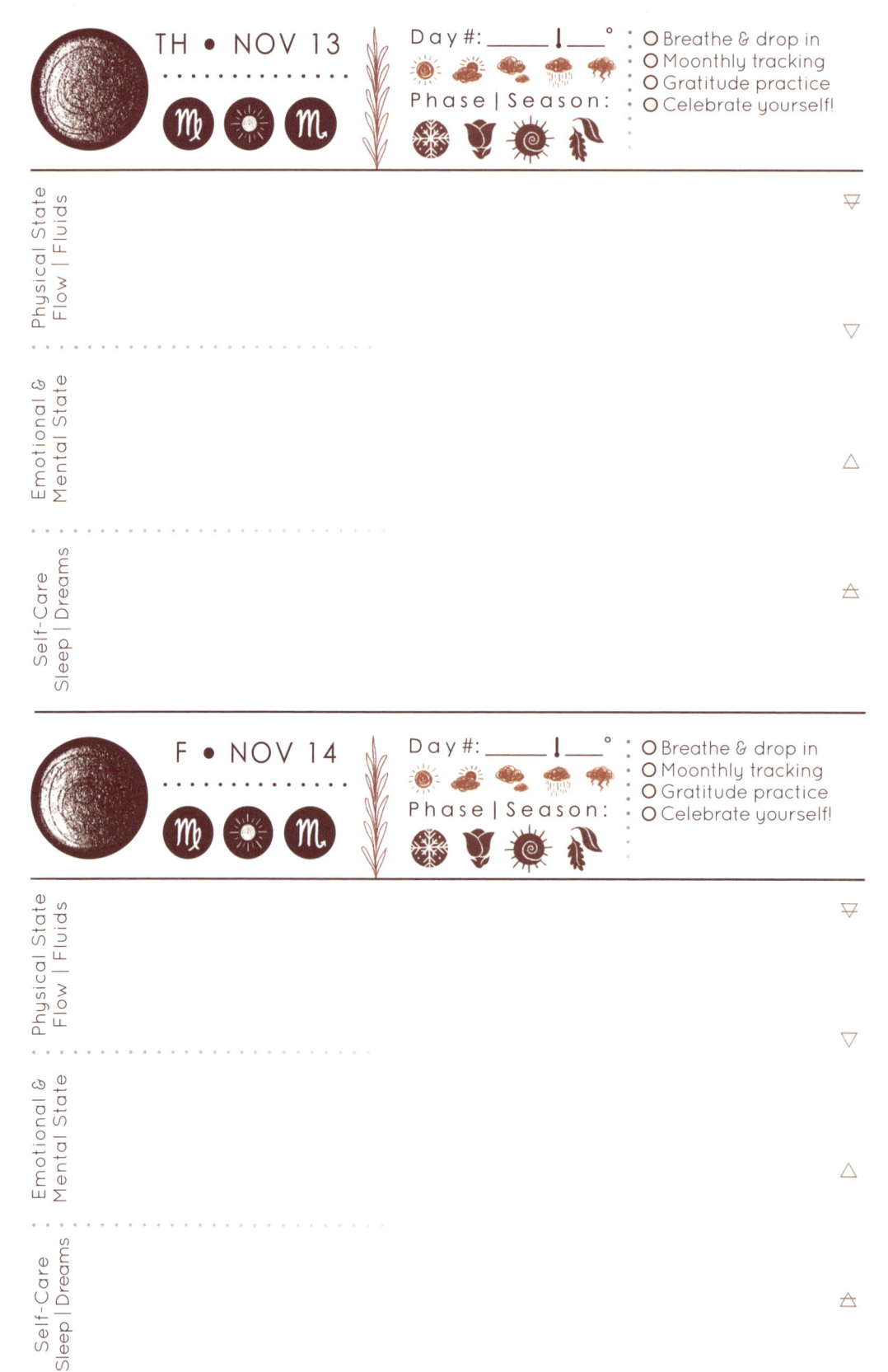

♍ ☼ ♏

Day #: _____ | _____°

Phase | Season:

- ○ Breathe & drop in
- ○ Moonthly tracking
- ○ Gratitude practice
- ○ Celebrate yourself!

Physical State / Flow | Fluids

Emotional & Mental State

Self-Care / Sleep | Dreams

F • NOV 14

♍ ☼ ♏

Day #: _____ | _____°

Phase | Season:

- ○ Breathe & drop in
- ○ Moonthly tracking
- ○ Gratitude practice
- ○ Celebrate yourself!

Physical State / Flow | Fluids

Emotional & Mental State

Self-Care / Sleep | Dreams

S • NOV 15

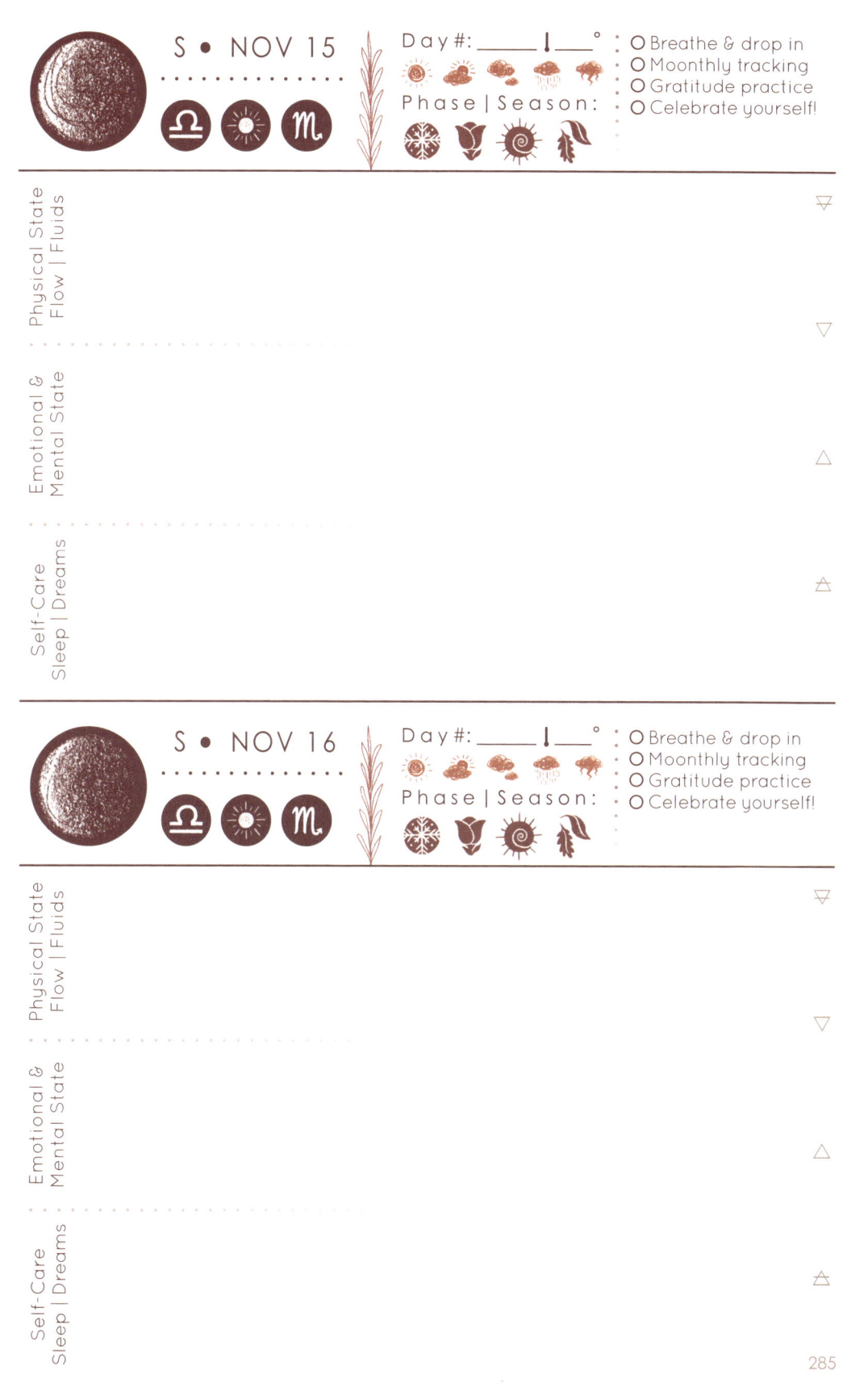

Day #: ____ | ____°

Phase | Season:

- ○ Breathe & drop in
- ○ Moonthly tracking
- ○ Gratitude practice
- ○ Celebrate yourself!

Physical State / Flow | Fluids

Emotional & Mental State

Self-Care / Sleep | Dreams

S • NOV 16

Day #: ____ | ____°

Phase | Season:

- ○ Breathe & drop in
- ○ Moonthly tracking
- ○ Gratitude practice
- ○ Celebrate yourself!

Physical State / Flow | Fluids

Emotional & Mental State

Self-Care / Sleep | Dreams

☾ 10th
10 | 21
11 | 19

CHECK IN & REFLECT

Use this space to reflect on your experiences & findings from this ending lunar cycle or your last menstrual cycle. Use cycle day #s if you bleed, or moon phases if you don't.

Last Cycle Day 1: _____

Last Cycle Length: _____

Circle the phase you bled near:

○ ☾ ☾ ☾ ☽ ● ● ● ☾ ☾ ☽ ☽ ○

Caution Days: (days I needed space)   **Bliss Days:** (days I felt great)

DAYS TO NOTE — Which cycle days stood out?

OBSERVATIONS — Notice any changes or patterns?

SELF-CARE — What was helpful & nourishing?

286

PLAN & PREPARE

Next Predicted Cycle:
🩸 ☾ _____

CHECKLIST

Add the following to any other planners or calendars for your next cycle, then check it off.

- ☐ Predicted "days to note" _____
- ☐ Days to slow down (pre-bleed) _____
- ☐ Rest day(s) (next bleed) _____
- ☐ Date with yourself _____
- ☐ _____

- ☐ Self chest/breast exam
- ☐ Meal plan with cycle
- ☐ _____
- ☐ _____
- ☐ _____

OPEN SPACE

Use this space how you wish, or print out one of our free templates to paste here for BBT charting, dream tracking, or something else:

Connect with Your Blood Through Self-Pleasure

by Gem Campbell (they/them) AKA The Blood Slut • Sexologist & Dietitian
Specialising in Labia Insecurity, PMDD + more • @thebloodslut • iamawildgem.com

Learn how to worship your menstrual blood to cultivate love for your bleeding body. Using blood during self-pleasure (sexual or not) is a magikal way to build a strong bond with your blood and cycle (with the added bonus of dissolving period and sexual shame). This can be used as a manifestation practice as well - your blood is a powerful manifestation tool. Have some menstrual blood at the ready.

1. Set up a sensual space: music, scented candles, decorate with crystals and rose petals.

2. Take deep inhales through the nose and primal vocal exhales out the mouth and activate your senses - what can you smell, hear and feel?

3. Hold your blood and meditate with it, tuning into its wisdom. Use blood collected in a menstrual cup or retrieve some with your fingers directly from your vagina.

4. In front of a mirror, intuitively begin painting your naked body with your blood using your fingers or a paint brush. Tune into every sensation you're experiencing and creatively explore your naked skin. If it feels good, dance and move your body to music as you do this.

5. If you feel sexually aroused, sit in front of a mirror and gaze at your vulva while you use the sensation of the blood on your skin to stimulate your erogenous zones (use coconut oil if desired). Common erogenous zones: vulva, breasts, feet, behind the knees, neck and anus. Explore different parts of the clitoris, such as the bulbs and glans clitoris (head). Arouse yourself further by massaging your labia majora - the glans clitoris isn't the only source of pleasure.

6. When you are ready to close the ritual, be sure to thank your womb, blood and pussy for this delicious experience and sit quietly for a few minutes to integrate. Take out your journal to reflect on the experience and write down any spiritual messages you received.

Here's a link to my Bleeding Pleasure playlist:

Phasic Overview & In-Betweens

Use this space to focus on the phases of the moonth and the in-betweens of the peak lunations.

One way of using this space is to designate one column for your goal-planning, intention-setting or focus per phase/week. Use the other column for reflections, dream themes, nutrition tracking, cards pulls, etc!

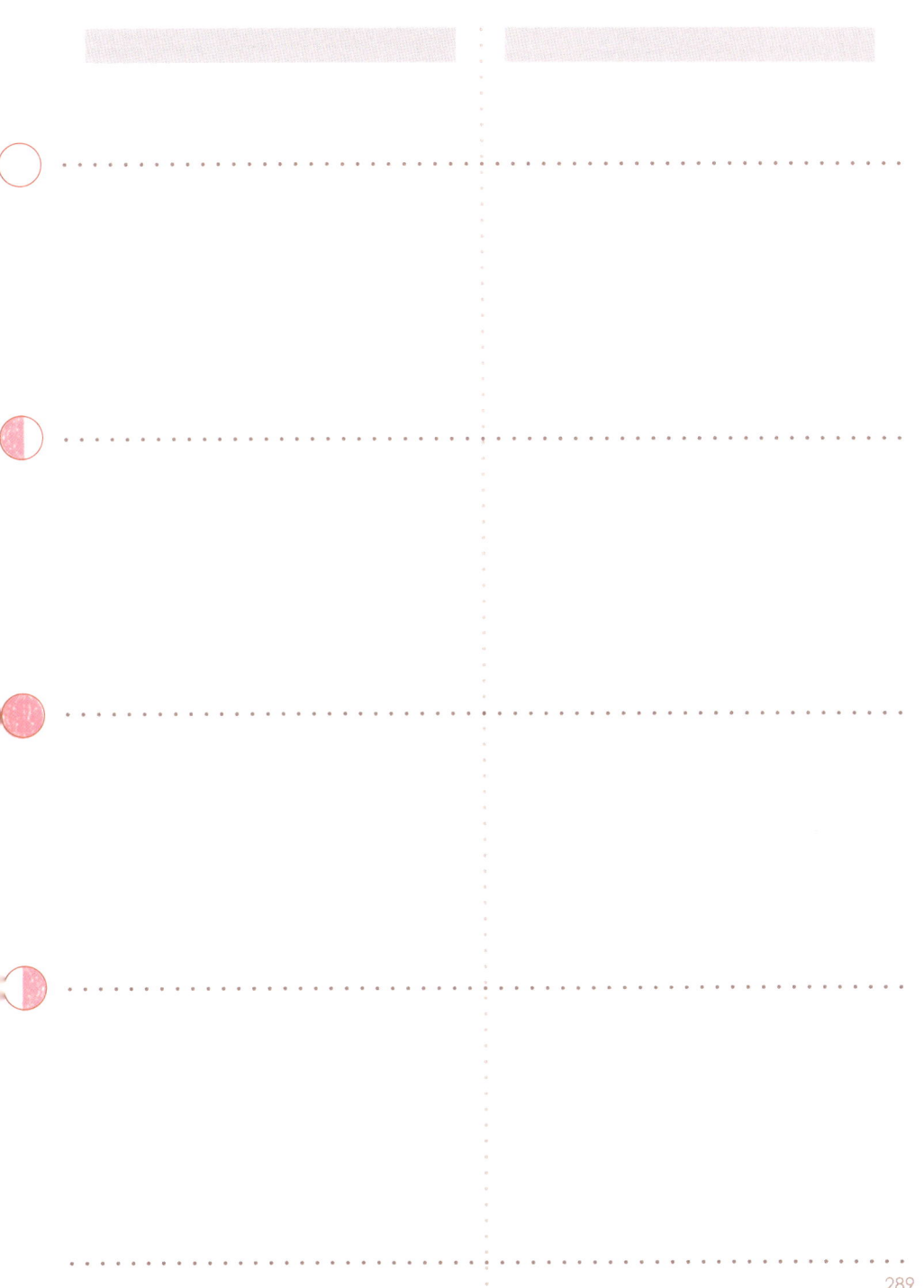

M • NOV 17

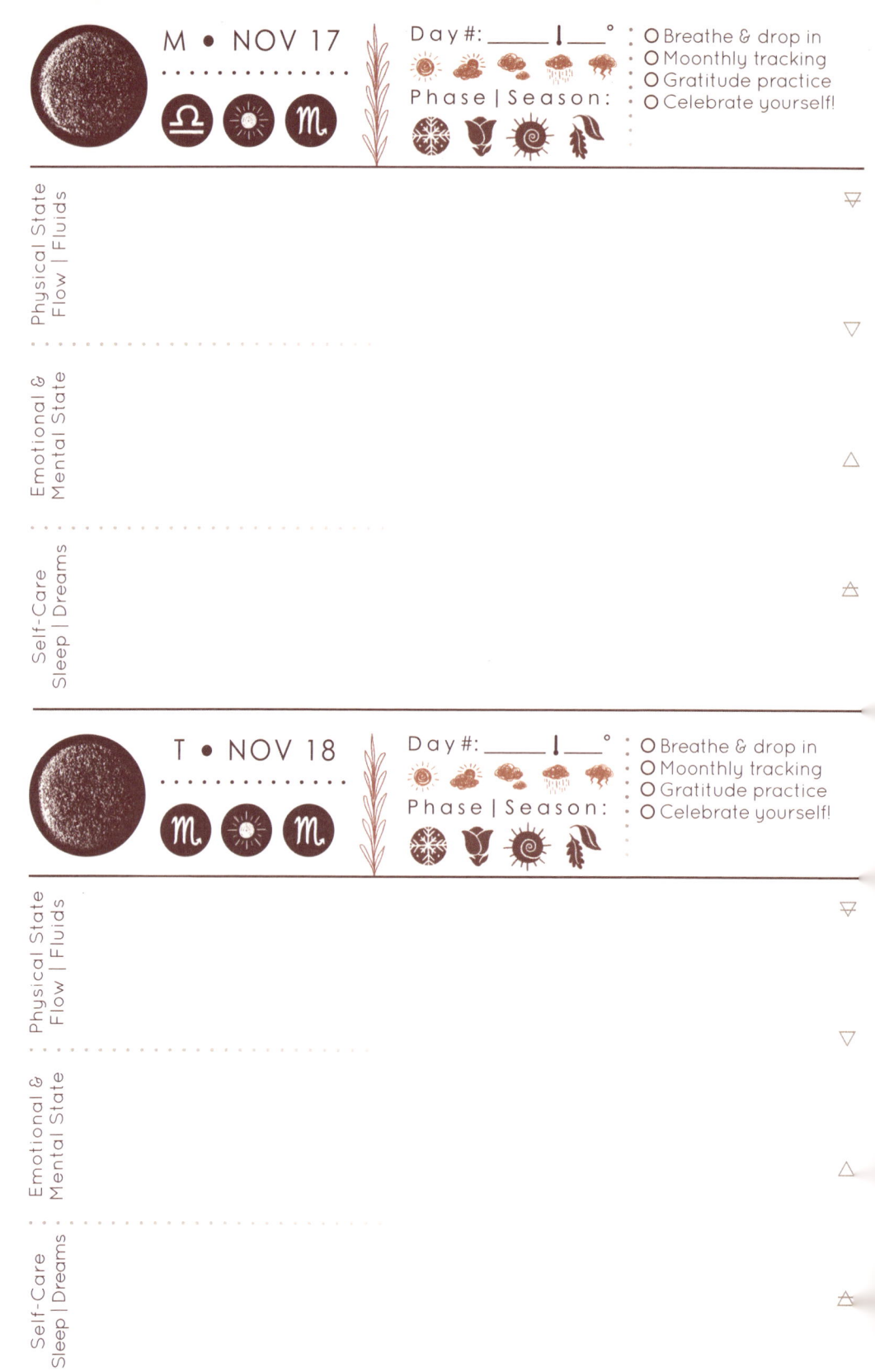

Day #: _____ | _____°

Phase | Season:

- ○ Breathe & drop in
- ○ Moonthly tracking
- ○ Gratitude practice
- ○ Celebrate yourself!

Physical State
Flow | Fluids

Emotional & Mental State

Self-Care
Sleep | Dreams

T • NOV 18

Day #: _____ | _____°

Phase | Season:

- ○ Breathe & drop in
- ○ Moonthly tracking
- ○ Gratitude practice
- ○ Celebrate yourself!

Physical State
Flow | Fluids

Emotional & Mental State

Self-Care
Sleep | Dreams

W • NOV 19

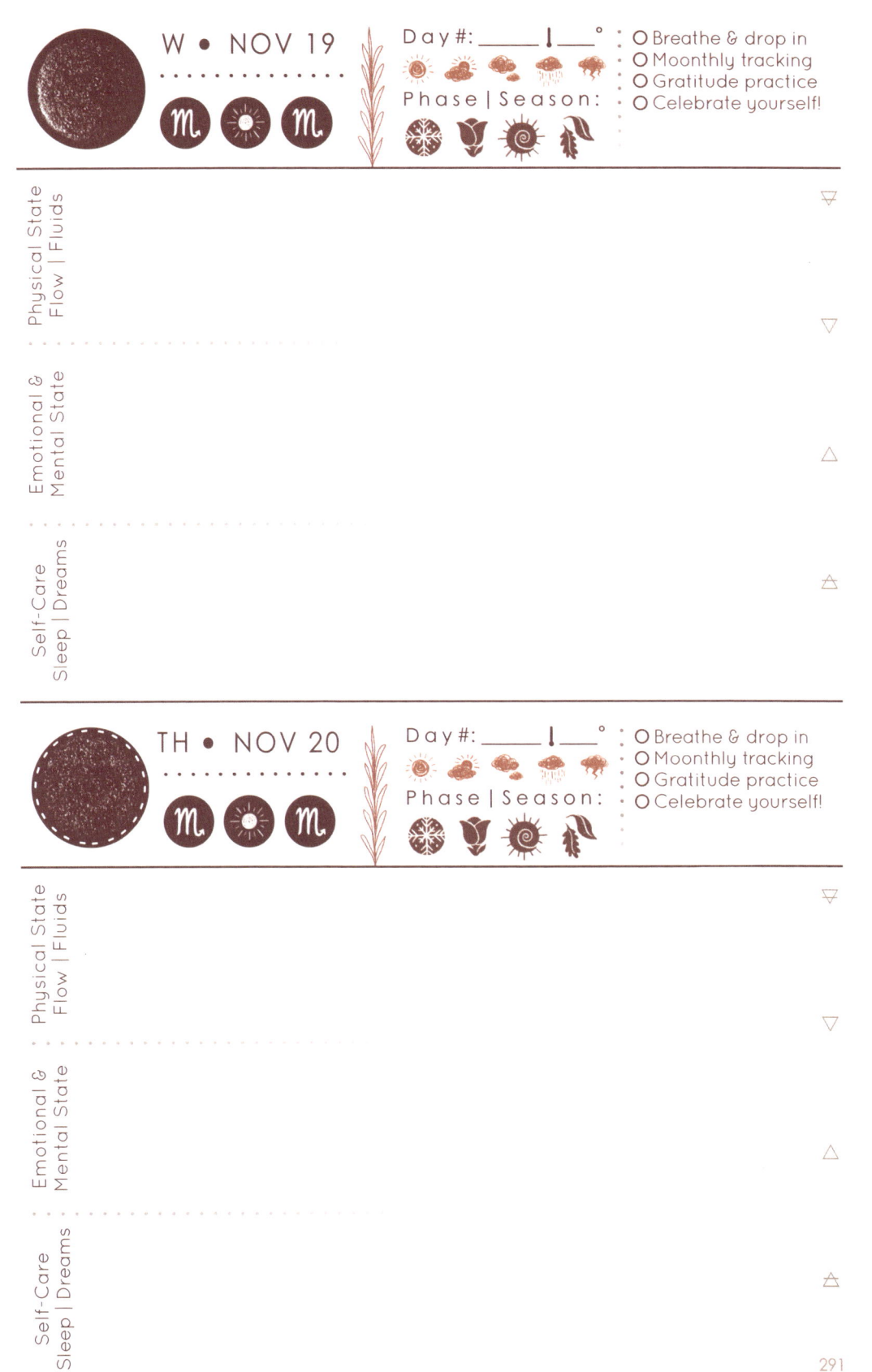

Day #: _____ | _____°

Phase | Season:

- ○ Breathe & drop in
- ○ Moonthly tracking
- ○ Gratitude practice
- ○ Celebrate yourself!

Physical State / Flow | Fluids

Emotional & Mental State

Self-Care / Sleep | Dreams

TH • NOV 20

Day #: _____ | _____°

Phase | Season:

- ○ Breathe & drop in
- ○ Moonthly tracking
- ○ Gratitude practice
- ○ Celebrate yourself!

Physical State / Flow | Fluids

Emotional & Mental State

Self-Care / Sleep | Dreams

NEW MOON IN SCORPIO

Breaking through the surface of a new chapter with an open mind

What do I want to grow & focus on during this lunar cycle?

How will I hold space for this?

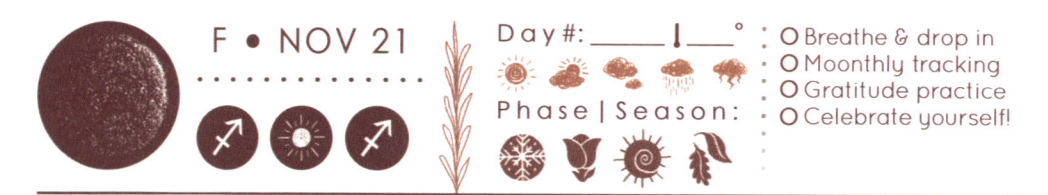

F • NOV 21

Day #: _____ | ___°

Phase | Season:

- ○ Breathe & drop in
- ○ Moonthly tracking
- ○ Gratitude practice
- ○ Celebrate yourself!

Physical State / Flow | Fluids

Emotional & Mental State

Self-Care / Sleep | Dreams

S • NOV 22

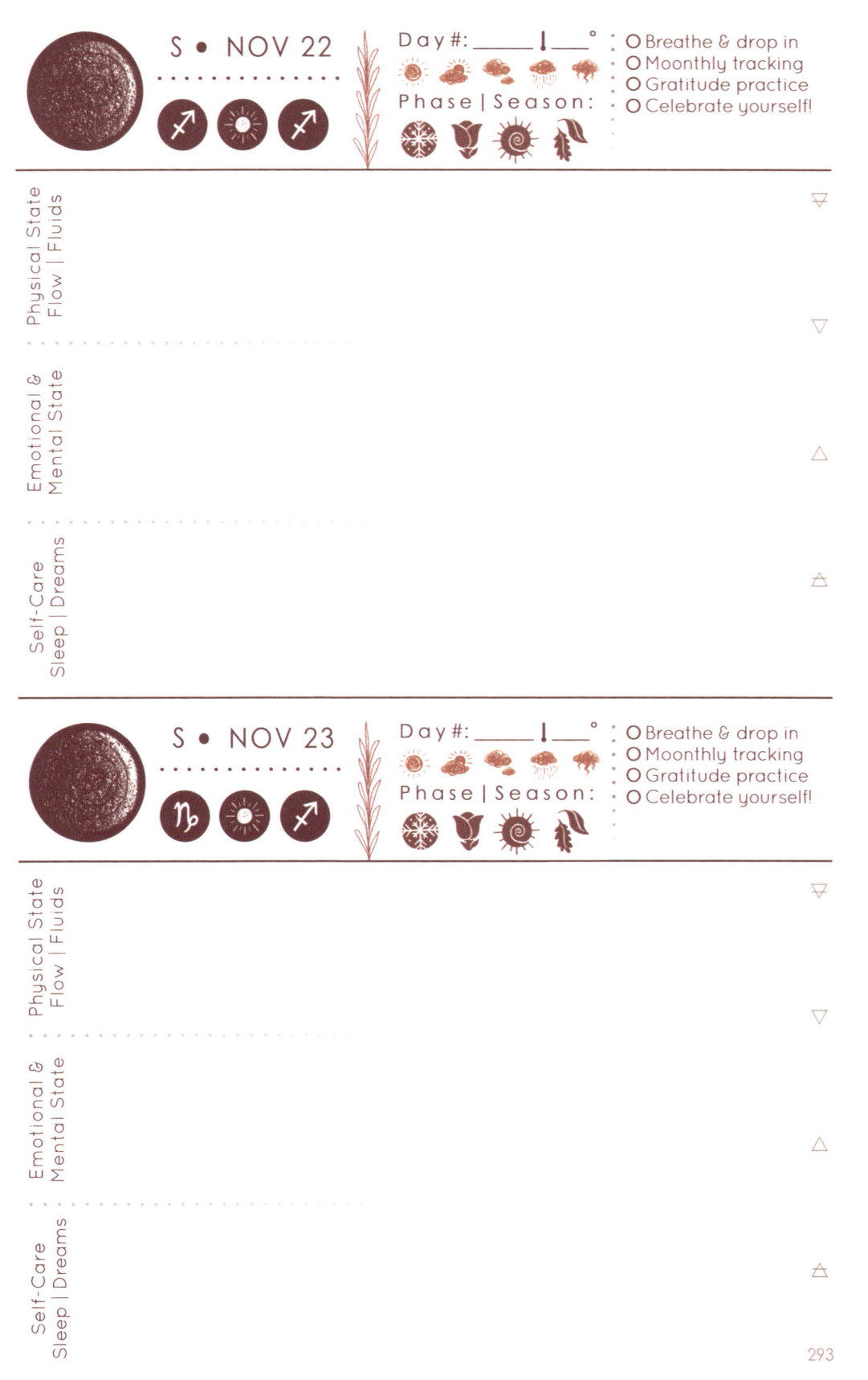

Day #: _____ | _____°

Phase | Season:

- ○ Breathe & drop in
- ○ Moonthly tracking
- ○ Gratitude practice
- ○ Celebrate yourself!

Physical State / Flow | Fluids

Emotional & Mental State

Self-Care / Sleep | Dreams

S • NOV 23

Day #: _____ | _____°

Phase | Season:

- ○ Breathe & drop in
- ○ Moonthly tracking
- ○ Gratitude practice
- ○ Celebrate yourself!

Physical State / Flow | Fluids

Emotional & Mental State

Self-Care / Sleep | Dreams

M • NOV 24

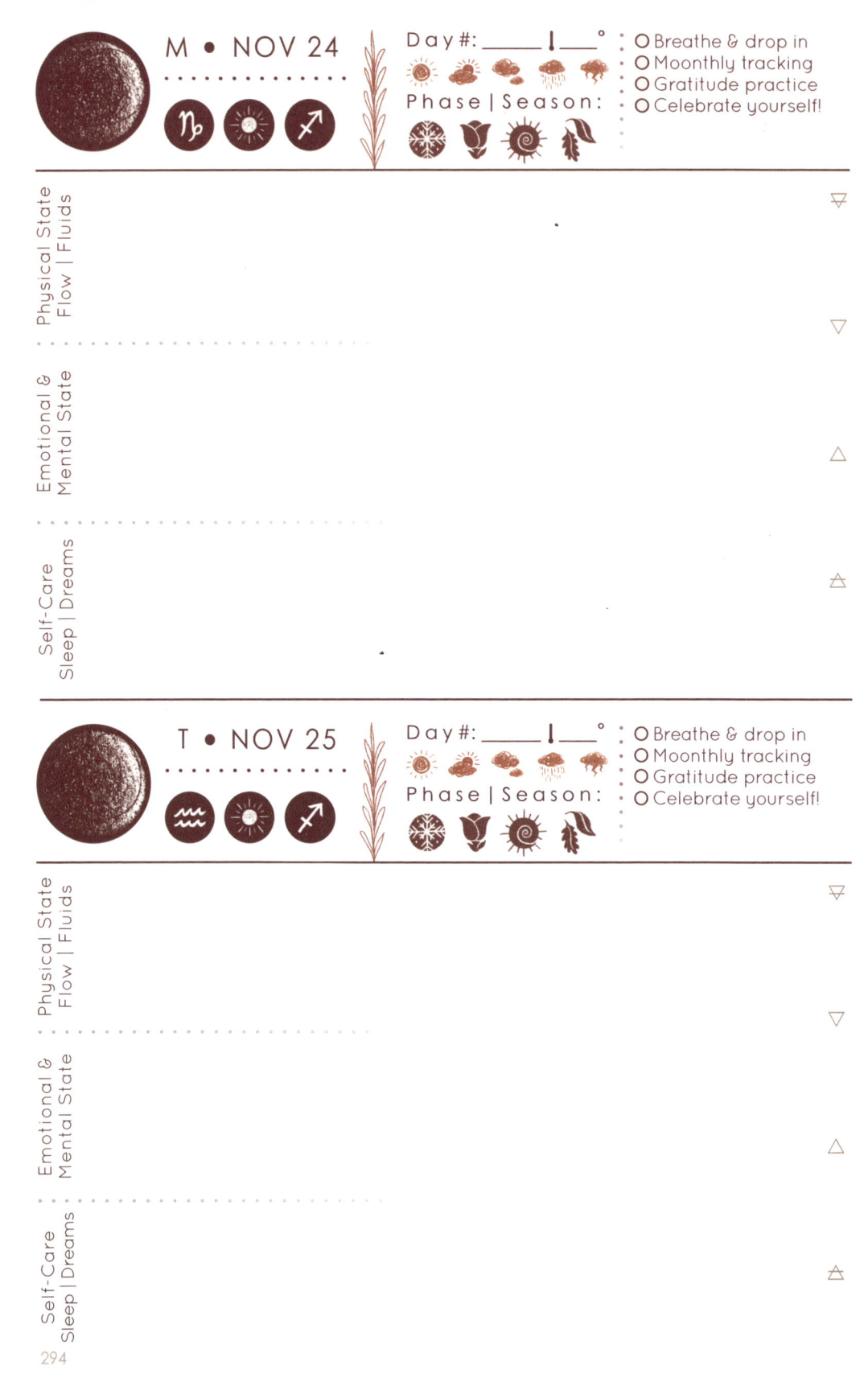

Day #: _____ | _____°

Phase | Season:

- ○ Breathe & drop in
- ○ Moonthly tracking
- ○ Gratitude practice
- ○ Celebrate yourself!

Physical State
Flow | Fluids

Emotional &
Mental State

Self-Care
Sleep | Dreams

T • NOV 25

Day #: _____ | _____°

Phase | Season:

- ○ Breathe & drop in
- ○ Moonthly tracking
- ○ Gratitude practice
- ○ Celebrate yourself!

Physical State
Flow | Fluids

Emotional &
Mental State

Self-Care
Sleep | Dreams

W • NOV 26

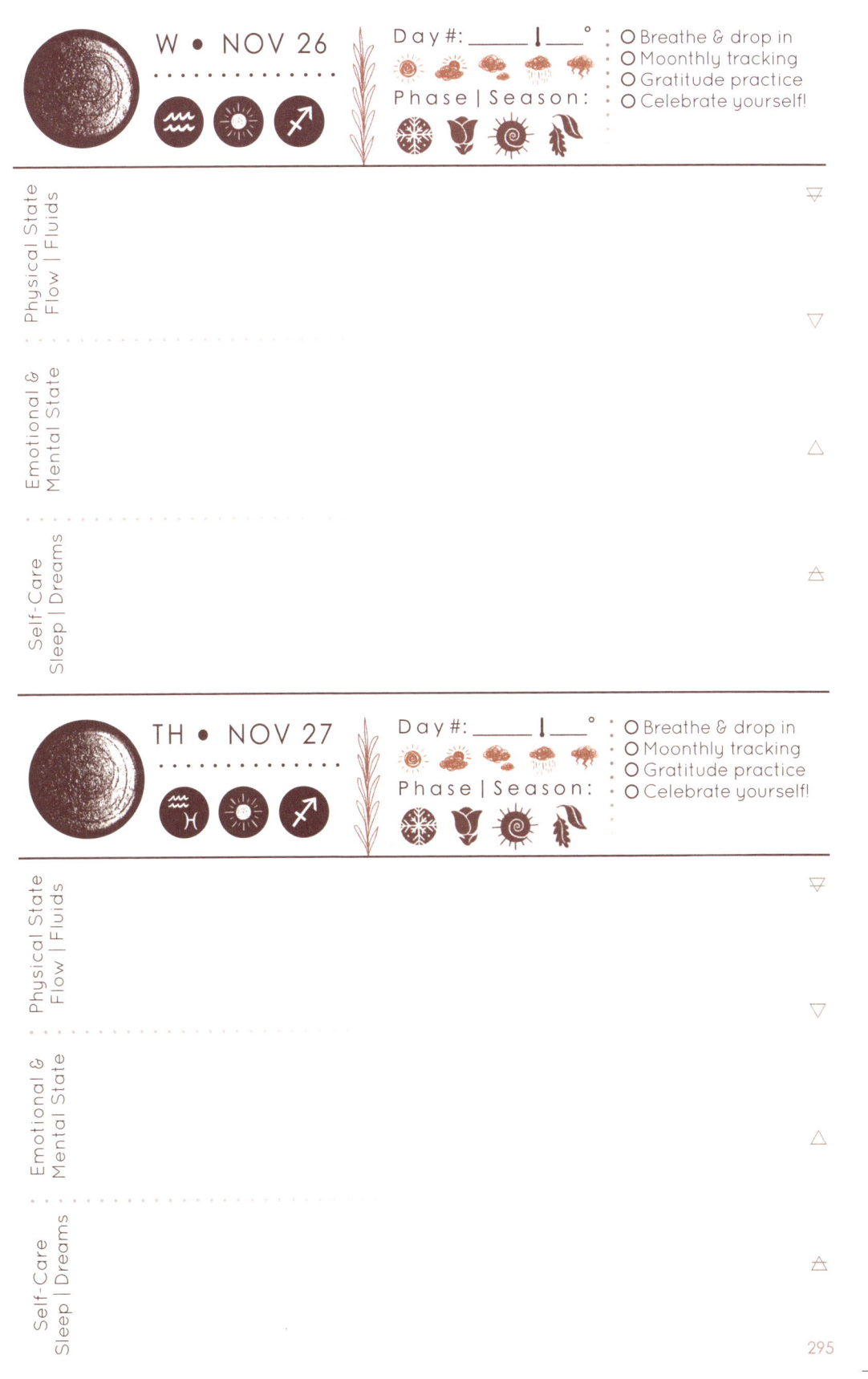

Day #: _____ | _____°

Phase | Season:

- ○ Breathe & drop in
- ○ Moonthly tracking
- ○ Gratitude practice
- ○ Celebrate yourself!

Physical State / Flow | Fluids

Emotional & Mental State

Self-Care / Sleep | Dreams

TH • NOV 27

Day #: _____ | _____°

Phase | Season:

- ○ Breathe & drop in
- ○ Moonthly tracking
- ○ Gratitude practice
- ○ Celebrate yourself!

Physical State / Flow | Fluids

Emotional & Mental State

Self-Care / Sleep | Dreams

F • NOV 28

Day #: ____ | ____°

Phase | Season:

- Breathe & drop in
- Moonthly tracking
- Gratitude practice
- Celebrate yourself!

Physical State / Flow | Fluids

Emotional & Mental State

Self-Care / Sleep | Dreams

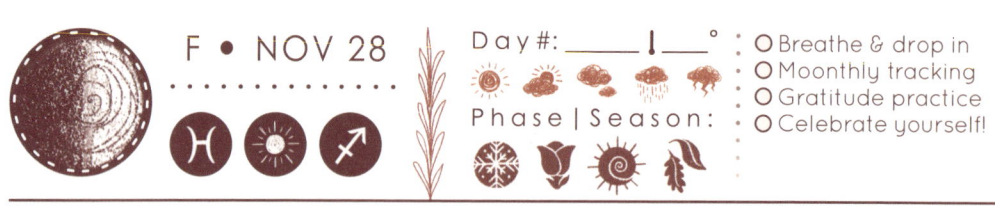

FIRST QUARTER IN PISCES

Surfacing from a dream-state to move forward with intention

What is sprouting & coming into awareness?

What can I release to make space for further growth & grounding?

S • NOV 29

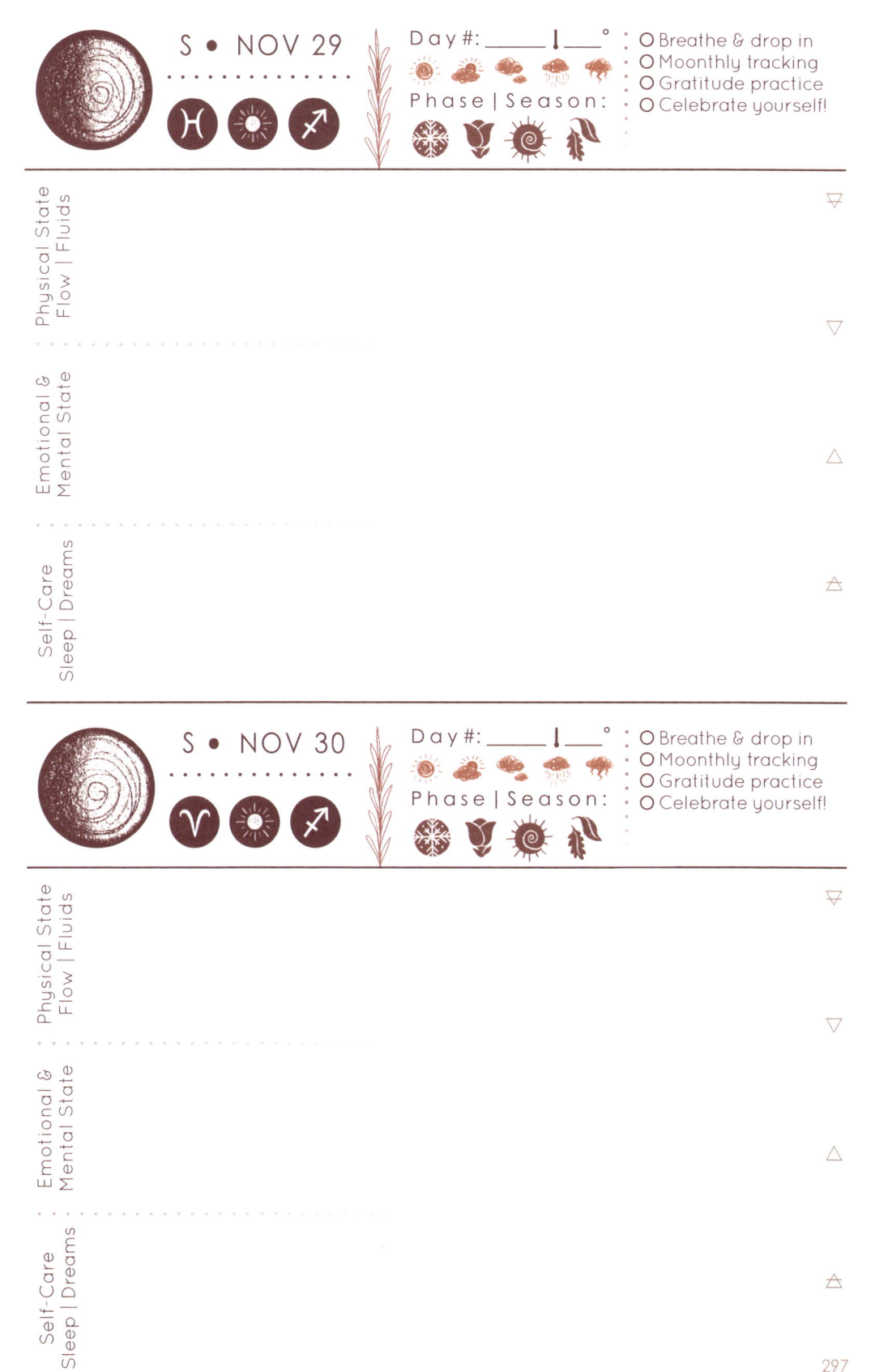

♓ ☀ ♐

Day #: _____ | ___°

Phase | Season:

- ○ Breathe & drop in
- ○ Moonthly tracking
- ○ Gratitude practice
- ○ Celebrate yourself!

Physical State
Flow | Fluids

Emotional & Mental State

Self-Care
Sleep | Dreams

S • NOV 30

♈ ☀ ♐

Day #: _____ | ___°

Phase | Season:

- ○ Breathe & drop in
- ○ Moonthly tracking
- ○ Gratitude practice
- ○ Celebrate yourself!

Physical State
Flow | Fluids

Emotional & Mental State

Self-Care
Sleep | Dreams

M • DEC 1

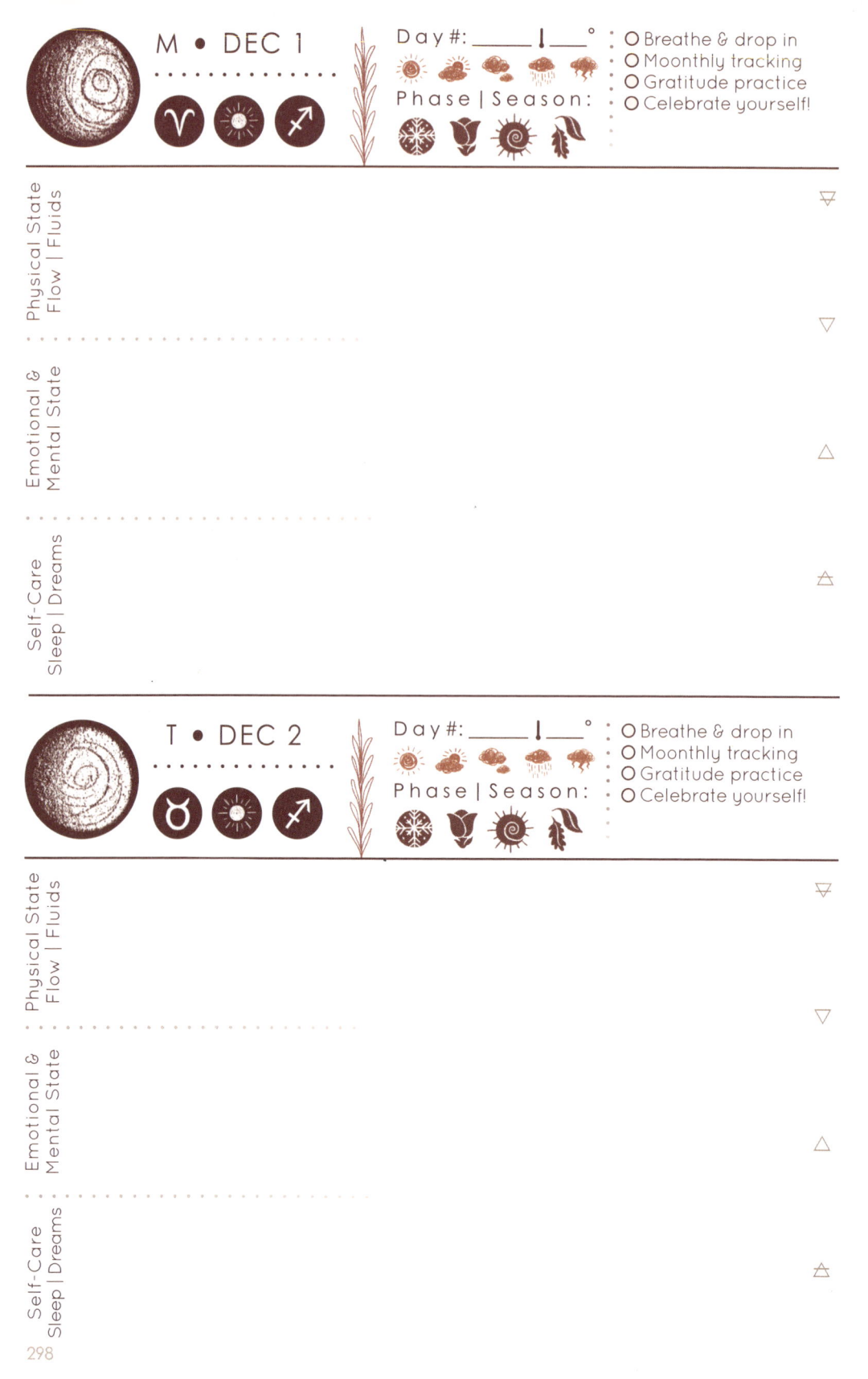

Day #: _____ | _____°

Phase | Season:

- ○ Breathe & drop in
- ○ Moonthly tracking
- ○ Gratitude practice
- ○ Celebrate yourself!

Physical State / Flow | Fluids

Emotional & Mental State

Self-Care / Sleep | Dreams

T • DEC 2

Day #: _____ | _____°

Phase | Season:

- ○ Breathe & drop in
- ○ Moonthly tracking
- ○ Gratitude practice
- ○ Celebrate yourself!

Physical State / Flow | Fluids

Emotional & Mental State

Self-Care / Sleep | Dreams

W • DEC 3

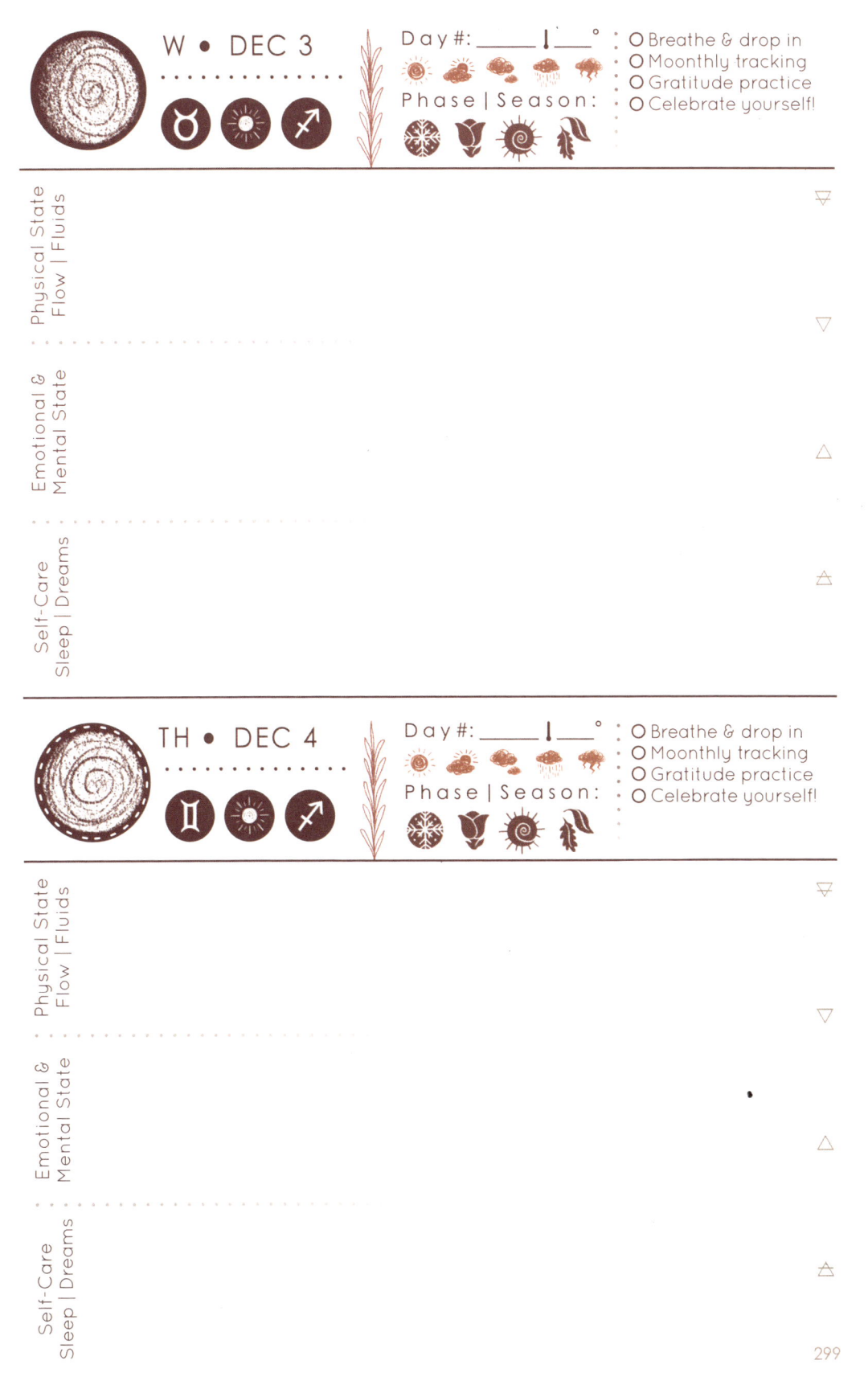

Day #: _____ | _____°

Phase | Season:

- ○ Breathe & drop in
- ○ Moonthly tracking
- ○ Gratitude practice
- ○ Celebrate yourself!

Physical State / Flow | Fluids

Emotional & Mental State

Self-Care / Sleep | Dreams

TH • DEC 4

Day #: _____ | _____°

Phase | Season:

- ○ Breathe & drop in
- ○ Moonthly tracking
- ○ Gratitude practice
- ○ Celebrate yourself!

Physical State / Flow | Fluids

Emotional & Mental State

Self-Care / Sleep | Dreams

FULL MOON IN GEMINI

Expanding mentally to awaken ever-greater potential

What is being illuminated?

I give gratitude for what is & what is becoming:

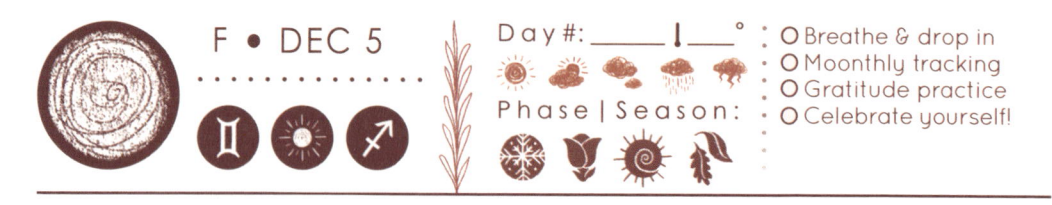

F • DEC 5

Day #: _____ | _____°

Phase | Season:

○ Breathe & drop in
○ Moonthly tracking
○ Gratitude practice
○ Celebrate yourself!

Physical State / Flow | Fluids

Emotional & Mental State

Self-Care / Sleep | Dreams

S • DEC 6

Day #: _____ | _____°

Phase | Season:

- ○ Breathe & drop in
- ○ Moonthly tracking
- ○ Gratitude practice
- ○ Celebrate yourself!

Physical State / Flow | Fluids

Emotional & Mental State

Self-Care / Sleep | Dreams

S • DEC 7

Day #: _____ | _____°

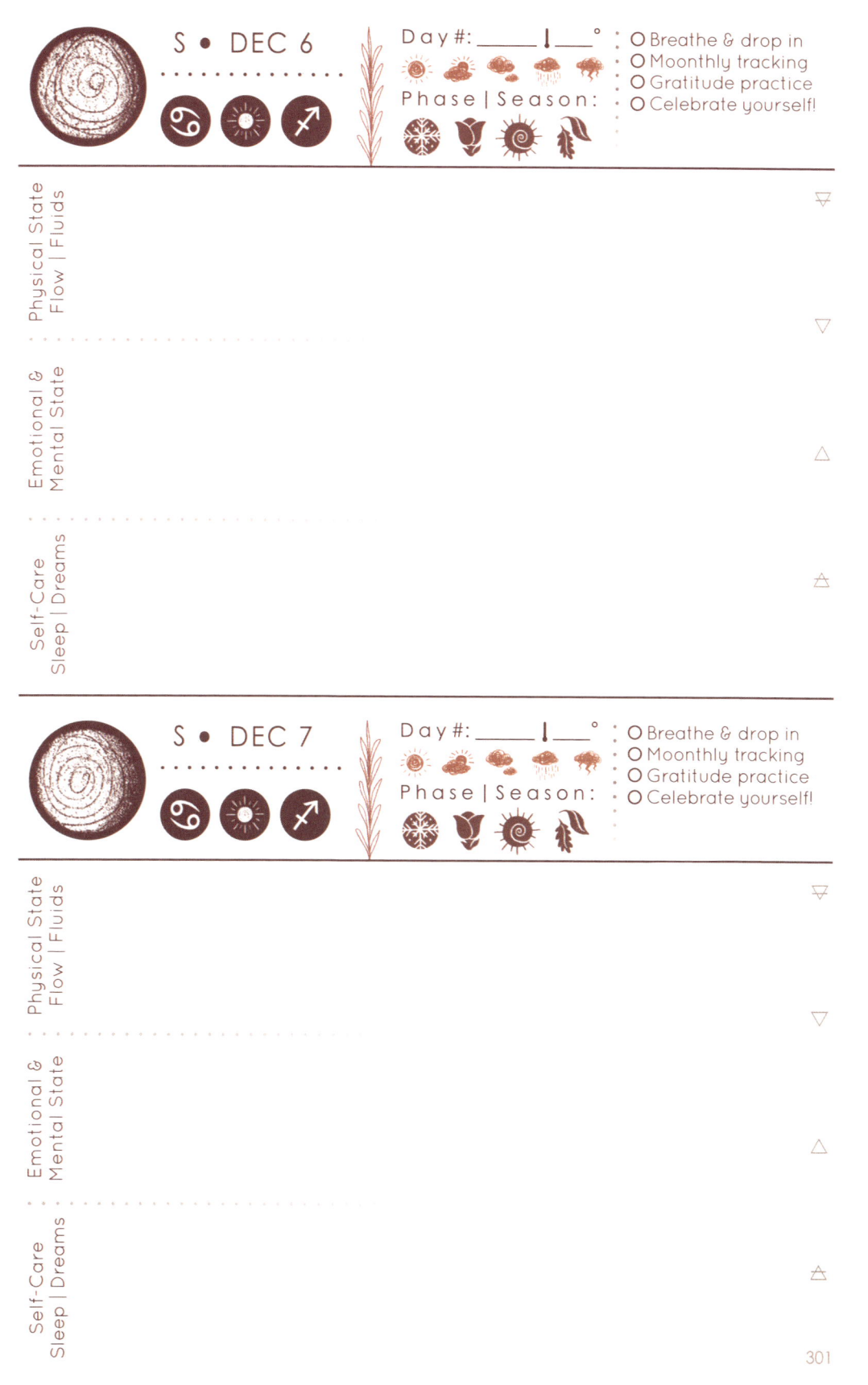

Phase | Season:

- ○ Breathe & drop in
- ○ Moonthly tracking
- ○ Gratitude practice
- ○ Celebrate yourself!

Physical State / Flow | Fluids

Emotional & Mental State

Self-Care / Sleep | Dreams

M • DEC 8

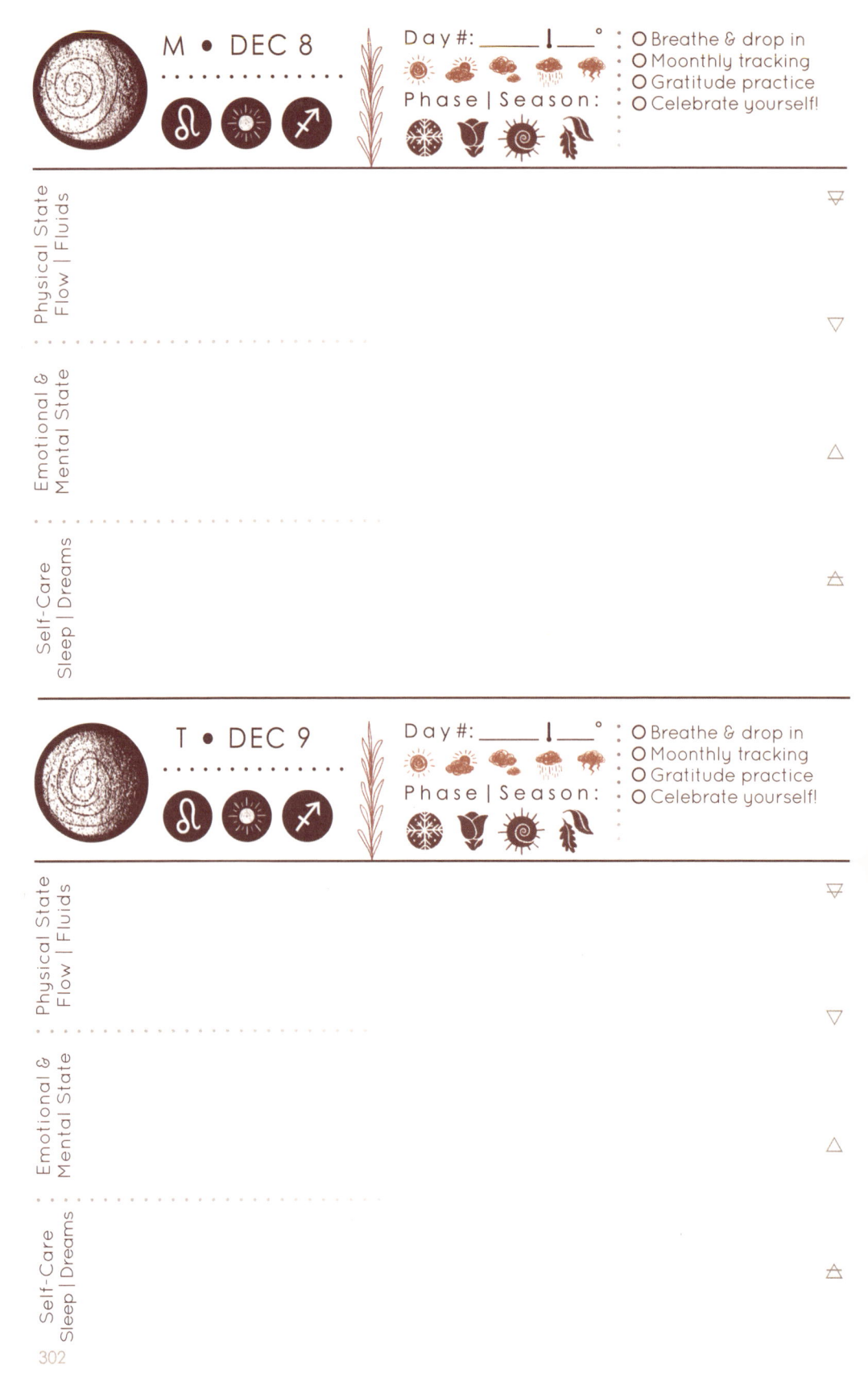

Day #: _____ | ___°

Phase | Season:

- Breathe & drop in
- Moonthly tracking
- Gratitude practice
- Celebrate yourself!

Physical State
Flow | Fluids

Emotional &
Mental State

Self-Care
Sleep | Dreams

T • DEC 9

Day #: _____ | ___°

Phase | Season:

- Breathe & drop in
- Moonthly tracking
- Gratitude practice
- Celebrate yourself!

Physical State
Flow | Fluids

Emotional &
Mental State

Self-Care
Sleep | Dreams

W • DEC 10

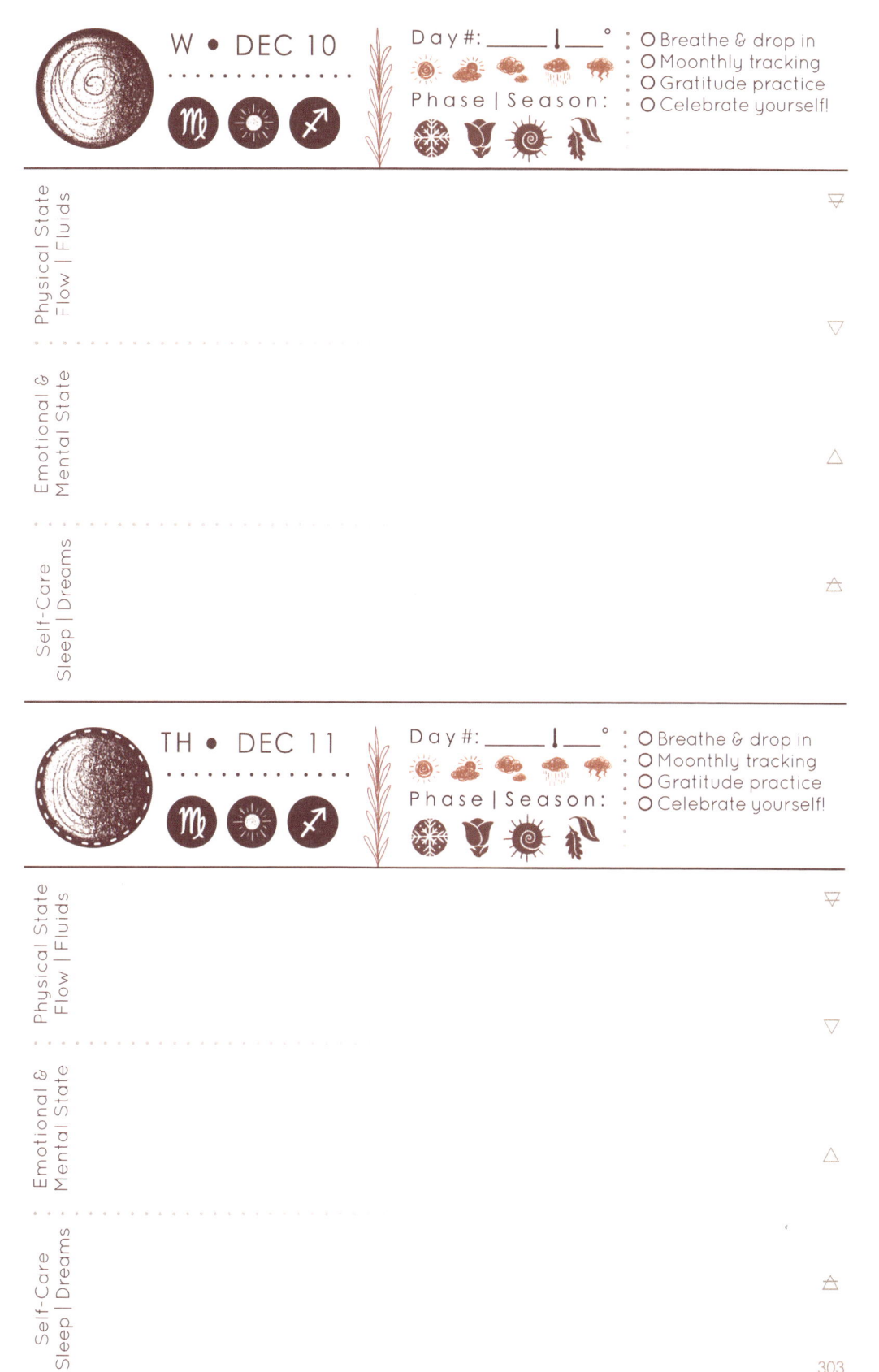

Day #: _____ | ____°

Phase | Season:

- ○ Breathe & drop in
- ○ Moonthly tracking
- ○ Gratitude practice
- ○ Celebrate yourself!

Physical State / Flow | Fluids

Emotional & Mental State

Self-Care / Sleep | Dreams

TH • DEC 11

Day #: _____ | ____°

Phase | Season:

- ○ Breathe & drop in
- ○ Moonthly tracking
- ○ Gratitude practice
- ○ Celebrate yourself!

Physical State / Flow | Fluids

Emotional & Mental State

Self-Care / Sleep | Dreams

LAST QUARTER IN VIRGO

Zooming out to see the bigger picture & accept all parts of the whole as is

What am I leaving behind this lunar cycle?

Where can I make more space for reflection &/or integration?

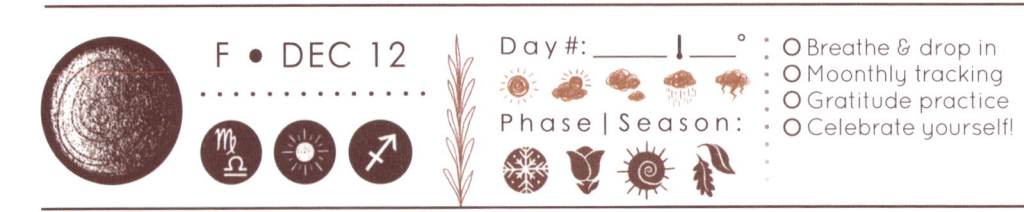

F • DEC 12

Day #: _____ | _____°

Phase | Season:

- ○ Breathe & drop in
- ○ Moonthly tracking
- ○ Gratitude practice
- ○ Celebrate yourself!

Physical State Flow | Fluids

Emotional & Mental State

Self-Care Sleep | Dreams

S • DEC 13

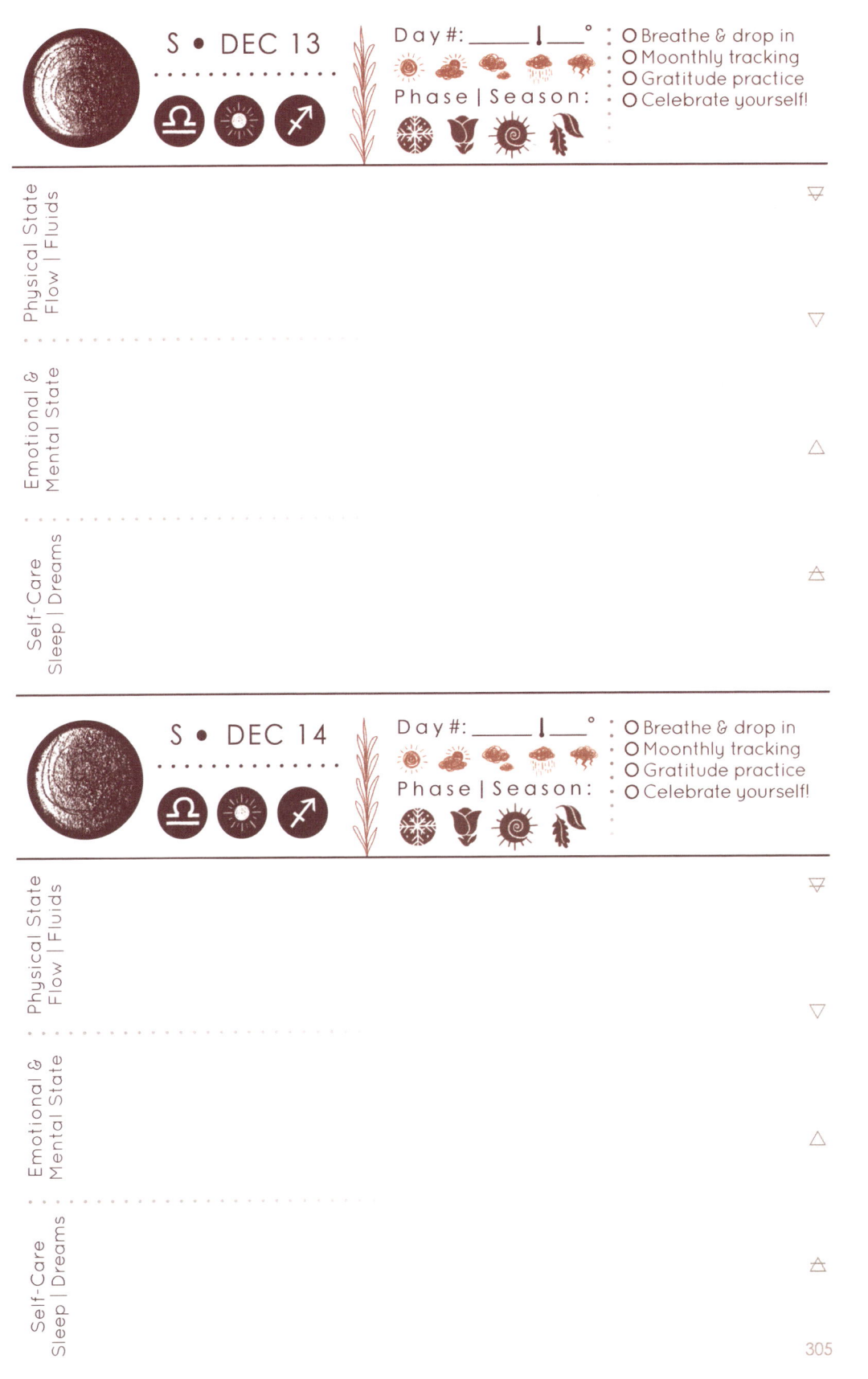

Day #: _____ | _____°

Phase | Season:

- ○ Breathe & drop in
- ○ Moonthly tracking
- ○ Gratitude practice
- ○ Celebrate yourself!

Physical State
Flow | Fluids

Emotional &
Mental State

Self-Care
Sleep | Dreams

S • DEC 14

Day #: _____ | _____°

Phase | Season:

- ○ Breathe & drop in
- ○ Moonthly tracking
- ○ Gratitude practice
- ○ Celebrate yourself!

Physical State
Flow | Fluids

Emotional &
Mental State

Self-Care
Sleep | Dreams

M • DEC 15

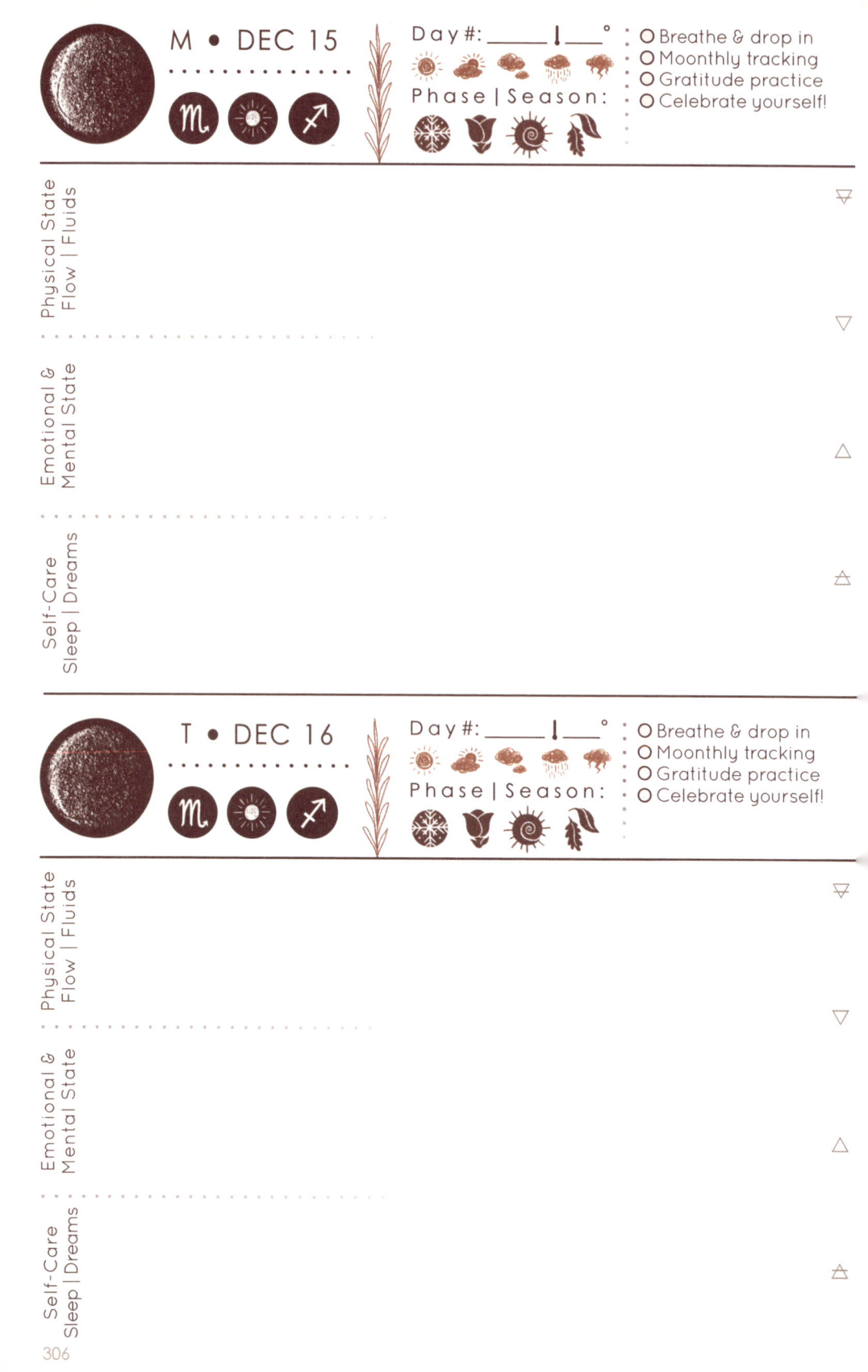

Day #: _____ | _____°

Phase | Season:

- ○ Breathe & drop in
- ○ Moonthly tracking
- ○ Gratitude practice
- ○ Celebrate yourself!

Physical State
Flow | Fluids

Emotional & Mental State

Self-Care
Sleep | Dreams

T • DEC 16

Day #: _____ | _____°

Phase | Season:

- ○ Breathe & drop in
- ○ Moonthly tracking
- ○ Gratitude practice
- ○ Celebrate yourself!

Physical State
Flow | Fluids

Emotional & Mental State

Self-Care
Sleep | Dreams

W • DEC 17

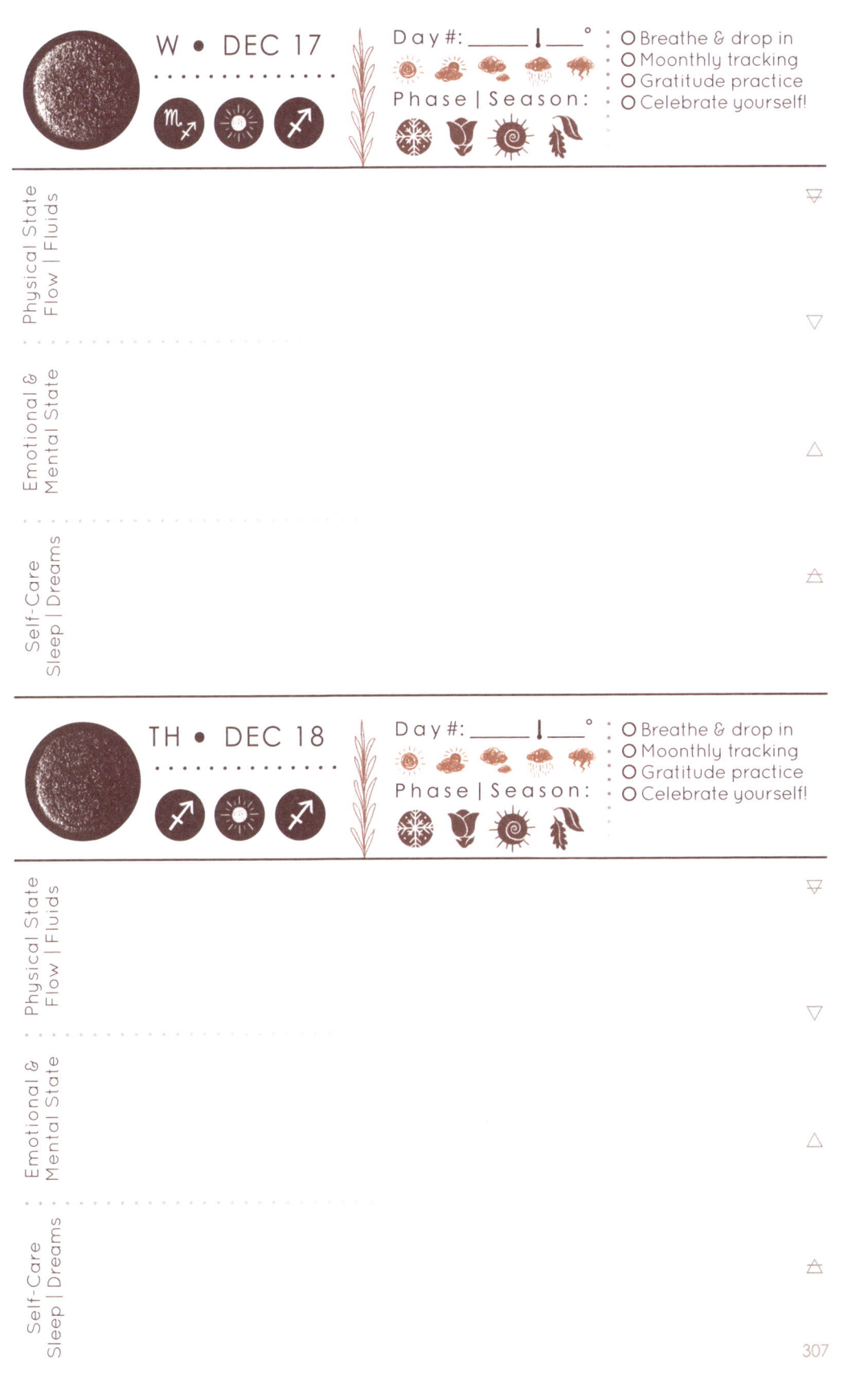

Day #: _____ | _____°

Phase | Season:

- Breathe & drop in
- Moonthly tracking
- Gratitude practice
- Celebrate yourself!

Physical State
Flow | Fluids

Emotional &
Mental State

Self-Care
Sleep | Dreams

TH • DEC 18

Day #: _____ | _____°

Phase | Season:

- Breathe & drop in
- Moonthly tracking
- Gratitude practice
- Celebrate yourself!

Physical State
Flow | Fluids

Emotional &
Mental State

Self-Care
Sleep | Dreams

☾ 11th
11 | 20
12 | 18

CHECK IN & REFLECT

Last Cycle Day 1: _____

Last Cycle Length: _____

Circle the phase you bled near:

○ ☾ ☾ ☾ ☽ ● ● ● ☾ ☾ ☾ ○

Use this space to reflect on your experiences & findings from this ending lunar cycle or your last menstrual cycle. Use cycle day #s if you bleed, or moon phases if you don't.

Caution Days: (days I needed space)

Bliss Days: (days I felt great)

DAYS TO NOTE — Which cycle days stood out?

OBSERVATIONS — Notice any changes or patterns?

SELF-CARE — What was helpful & nourishing?

PLAN & PREPARE

Next Predicted Cycle:
🩸 ☾ _____

CHECKLIST

Add the following to any other planners or calendars for your next cycle, then check it off.

- ☐ Predicted "days to note" _____
- ☐ Days to slow down (pre-bleed) _____
- ☐ Rest day(s) (next bleed) _____
- ☐ Date with yourself _____
- ☐ _____

- ☐ Self chest/breast exam
- ☐ Meal plan with cycle
- ☐ _____
- ☐ _____
- ☐ _____

OPEN SPACE

Use this space how you wish, or print out one of our free templates to paste here for BBT charting, dream tracking, or something else:

Love Letters From The Land

by Billimarie (she/her) For Every Star, A Tree • Poet & Earthworker •
@ForEveryStarATree • foreverystaratree.com •

"Dear You,

I am writing you from our tiny house near our tiny forest in the middle of a vast desert.

This morning, I woke from a strange dream where I was standing beneath a large pomegranate bush. It did not feel like a dream--it felt like deja vu. Like I was living a future memory. I could see with perfect clarity the exact spot in the desert where we planted this pomegranate bush, back in 2022.

Only this time, it was towering over me like a tree."

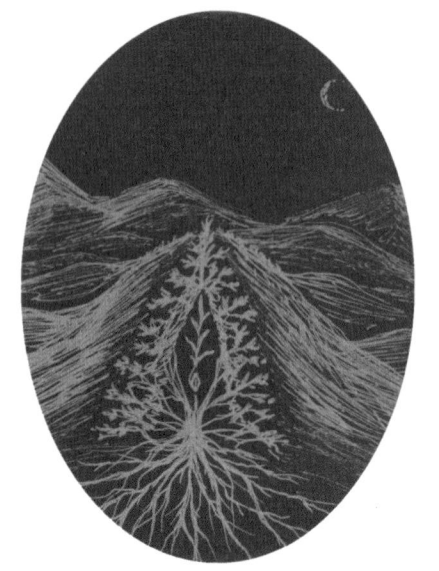

I have been sending these Love Letters to people all over the world.

To access these memories, I take a barefoot walk in our Tiny Forest. We planted native trees, flowers, herbs, and shrubs with the help of volunteers from our local community. Every week, I water it--normally at night.

There is something about being outside, underneath a blanket of stars, your bare feet digging into the earth, and the silence of the moon reflecting the water that pools around each tiny patch of garden.

You can join our letter community by donating a plant to our Tiny Forest on our website.

In the meantime, here is a dream prompt for you to consider:

Step outside, preferably without shoes, and find somewhere to steep your fingers into the earth. This can even be a small planter, if you are surrounded by concrete. (I have noticed there is always someone growing a plant, regardless of limitations.)

Breathe in the earth. Imagine each tiny microbe drifting into you, filling you with warm thoughts about home, love, and bliss.

Then, write in the space below a dream--or a memory--that you know for certain was sent to you by a tree, a flower, an herb, or any other plant.

Phasic Overview & In-Betweens

Use this space to focus on the phases of the moonth and the in-betweens of the peak lunations.

One way of using this space is to designate one column for your goal-planning, intention-setting or focus per phase/week. Use the other column for reflections, dream themes, nutrition tracking, cards pulls, etc!

F • DEC 19

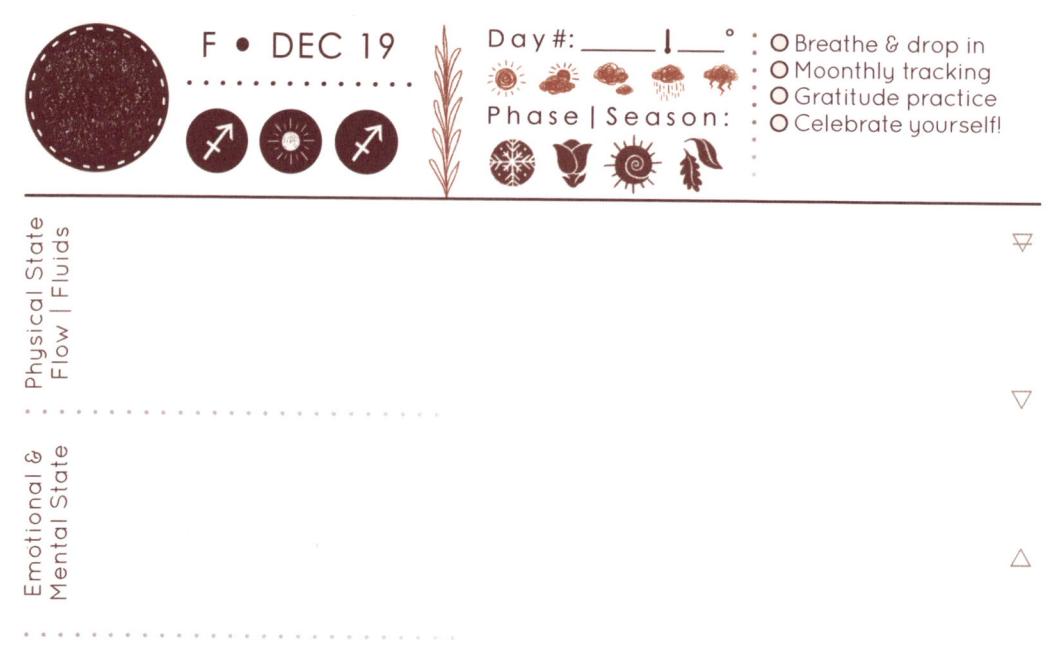

Day #: ____ | ____°

Phase | Season:

- ○ Breathe & drop in
- ○ Moonthly tracking
- ○ Gratitude practice
- ○ Celebrate yourself!

Physical State / Flow | Fluids

Emotional & Mental State

Self-Care / Sleep | Dreams

NEW MOON IN SAGITTARIUS

Breaking through the surface of a new chapter with an open mind

What do I want to grow & focus on during this lunar cycle?

How will I hold space for this?

S • DEC 20

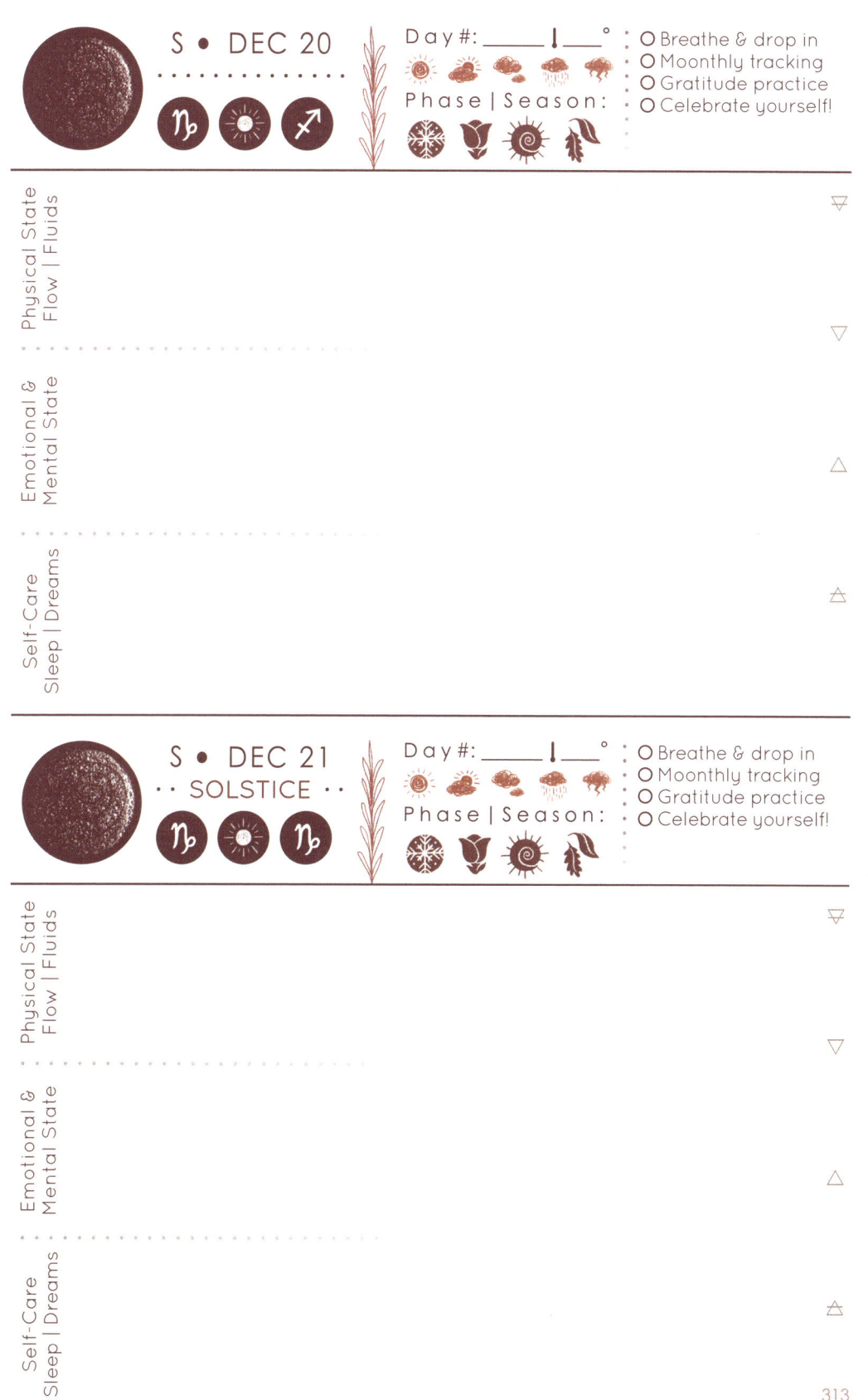

Day #: _____ | ___°
Phase | Season:

- O Breathe & drop in
- O Moonthly tracking
- O Gratitude practice
- O Celebrate yourself!

Physical State
Flow | Fluids

Emotional & Mental State

Self-Care
Sleep | Dreams

S • DEC 21
·· SOLSTICE ··

Day #: _____ | ___°
Phase | Season:

- O Breathe & drop in
- O Moonthly tracking
- O Gratitude practice
- O Celebrate yourself!

Physical State
Flow | Fluids

Emotional & Mental State

Self-Care
Sleep | Dreams

M • DEC 22

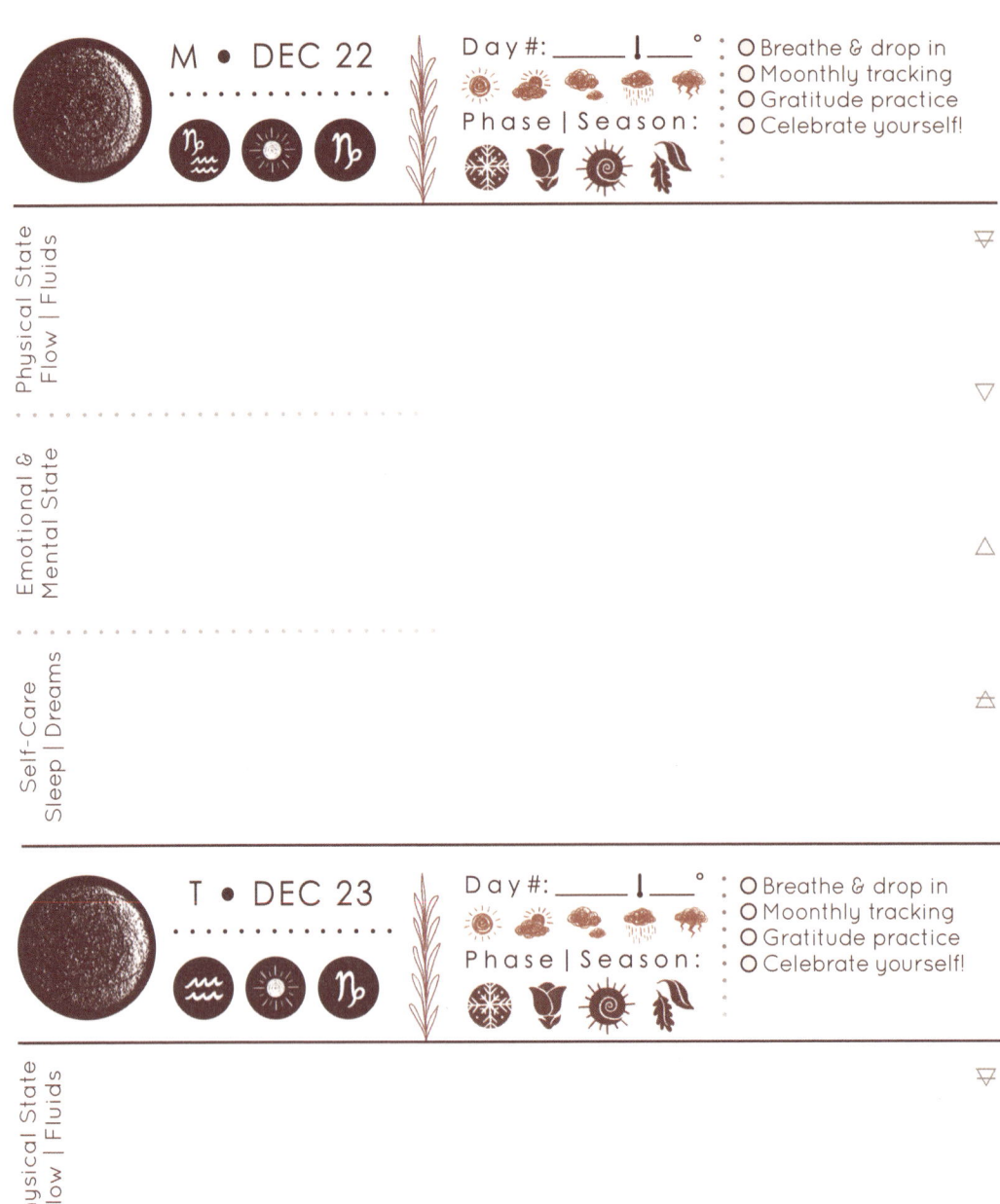

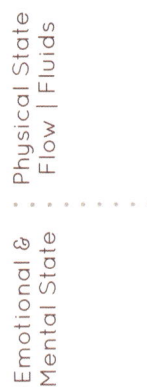

Day #: _____ | _____°

Phase | Season:

- ○ Breathe & drop in
- ○ Moonthly tracking
- ○ Gratitude practice
- ○ Celebrate yourself!

Physical State / Flow | Fluids

Emotional & Mental State

Self-Care / Sleep | Dreams

T • DEC 23

Day #: _____ | _____°

Phase | Season:

- ○ Breathe & drop in
- ○ Moonthly tracking
- ○ Gratitude practice
- ○ Celebrate yourself!

Physical State / Flow | Fluids

Emotional & Mental State

Self-Care / Sleep | Dreams

W • DEC 24

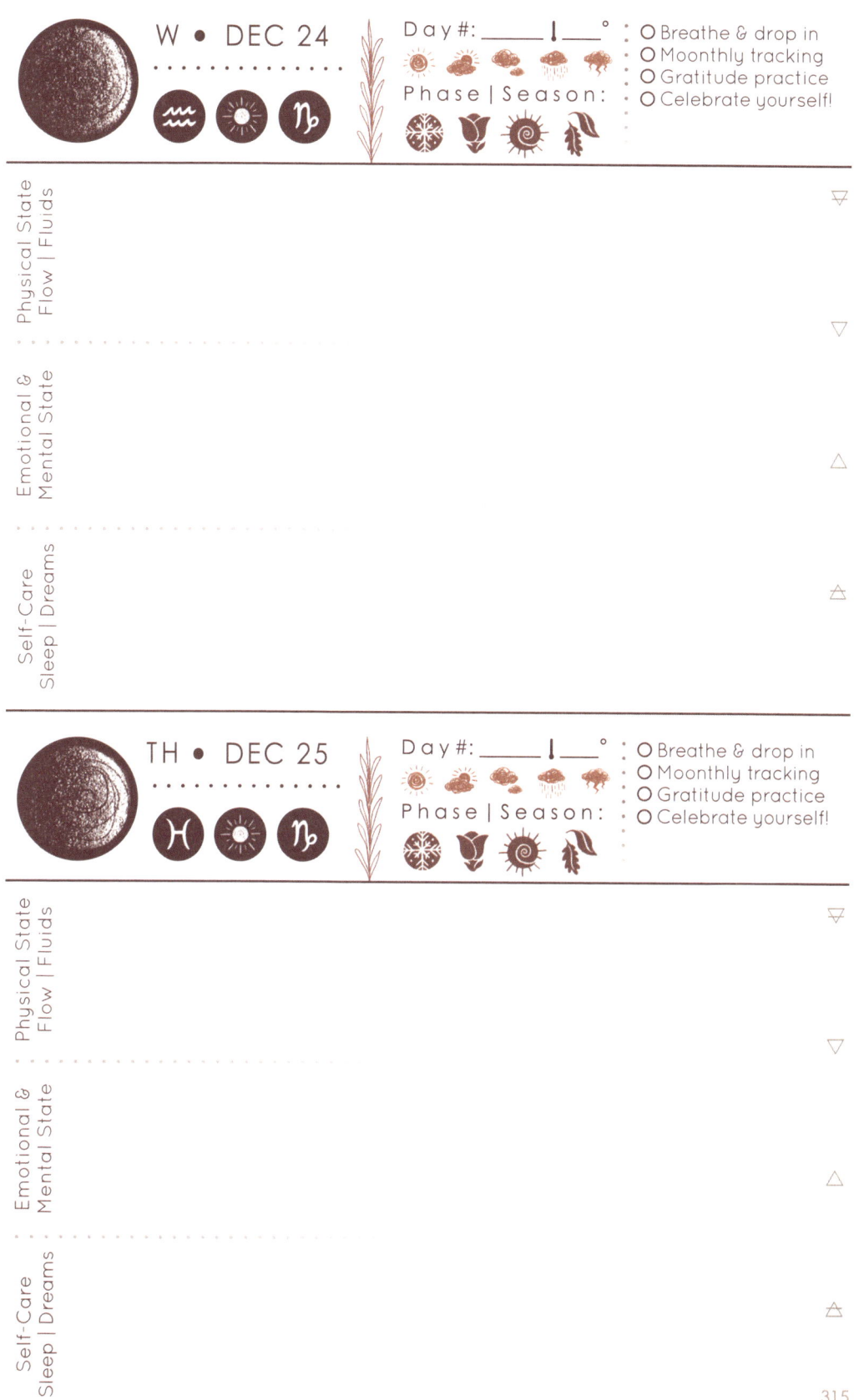

Day #: _____ | _____°

Phase | Season:

- ○ Breathe & drop in
- ○ Moonthly tracking
- ○ Gratitude practice
- ○ Celebrate yourself!

Physical State
Flow | Fluids

Emotional & Mental State

Self-Care
Sleep | Dreams

TH • DEC 25

Day #: _____ | _____°

Phase | Season:

- ○ Breathe & drop in
- ○ Moonthly tracking
- ○ Gratitude practice
- ○ Celebrate yourself!

Physical State
Flow | Fluids

Emotional & Mental State

Self-Care
Sleep | Dreams

F • DEC 26

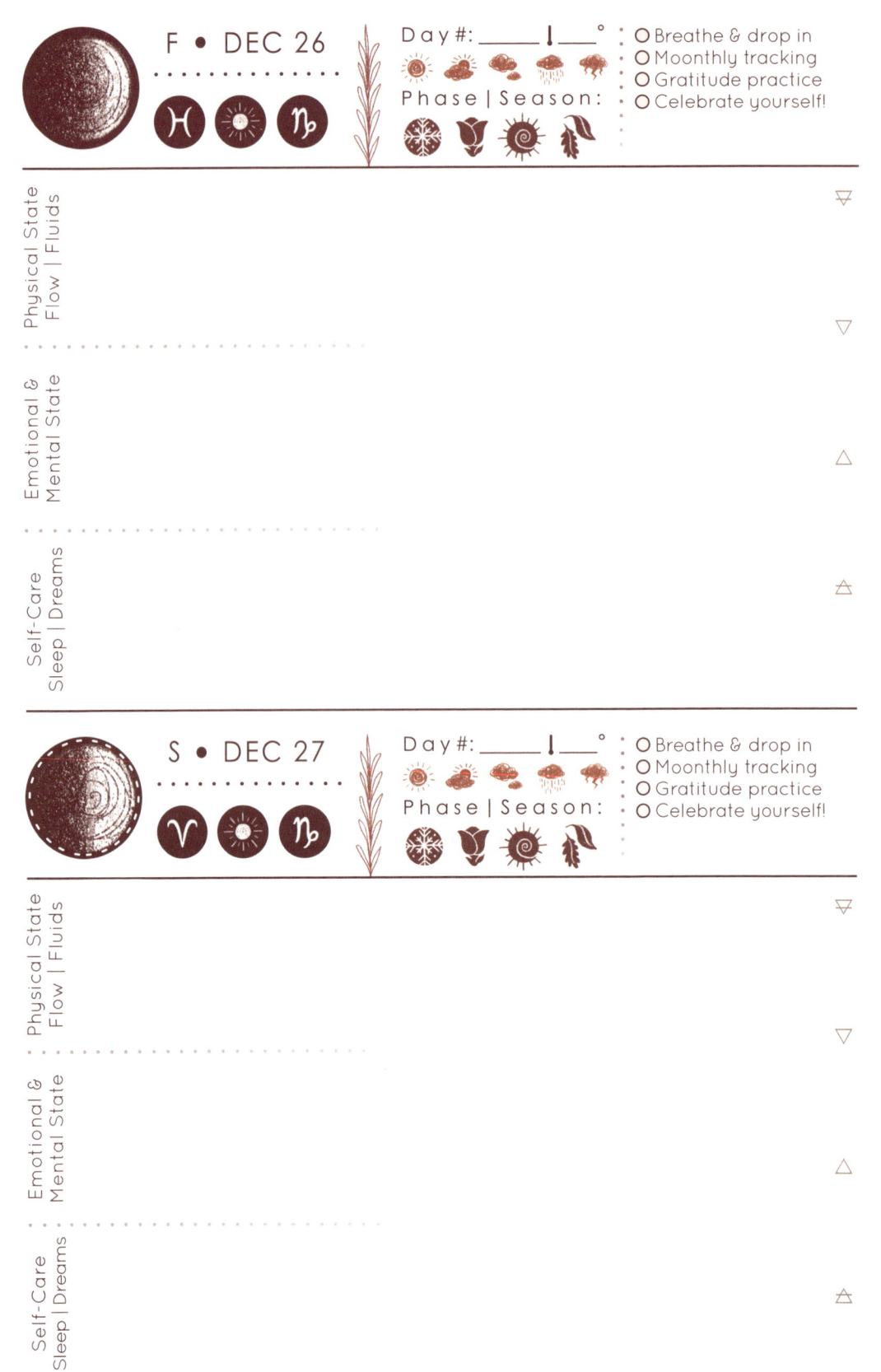

♓ ☉ ♑

Day #: _____ | _____°

Phase | Season:

- ○ Breathe & drop in
- ○ Moonthly tracking
- ○ Gratitude practice
- ○ Celebrate yourself!

Physical State | Flow | Fluids

Emotional & Mental State

Self-Care | Sleep | Dreams

S • DEC 27

♈ ☉ ♑

Day #: _____ | _____°

Phase | Season:

- ○ Breathe & drop in
- ○ Moonthly tracking
- ○ Gratitude practice
- ○ Celebrate yourself!

Physical State | Flow | Fluids

Emotional & Mental State

Self-Care | Sleep | Dreams

FIRST QUARTER IN ARIES

Allowing expansive presence within forward-movement

What is sprouting & coming into awareness?

What can I release to make space for further growth & grounding?

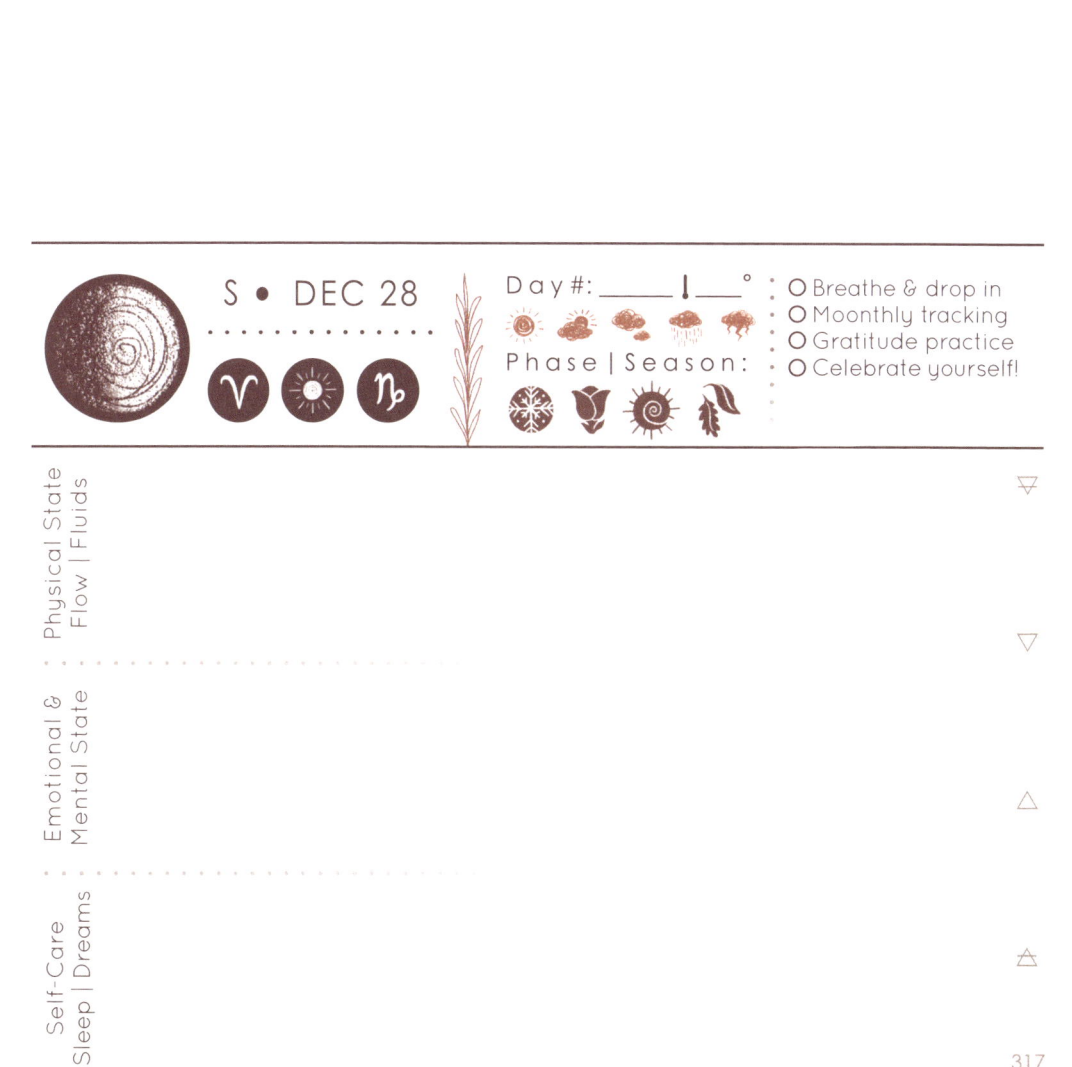

S • DEC 28

Day #: _____ | _____°

Phase | Season:

- ○ Breathe & drop in
- ○ Moonthly tracking
- ○ Gratitude practice
- ○ Celebrate yourself!

Physical State
Flow | Fluids

Emotional &
Mental State

Self-Care
Sleep | Dreams

M • DEC 29

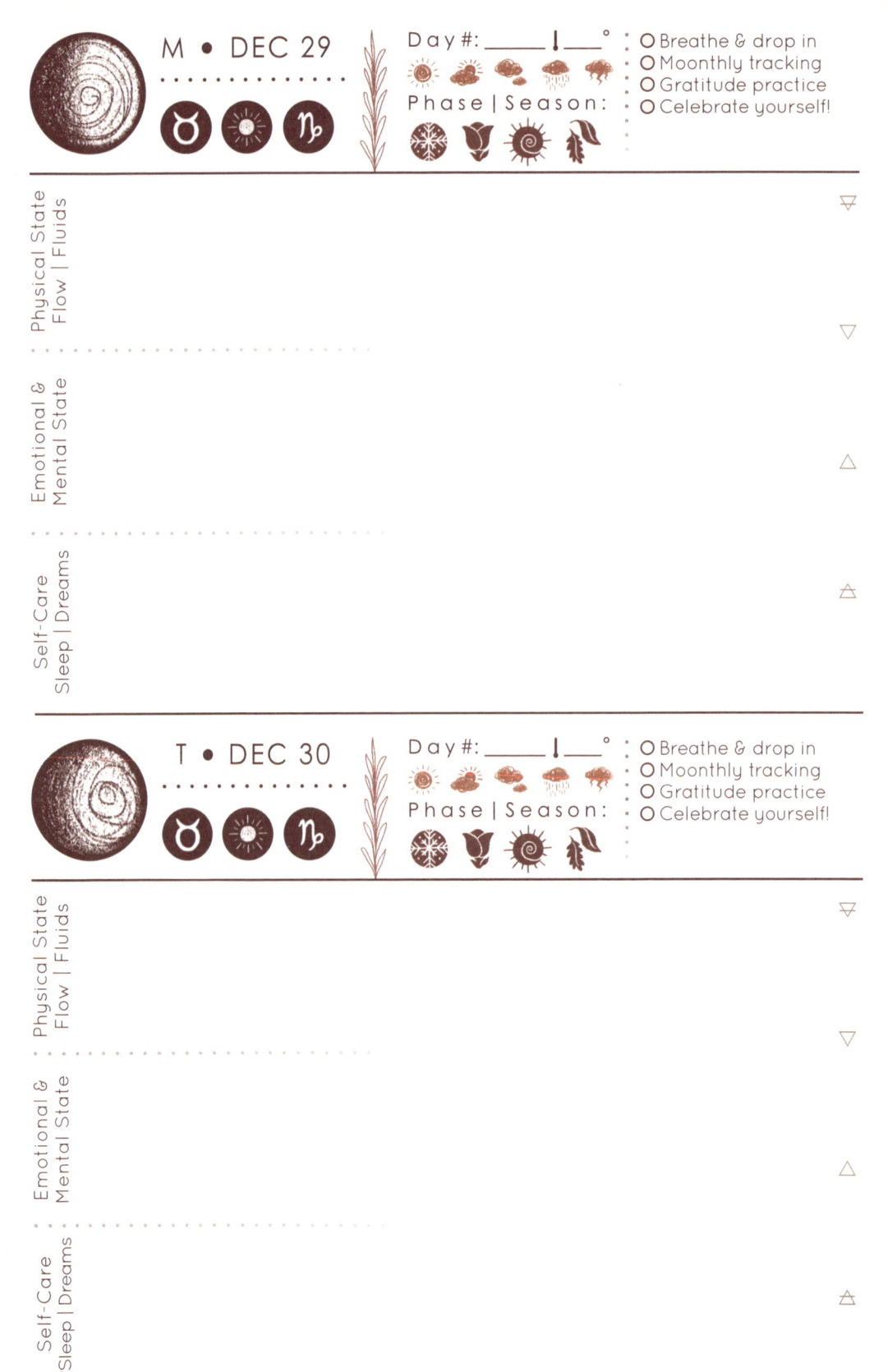

Day #: _____ | _____°
Phase | Season:

○ Breathe & drop in
○ Moonthly tracking
○ Gratitude practice
○ Celebrate yourself!

Physical State / Flow | Fluids

Emotional & Mental State

Self-Care / Sleep | Dreams

T • DEC 30

Day #: _____ | _____°
Phase | Season:

○ Breathe & drop in
○ Moonthly tracking
○ Gratitude practice
○ Celebrate yourself!

Physical State / Flow | Fluids

Emotional & Mental State

Self-Care / Sleep | Dreams

W • DEC 31

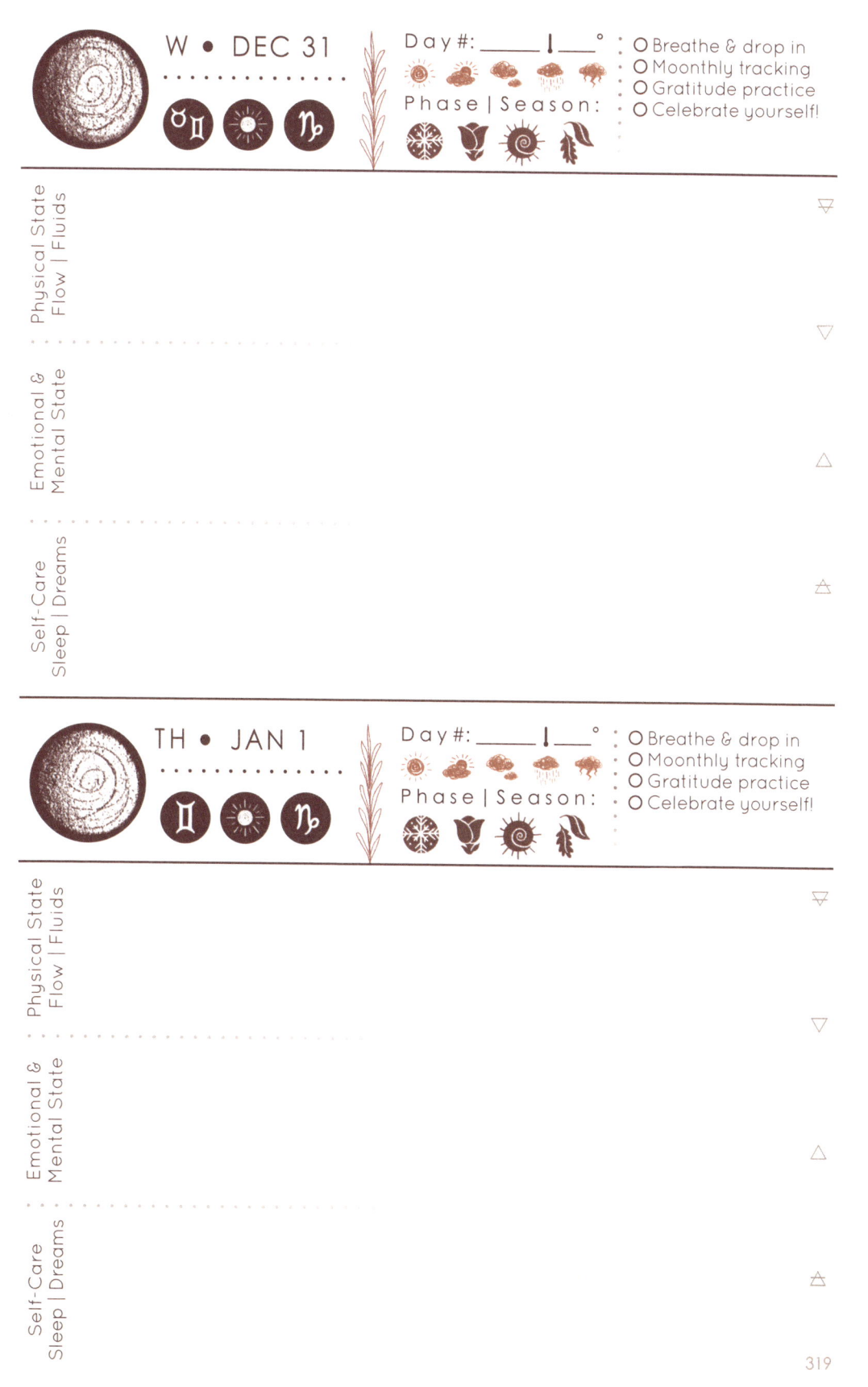

Day #: _____ | _____°

Phase | Season:

- ○ Breathe & drop in
- ○ Moonthly tracking
- ○ Gratitude practice
- ○ Celebrate yourself!

Physical State / Flow | Fluids

Emotional & Mental State

Self-Care / Sleep | Dreams

TH • JAN 1

Day #: _____ | _____°

Phase | Season:

- ○ Breathe & drop in
- ○ Moonthly tracking
- ○ Gratitude practice
- ○ Celebrate yourself!

Physical State / Flow | Fluids

Emotional & Mental State

Self-Care / Sleep | Dreams

A letter of gratitude to yourself for how far you've come;

Dear _____,
        (your name here)

I am so proud of you – I mean, look how far you've come! We've been on this journey together for some time now, but this has been a year of beautiful progress.

You are whole & amazing no matter how many pages you missed, no matter how many rough days there were – the point is you are here. We learned so much about one another, and this isn't the end.

I'm grateful for this time together that has only brought us closer through understanding. I intend to continue to heal with you and give you all that you deserve & ask for.

The deeper we go, the more I realize that our hardships are just learning curves. Our high tides are just a ride to calmer waves. The more I remember our unity, the easier the trip gets. I'm excited to see where it takes us next.

I love every part of you even when I may not understand you. I look forward to continuing to get to know you better & find ways to make our life more blissful.

As we prepare for a new year, I promise to continue to . . .

Love,

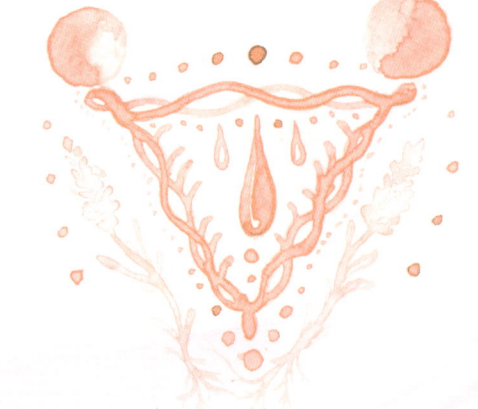

_____
      (your name here)

*Once you've completed adding your own words to this letter,
read it out loud while facing yourself in a mirror & then sign + date at the bottom.*

Reflect on how far you've come...

What patterns have you discovered this year?

What has shifted in your body?

Is there anything you discovered that you're seeking a deeper understanding of?

Is there anything that became clearer & revealed to you?

How has your self-care practice changed since beginning this journal?

How do you feel about your body & menstrual cycle after all you've uncovered?

How will you continue this journey & practice into next year?

My Healing Toolkit

Record your favorite resources, rituals, practices, tools and words on this page. Return here whenever you feel stuck & need a reminder of what helps you most.

Some Suggestions:

- *Take a Nature walk*
- *Drink water (charge it with a flower essence or intention)*
- *Inhale for 4 count, hold for 2, exhale for 4, repeat.*
- *Pull a tarot or oracle card*
- *Look up at the sky*
- *Place a hand on your heart*
- *Take a bath or shower or dip in a natural water body*
- *Hum or sing*
- *Move, stretch, shake or dance*
- *Practice meditation*
- *Reach out to a loved one*
- *Draw or write to release*
- *Make some herbal tea or an elixir*
-
-
-
-

◁◁◁●● Healing Resource Directory ●▷▷▷

Complied within these next pages are aligned healers, guides & resources that are ready to support your continual + expansive healing journey.

Healing Arts & Services

Adriana Rose | MysticIntimacy
Feminine Embodiment and Sacred Intimacy Guide for Women

- @intimacygoddess
- mysticintimacy.com

Alia Alsaif Spiers | Alchemic Vigor
Oracle Reader, Spiritual Alchemist, Holistic Life Coach, and Artist

- @alchemicvigor
- alchemicvigor.square.site

Amy Heneveld | Enosburgh Essences
Flower Essences & Creative Coaching with the Flowers

- @amysheneveld
- enosburghessences.com

Cole Lopez | Enter the Portal
DIVINATION : AstroHerbalism & Tarot | WOMB Awakening

- enter-the-portal.com

Jade Fearn | Grief & Gratitude Co.
Grief Coach & Support Specialist

- griefandgratitudeco.com

Jenna Handloff : Aspen Botanicals Apothecary
Womb Wellness Educator, Herbalist, Ceremonialist, Tarot Enthusiast

- @aspenbotanicals
- aspenbotanicals.com

Maya Rain
Intuitive Therapist, Spiritual Coach, Shamanic Practitioner

- @mayarain
- mayarain.com

Megan Embodied | Cycle Sync Psychic
Certified Psychic Reader & Energy Healer, Somatic Embodiment Mentor, Cycle Sync Educator

- @meganembodied
- stan.store/meganembodied

OUR EXTENDED DIRECTORY: CYCLESJOURNAL.COM/HEALINGRESOURCES

APPLY TO BE HERE NEXT YEAR: CYCLESJOURNAL.COM/SPONSOR

Healing Arts & Services (Cont'd)

Regina Verret Foster: The Celestial Womb LLC
Astrologer, Birth Coach, & Ceremonialist of Conscious Transformation for Women, Parents, & Families.

@thecelestialwomb
thecelestialwomb.love

Vanessa Wells | Dark Hearts Healing Arts
Self-Connection Coach, Authenticity Alchemist, & Integrative Intuitive Healing Artist.

@darkheartshealingarts
darkheartshealingarts.com

Xeres Villanueva The Estuary Moments
Soul Vocation Guide, Spiritual Director and Divination Ritualist

@the_estuary_moments
linktr.ee/xvilla1228

Menstrual Health & Cycle Education

Abigail Maxon | Rhythmic Renewal
Herbal Medicines, Intuitive Somatics, & Nature Based Menstrual Empowerment

@rhythmic_renewal
rhythmicrenewal.com

Briana Villegas | Embracing Cyclical
Menstrual Cycle Coach Specilizing in Holistic PMDD Support

@brianavillegascoaching
brianavillegas.com

Gem Campbell AKA the Blood Slut
Sexologist & Dietitian Specialising in Labia Insecurity, PMDD, Cyclical Living + more

@thebloodslut
iamawildgem.com

Kelly Dobrin | Self Healing Wellness
Certified Fertility Awareness Instructor - Handmade & Wildcrafted Gifts - Flow Arts Guide

@selfhealingwellness
selfhealingwellness.com

Leila Madeline | R E W I L D I N G
Cycle Reclamation for Decolonising the Mind and Finding Our Role in the Revolution

@leilamadeline___
leilamadeline.com/rewilding

OUR EXTENDED DIRECTORY: CYCLESJOURNAL.COM/HEALINGRESOURCES

Natural Medicine & Holistic Healing

Andrea Webb | Every Light Wellness
Divergent Astroherbalism for Human Souls and the Bodies We Haunt

- @everylightwellnessllc
- everylightwellness.squarespace.com

Angela Hayes | Modern Journey
Integrative Wellness Coach for Women's Health through Embodiment, Self Care & Cyclical Living

- @modernjourneywellness
- modernjourneywellness.com

Azaria Glover | Azaria's Apothecary
Womb-Centered Herbal Offerings Beneficial to the Cyclical Nature of Women

- @azariasapothecary @earthwitch
- azariasapothecary.etsy.com

Luminous Creatrix Theresa Swan BA, DKATI, PHE, PHC
Certified Peristeam Hydrotherapist. Pelvic Health: Menstrual Irregularities, Fertility, Postpartum & More!

- @luminouscreatrix
- luminouscreatrix.com

Luna Xóchitl Botánica
Folk Herbalist, Yoga + Meditation Teacher, Curanderismo Student, Brujx, Cannabis Extractor

- @lunaxochitl_
- lunaxochitl.com

Mandy Rother | Reveal Functional Nutrition
Functional Dietitian Specializing in Holistic Approach to Premenstrual Dysphoric Disorder (PMDD)

- @mandyrother.rd
- revealfunctionalnutrition.com/PMDD

Nikki Renee | Elevated Ananda Collective
Certified Cannabis Wellness Coach and Educator. Community, Yoga, Meditation, Ritual, Lunar Living

- @elevated_ananda
- linktr.ee/elevated_ananda

Nimisha Gandhi | Moon Cycle Nutrition
Ayurvedic & Functional Nutritionist and Yoni Shakti Practitioner

- @mooncyclenutrition
- mooncyclenutrition.com

Reiki for Today & Befriend Your Grief
Animal Reiki & Chaplaincy, Reiki for People, Grief Support after Suicide Loss

- @reikifortoday
- reikifortoday.com

Apply to be here next year: cyclesjournal.com/sponsor

Natural Medicine & Holistic Healing (Cont'd)

Sarah Marcus | White Horse Healing
Reiki Teacher/Master - Holding Space via Distance & In-Person Healing Sessions + Classes

@whitehorsehealing_idaho
whitehorsehealing-idaho.com

Visual Arts & Physical Wares

Hannah Shenton | Hart Skincare
Cyclical Skincare | Natural + Holistic

@hartskincare
hartskincare.com.au

Womb Healing & Ritual Facilitators

Desert Bloom
Integrative Pelvic Therapist & LMT
Virtual Somatic Womb Focused Healing

@desertbloommt
desertbloommassage.org

Josephine Loha | Temple of Loha
Embodiment Guide, Somatic Sexologist & Eros Priestess

@templeofloha
cur8chicago.com

OUR EXTENDED DIRECTORY: CYCLESJOURNAL.COM/HEALINGRESOURCES

Cycles Journal would not be possible without our Amazing Sponsors...

As an independent publication, we are 100% community-funded through sponsors & pre-sales each year.

Thank you to all who helped make this edition of Cycles Journal possible!

- Our Featured Collective – Wisdom Offerings Article Pages
- All in the Healing Resource Directory
- All who have helped us spread & share the mission!

We are eternally grateful for your support. Without you, this journal would not be in the hands of thousands of cyclical beings.
You are an essential part of our whole!

Each year we have a limited number of spaces inside our journal that we offer up for an exchange of reciprocal support.

Browse our current offerings & inquire within March of the upcoming year to be featured inside our next Cycles Journal and/or online. We have a limited # of scholarships reserved for BIPOC individuals.

Learn more about how to join our collective of reciprocal support;

It takes a hive...

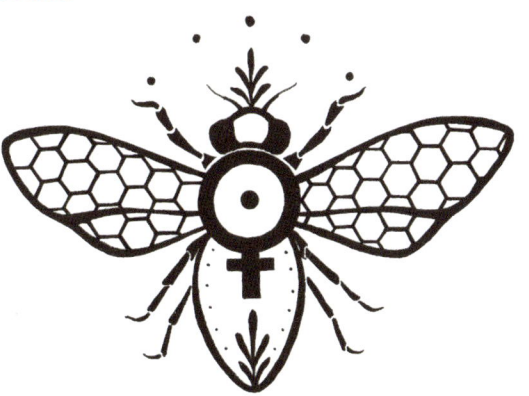

Thank you to all who help make this annual publication happen through community contribution, sharing & funding.

GRATITUDE

This journal would not be in existence without ...

My loving partner & his endless support, patience, & trust.
Beloved friends, family, community, & loved ones for all their support & love.
This amazing tiny team behind Cycles Journal & the mentors who have supported.
Mother for birthing me, believing in me, & being the definition of compassion.
Father for being a part of my evolvement too, & for teaching me ambition.
Ancestors & guides for empowering this path & providing wisdom.
Earth for holding us. Spirit for being. The land & Indigenous people who we honor.
All who are on this path of collective healing.
&
All of the cyclical beings including YOU
who supported this project & are living its mission.
All of the Featured Collective Sponsors who are a part of this journal.
Thank you, thank you to those who supported this project from early on —
for trusting my vision & its purpose to serve a bigger purpose.

Love, Rachael Amber

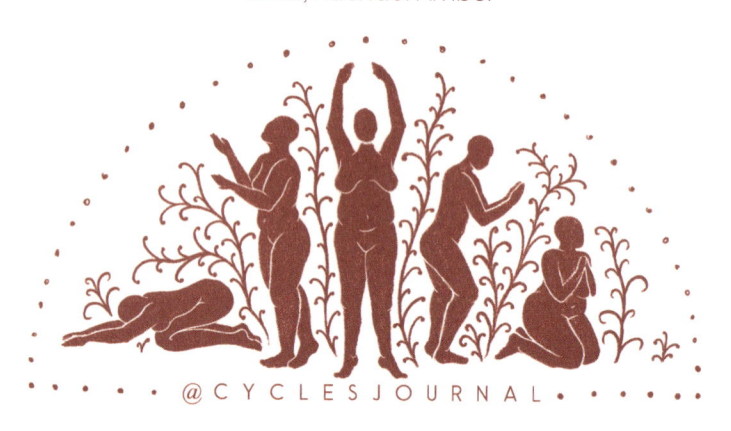

· @ C Y C L E S J O U R N A L ·

How to Reuse & Recycle Your Journal

You now hold more than a journal & guide in your hands; you hold a priceless record of yourself. This journal is now part of your sacred space.

Consider its value in your immediate & distant future as it not only holds memories & wisdom translated from your body, but it also holds records of your health. This vital information is still relevant to the next few or many years of your life as you develop and analyze patterns over time.

I recommend storing this journal in a special space or on your frequented bookshelf. Use it like you would any other reference book. Use it as a place to derive inspiration from when you're feeling disconnected.

If at some point you choose to part with this journal, you can recycle it as you would paper. Or you can burn it ceremonially and scatter the ashes onto Earth.

Cycles Journal® is created by Rachael Amber

who designs, illustrates, & curates each edition, with the help of editors, featured writers + sponsors, & a small but mighty team that helps get the word out! It's an ever-evolving grassroots effort of love & care.

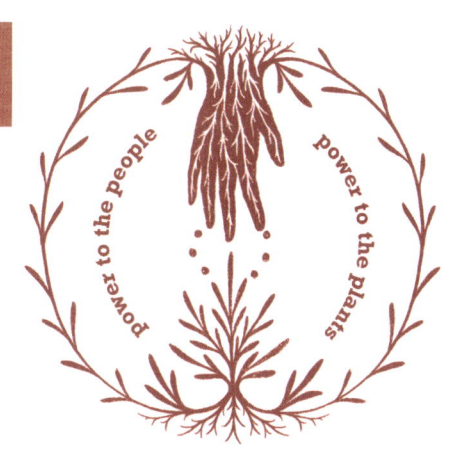

power to the people · power to the plants

Rachael (they/she) is a queer, intuitive artist, writer & designer who is deeply focused on our embodiment as beings of nature. They channel artwork + supportive structures in collaboration with Earth & Spirit to help our wholistic healing & awareness journeys. They are devoted to paths of deep ecology, mindfulness, and other realms of Earth-based healing lineages.

All of the artwork in this journal was created by Rachael.

Find more on Rachael's artwork:

- @ rachael.amber
- www.rachaelamber.com

Prints & Products of the Art in Cycles Journal...

Bring the art in the journal into your home life & sacred space – visit our shop:

Inquire about usage + licensing, all at cyclesjournal.com/art

WHAT'S NEXT? STAY CONNECTED ...

On to Cycles Journal® 2026

Cycles Journal® 2026 will be available for pre-order in summer 2025 & available in autumn 2025. We rely on pre-orders to keep this self-funded publication going!

Each edition contains new wisdom, rituals, & illustrations from our featured collective sponsors to keep you inspired & in the flow.

FOR FUTURE UPDATES:

If you'd like to be among the first to know about early bird pre-sale specials, to be a part of future online events, and to receive future perks, freebies, prompts & more — join our newsletter at cyclesjournal.com/moonletters

Find it all online by scanning this code:

You're invited to join our online community!

A safe, free space to connect, share, & support one another on our journeys

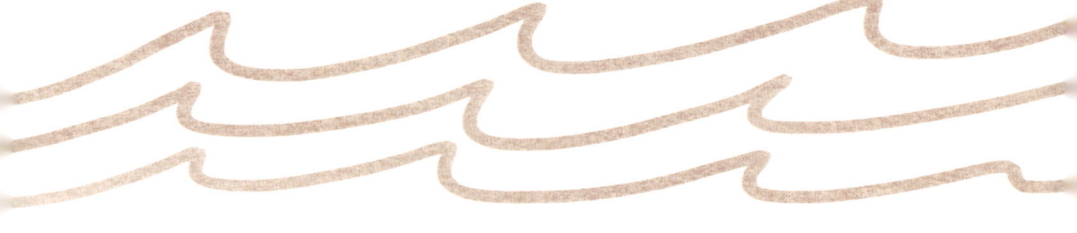

See you next year!
Stay well, cyclical one.

www.cyclesjournal.com | @cyclesjournal

9 781735 712765